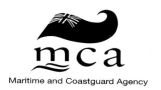

Maritime and Coastguard Agency

The Ship Captain's
MEDICAL
GUIDE

London: The Stationery Office

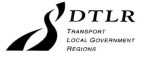

DTLR
TRANSPORT
LOCAL GOVERNMENT
REGIONS

Executive Agency of the Department for Transport, Local Government and Regions (DTLR)

Twenty-second edition first published 1999
Second impression 2001

ISBN 0 11 551658 1

*Cover: Top photograph of fishing vessel supplied
courtesy of the Scottish Fishermen's Federation*

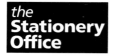

Published by The Stationery Office and available from:

The Stationery Office
(mail, telephone and fax orders only)
PO Box 29, Norwich NR3 1GN
General enquiries/Telephone orders 0870 600 5522
Fax orders 0870 600 5533

www.thestationeryoffice.com

The Stationery Office Bookshops
123 Kingsway, London WC2B 6PQ
020 7242 6393 Fax 020 7242 6394
68–69 Bull Street, Birmingham B4 6AD
0121 236 9696 Fax 0121 236 9699
33 Wine Street, Bristol BS1 2BQ
0117 926 4306 Fax 0117 929 4515
9–21 Princess Street, Manchester M60 8AS
0161 834 7201 Fax 0161 833 0634
16 Arthur Street, Belfast BT1 4GD
028 9023 8451 Fax 028 9023 5401
The Stationery Office Oriel Bookshop
18–19 High Street, Cardiff CF1 2BZ
029 2039 5548 Fax 029 2038 4347
71 Lothian Road, Edinburgh EH3 9AZ
0870 606 5566 Fax 0870 606 5588

The Stationery Office's Accredited Agents
(see Yellow Pages)
and through good booksellers

Contents

Contributors

Mr C J Cahill Consultant in Accident & Emergency Medicine

Mr G A Carrs Consultant in Accident & Emergency Medicine

Mr S T H Mullett Consultant in Accident & Emergency Medicine

Dr R Brindle Consultant Medical Microbiologist

Dr J Kitching Specialist Registrar in Accident & Emergency Medicine

Mr M A Howell Specialist Registrar in Accident & Emergency Medicine

Dr K Hartington Specialist Registrar in Accident & Emergency Medicine

Dr M Saunders Principal in General Practice

Mr A Dobson Accident & Emergency Clinical Nurse Manager

Miss D Rock Senior Sister in Accident & Emergency & Nurse Practitioner

Mrs P Hutchings Community Psychiatric Nurse Manager (Deliberate Self Harm)

Preface

The Ship Captain's Medical Guide is primarily intended for use on ships not carrying a doctor. The recommended measures of prevention and treatment are therefore confined to those which can reasonably be expected of the ship's officers.

The First edition of the Guide was compiled in 1868 by Dr Harry Leach, Medical Officer of Health of the Port of London. The Twentieth edition was published nearly 100 years later in 1967. The Twenty First edition was a major revision, first published in 1983, and reprinted no fewer than seven times, with some amendments, between then and 1993. It stood the test of time well but has inevitably become outdated in some aspects.

This, the Twenty Second edition, is a further major revision of the text aimed at bringing the recommended actions and treatments in line with current medical practice and medical stores regulations. Where necessary the text has been re-written and the information re-arranged to improve accessibility. It is hoped that this revised text will prove 'user friendly' and will become, like its predecessor, a trusted and long lived publication.

The Guide is designed to be used in conjunction with Merchant Shipping Notice MSN 1726 (M & F), or any subsequent update, which sets out the medical stores which are required under the Merchant Shipping and Fishing Vessels (Medical Stores) Regulations 1995 SI No. 1802 (as amended by 1996 SI No. 2821). It is recommended this Merchant Shipping Notice is kept with the guide, in the pocket provided, for immediate reference.

The Maritime and Coastguard Agency (MCA) acknowledges the contributions of the working group from the Queen Alexandra Hospital, Cosham, Portsmouth, Hampshire.

Grateful acknowledgements are also due to Dr PAM Diamond, Dr DB Carron and Mr DC Cahill for invaluable additional advice.

Time, medical science and technology will not stand still after the publication of this Twenty Second edition. As updating is required, it is hoped to be able to incorporate amendments to reflect advances and changes in medical knowledge and practice, and to improve the guide. To this end the MCA would welcome suggestions for improvements or changes at any time. These should be sent to: Maritime and Coastguard Agency, Bay 2/1, Spring Place, 105 Commercial Road, Southampton, SO15 1EG.

Introduction: How to use this guide

The three functions of this Guide are:

■ to enable you to diagnose and treat injured and sick seafarers;

■ to serve as a text book for Medical First Aid and Proficiency in Medical Care courses; and

■ to help you give some training to your crew.

The Guide should be kept in the ship's medical cabinet.

All members of your crew should be encouraged to learn the immediate life-saving measures described in the first part of Chapter 1.

Casualties

The first aid treatment for casualties is given in Chapter 1 or, in the case of toxic hazards, Chapter 2 and the Medical First Aid Guide for Use in Accidents involving Dangerous Goods (MFAG) 1994 and subsequent amendments. Chapter 4 describes how to give any necessary further treatment for wounds and other injuries following first aid and removal to the ship's hospital or a cabin.

Illnesses

When a person falls sick the first step is diagnosis. Some diseases and medical problems are relatively easy to diagnose, others may be much more difficult.

Diagnosis of the common diseases need not be difficult if you are methodical and make plenty of legible notes. One approach is to use a check list based on the format recommended for requesting Radio Medical Assistance. The list will both serve as a guideline for diagnosis and be useful if you have to request Radio Medical Advice or to send the patient to a hospital ashore.

Ask the patient when he first felt ill and what he feels is wrong with him. Obtain the full history of the complaint and also ask about his past medical history including drug treatment and allergies. Always listen carefully to everything the sick person has to say, and to his (and others') recollections of recent relevant events, e.g. has he been drinking, has he eaten something which has disagreed with him?

Note his general appearance, (is he flushed, pale, sweating, anxious, etc.?) Depending on the complaint, get the patient to remove his clothing and examine him thoroughly. Look for rashes, bad breath, tender areas, etc. Take his temperature, pulse rate and respiration rate and examine his urine, faeces, sputum and other discharges when necessary.

You should now have in front of you a list of symptoms, your findings and the patient's temperature, pulse and respiration rates. Reference should then be made where appropriate to the following sections:

■ Probable causes of abdominal pain – chart

■ Probable causes of chest pain – chart

■ Diagnostic signs associated with unconsciousness – chart

■ Descriptions of diseases in Chapters 6, 7, 8 and 9

Consider this example of how a diagnosis is established. The patient complains that he has had abdominal pain for a few hours. This started around the navel but has now settled in the right lower quarter of the abdomen. He has felt sick and has now begun to vomit. He has vomited on two occasions.

You find out by questioning him that the pain at first was spasmodic but, since it passed downwards into the lower abdomen, it has become a steady but not severe pain. He has not had diarrhoea, but is rather constipated. Examination shows that he has a temperature of 37.4°C, his pulse is 86 per minute, his tongue is furred and his breath is foul. There is tenderness in the right side of the lower abdomen, maximal at a point about half way between the navel and the upper bony part of the pelvis. There is no protein in the urine.

To establish a diagnosis, turn to the index and consult the section on the abdominal system. Compare the symptoms and signs with your findings.

The diagnosis in the example above should be one of acute appendicitis. If the patient is female, think also of ruptured ectopic pregnancy and of salpingitis. Check as part of your history-taking when her last menstrual period occurred. Then read the relevant section. You should be able to exclude these problems. Should you not be able to exclude a right sided salpingitis, then do not be concerned, as the treatment suggested for appendicitis would be effective in salpingitis as well.

A simpler method of establishing the diagnosis may be to study the diagrams and the table on the probable causes of abdominal pain in the abdominal pain chart. There you will see that the pattern of pain in Diagram 5 follows that which you have obtained in your history-taking and that the symptoms and signs which you have recorded confirm that the diagnosis is one of appendicitis.

A similar method should be used in all cases of illness. Chest pains can be diagnosed from the chest pain chart.

When you have made your initial diagnosis, follow the treatment recommended for that particular illness. Carefully monitor and record the patient's progress. If other symptoms arise, check again to see whether your initial diagnosis was correct. If you are unsure of the diagnosis and the patient does not appear to be very ill, treat the symptoms only, (e.g. paracetamol for pain or fever) and allow the patient to rest in bed. See how the illness progresses. If the symptoms disappear you are on safe ground. If they do not you will normally find that by the second or third day of the illness, the symptoms and signs are sufficient to allow you to make a diagnosis. If the patient's condition worsens and you are still unable to make a diagnosis, seek RADIO MEDICAL ADVICE.

General advice on nursing the patient while he has to remain in bed will be found in Chapter 3. Advice on precautions to be taken in giving antibiotics, pain-killers and all medicines and information about their side-effects are given in the drug supplement. Finally, if you have to obtain radio medical advice or evacuate the patient, you should read Chapter 13. In seeking advice from a radio doctor it may help to refer also to Annex I which describes briefly how the body works and gives the names of the main bones, muscles, etc. and the position of the main organs.

The dying and the dead

Chapter 12 tells you how to care for patients who may be dying, how to decide if a patient is dead, and what to do if he does die.

Causes and prevention of disease and medical problems

Prevention is always better than cure. Every master should therefore take heed of the advice in Chapter 5 about such matters as the cleanliness of the ship, ensuring that the food and water can be safely consumed, and isolating a patient who has an infectious disease.

Medical stores

Merchant Shipping Notice MSN 1726 (M & F) (or any subsequent update) sets out the statutorily required medical stores, according to the category of vessel. The Guide is intended for use with these medicines and equipment, and regular checks on stocks of medicines and their expiry dates should be carried out.

Introduction

When a ship is in port, or near to port where hospital and other expert medical attention are available, the first aid treatment necessary aboard ship is similar to that practised ashore. At sea, in the absence of these facilities, trained ships' officers are required to give types of treatment beyond that accepted as normal first aid.

The content of this chapter covers the knowledge of first aid necessary for the safe and efficient immediate treatment of casualties before they are transported to the ship's hospital or to a cabin for any necessary definitive treatment of the type described in Chapter 4.

However, anyone aboard ship may find a casualty and every seaman should know three basic life-saving actions to be given immediately while waiting for trained help to arrive. These are:

- to give artificial respiration by the mouth to nose/mouth method;
- to place an unconscious casualty in the unconscious position;
- to stop severe bleeding.

Priorities

On finding a casualty:

- ensure your own safety;

if necessary, remove the casualty from danger or danger from the casualty (but see the note below on enclosed spaces);

- give immediate treatment to the casualty who is not breathing and/or whose heart has stopped, is bleeding severely or unconscious – others can be treated later;
- send for help.

If there is more than one unconscious or bleeding casualty:

- send for help;
- treat the most serious injury first in the order of:
  - not breathing and/or heart stopped;
  - unconsciousness.
  - serious bleeding;

If the casualty is in an ENCLOSED SPACE:

- DO NOT enter the enclosed space unless you are a trained member of a rescue team acting under instructions;
- send for help and inform the master.

It must be assumed that the atmosphere in the space is hostile. The rescue team MUST NOT enter unless wearing breathing apparatus which must also be fitted to the casualty as soon as possible. The casualty must be removed quickly to the nearest safe adjacent area outside the enclosed space unless his injuries and the likely time of evacuation makes some treatment essential before movement.

General principles of first aid on board ship

The general principles are:

■ make a rapid examination of the patient to assess responsiveness and the extent of the injury;

■ check breathing, heart and look for serious bleeding;

  • if breathing has stopped, give artificial respiration;

  • if the heart has stopped, give heart compression and artificial respiration;

  • arrest serious bleeding;

■ handle the patient as little and as gently as possible so as to:

  • prevent further injuries; and

  • prevent further shock;

■ see that the patient is put in the most comfortable position possible and loosen tight clothing so that he can breathe easily;

■ do not remove more clothing than is necessary and, when you do, remove it gently. With an injured limb, get the sound limb out of the clothing first and then peel the clothes off the injured limb, which should be supported by another person during the process. If cutting clothes is indicated to expose the injured part, do so. In removing a boot or shoe remove the lace and, if necessary, cut the upper down towards the toecap; keep onlookers away.

■ always remember that shock can be a great danger to life and one of the main objects of first aid is to prevent this;

■ you may have to improvise splints, bandages etc. (Figure 1.23);

■ do not give alcohol in any form;

■ do not move the patient until he is fit to be moved. Bleeding should be arrested, fractures immobilised and shock treated. See that the necessary personnel and equipment for smooth and efficient transport are available;

■ never consider anyone to be dead until you and others agree that:

  • breathing has stopped;

  • no pulse is felt and no sounds are heard when the examiner's ear is put to the chest;

  • the eyes are glazed and pupils are dilated;

  • there is a progressive cooling of the body.

(For a further description of the diagnosis of death Chapter 12).

General assessment of the situation

Once it has been established that there is no immediate threat to life there will be time to take stock of the situation. Reassurance and quick and effective attention to injuries and compassionate treatment of the injured person will alleviate his condition. Remember:

■ a calm and systematic approach should be adopted;

■ give nothing by mouth;

■ protect the casualty from heat or cold, remembering that in the tropics open steel decks can be very hot;

■ never underestimate and do not treat as minor injuries:

  • unconsciousness

  • suspected internal bleeding

  • stab or puncture wounds

  • wounds near joints (see fractures);

  • possible fractures

  • eye injuries

Dressings, bandages, slings and splints

Standard dressing

A standard dressing consists of a thick pad of gauze which is attached to a bandage, leaving about 30cm of tail. The dressing is packed in a paper cover and is sterile. Therefore, when the package is opened, it is important that the gauze pad should not be allowed to touch anything (including your fingers) before it is applied to the wound.

Standard dressings are available in three sizes:
Small Gauze pad measures 7.5 cm by 10 cm.
Medium Gauze pad measures 10 cm by 15 cm.
Large Gauze pad measures 15 cm by 20 cm.

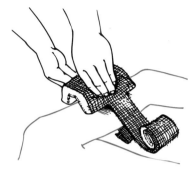

Always select a dressing with a pad which is larger than the wound which you have to cover up.

In use the pad is placed upon the wound, the tail is taken round the limb and held, the bandage is held taut as it is taken round the affected part so as to 'lock' the tail in position. The bandaging can then be continued to hold the dressing firmly in place by making turns above and below the pad so that they overlap it (Figure 1.1).

Figure 1.1

Bandages

Bandages are required to apply and maintain pressure on a wound to stop bleeding, to keep a dressing in place, to provide support, and to prevent movement. Wherever a standard dressing is not used it is customary to cover a wound in the following ways:

- dry dressing – sterile gauze or lint covered by a layer of cotton wool and held in place by a roller or triangular bandage;

- non-stick dressing – sterile paraffin gauze covered by sterile gauze or lint and cotton wool and held in place as above.

NOTE: Never use cotton wool as the first layer of a dressing. When using lint always put the smooth surface next to the skin.

Tube gauze finger bandage

Cut off a piece of tube gauze bandage 60 cm long. Lay this on a flat surface and make a longitudinal cut at one end 10 cm long through both thicknesses of the bandage (Figure 1.2). The tails so formed, 'B', will be used to secure the bandage.

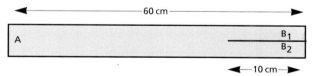

Figure 1.2

Insert the applicator into the bandage at end 'B', then push all the bandage on to it. Then pull 2.5 cm of the bandage off the end of the applicator (Figure 1.3). Tuck this inside.

Hold the finger dressing in place. Insert the finger into the applicator and push it gently towards the base of the finger. Hold the bandage in place with your thumb and withdraw the applicator with a slight turning motion. The bandage will slip off the applicator and will mould firmly to the finger (Figure 1.4).

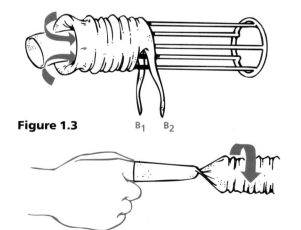

Figure 1.3   B₁ B₂

Figure 1.4

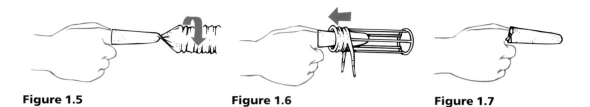

Figure 1.5   **Figure 1.6**   **Figure 1.7**

When the applicator comes off the finger, hold the bandage and the applicator firmly and turn through 360 degrees (Figure 1.5).

Re-insert the tip of the finger into the applicator and push it once again to the base of the finger (Figure 1.6).

Repeat the complete manoeuvre until the bandage is all used up. Then tie loosely at the base of the finger (Figure 1.7). Tape the base of the dressing avoiding encircling the finger.

Triangular bandage

This is the most useful bandage in first aid. It can be used as a broad or narrow fold bandage to hold dressings in place. It can also be used for immobilising limbs or as a sling. It is made from calico or similar material by cutting diagonally across a square of material having 1 metre sides. The ends should always be tied with a reef knot.

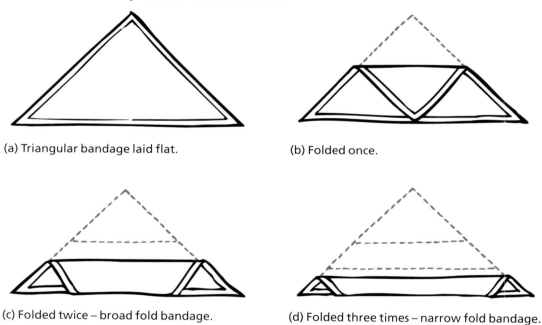

(a) Triangular bandage laid flat.   (b) Folded once.

(c) Folded twice – broad fold bandage.   (d) Folded three times – narrow fold bandage.

Figure 1.8 Broad and narrow fold bandages.

Broad and narrow fold bandages

Figure 1.8 shows how to make a broad and a narrow fold bandage.

The main ways in which a triangular bandage can be used, either as a temporary dressing or to secure or cover a proper dressing, are as follows:

Hand bandage

See Figure 1.9

Wrist and palm bandage

Place palm on the middle of a narrow fold bandage. Take the ends and cross the bandage at the back of the hand, leaving out the thumb. Take turns of the bandage round and round the wrist and tie off at the back (Figure 1.10).

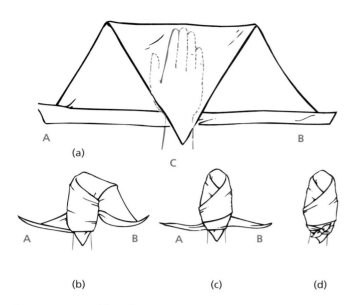

Figure 1.9 Hand bandage

(a) Place the hand on the bandage. Bring down point 'C' over the back of the hand to the wrist

(b) Turn 'A' over the back of the hand, under 'B' and half around the wrist.

(c) Turn 'B' over the back of the hand, over 'A' and half around the wrist.

(d) Take turns with 'A' and 'B' round the wrist and tie off.

Elbow bandage

Fold over the base of the bandage and place the back of the elbow in the middle of the bandage so that the point lies at the back of the upper arm. Take the ends of the bandage round the forearm, cross them in the bend of the elbow, and then take them round the upper arm – to make a 'figure of eight'. Tie off at the back of the arm about 10 cm above the elbow. Fold down the point and fix it with a safety pin (Figure 1.11).

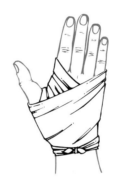

Figure 1.10

Shoulder bandage

Stand facing the casualty's injured side. Place the centre of an open bandage on his shoulder with the point running up the side of the neck (Figure 1.12a). Fold a hem inwards along the base, carry the ends round the middle of the arm, cross and tie them on the outer side (Figure 1.12b). This will secure the lower border of the bandage. Apply an arm sling. Turn the point of the shoulder bandage already applied down over the knot of the arm sling. Pull it tight and pin it in place (Figure 1.12c).

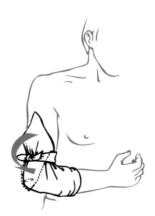

Figure 1.11

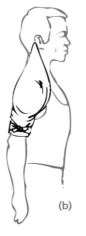

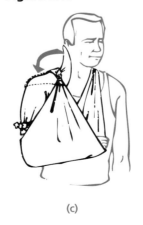

Figure 1.12

Crutch bandage

Tie a narrow fold bandage round the waist; at the middle of the back pass another one under it and allow ends to hang down at the same level. Grasp both these ends and bring them forward under the crutch. Pass one end under the waist bandage in front and tie off (Figure 1.13).

Hip bandage

Tie a narrow fold bandage round the waist with the knot on injured side. Pass the point of another bandage up under the knot, turn a fold at the base of the bandage and bring the ends round the thigh to tie off on the outer side. Pull the point up to remove creases and then fold it down over the knot and fix with safety pin (Figure 1.14).

Knee bandage

Place the point of the bandage in the front of the middle of the thigh, turn a fold at the base of the bandage so that it is about 10 cm below the kneecap. Take the ends round the back of the joint in a figure-of-eight and tie off in front well above the kneecap. Fold the point down over the knot and fix with safety pin (Figure 1.15).

Foot bandage

Lay the foot flat on the bandage. Bring point 'A' up over the foot in front of the ankle. Take 'B' over the foot and behind the ankle. Do the same with 'C'. Knot in front of the ankle (Figure 1.16).

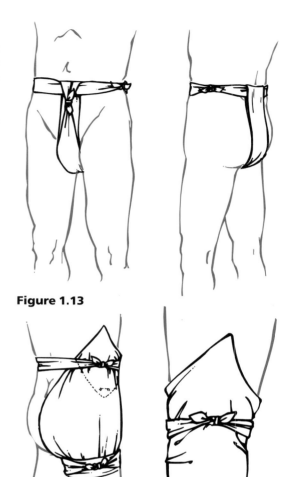

Figure 1.13

Figure 1.14   **Figure 1.15**

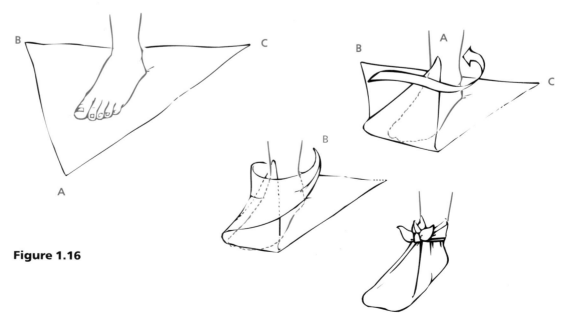

Figure 1.16

Eye bandage

Place the middle of a narrow fold bandage diagonally across the affected eye so as to cover the dressing. Take both ends round the head, cross them at the back and bring them forward again. Tie off over the forehead but not over the eye (Figure 1.17).

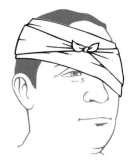

Figure 1.17

Head and scalp bandage

Figure 1.18 is self-explanatory. It is important that the bandage is placed just above the eyebrows. The tails 'B' and 'C' should be taken well under the occiput (the bump on the back of the head where the neck joins the head), and pulled fairly tight before taking them round to the front to be tied off. Failure to do this will result in the bandage falling off, if the patient should bend over (Figure 1.18).

Ring pad

Spread all the fingers of one hand to form a rough circle of the required size. Make two turns of a narrow fold bandage round the ends of the fingers. Twist the remainder of the bandage round the circle so formed to make a grommet (Figure 1.19).

To pass a narrow-fold bandage under the legs or body when the casualty cannot be moved –

Obtain a long piece of wood or a splint. Lay the narrow fold bandage on a flat surface. Place the splint on top of it. Then fold about 22 cm of the bandage back over the splint. Holding the splint and the bandage firmly, gently push the whole under the patient where it is required and carry on pushing until the end comes out on the opposite side. Free the bandage and draw it through. Withdraw the splint. Make the necessary tie.

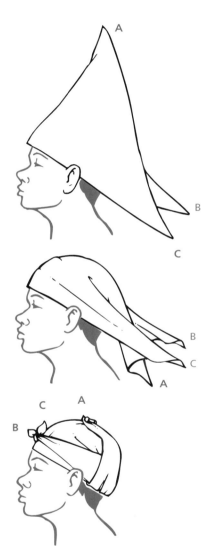

Figure 1.18

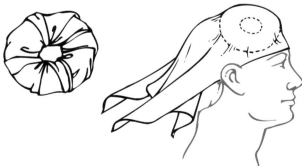

Figure 1.19

Slings

Slings are usually made from triangular bandages, or they can be improvised. The main ways in which to make a sling are as follows:

Large arm sling

Place the triangular bandage on the chest, carrying the point behind the elbow of the injured arm. One end is then placed over the shoulder of the uninjured side and the other hangs down. Gently settle the arm across the bandage, turn up its lower end over the forearm and tie it over the shoulder of the uninjured side so that it fully takes the weight of the forearm. Finally fold the point over the elbow and pin it in place (Figure 1.20).

Collar and cuff sling

This is used to support the wrist. To apply a collar and cuff sling, bend the casualty's elbow to a right angle. Pass a clove hitch round his wrist. Move his forearm across his chest with his fingers touching his opposite shoulder. Tie the ends of the bandage in the hollow just above the collarbone (Figure 1.21).

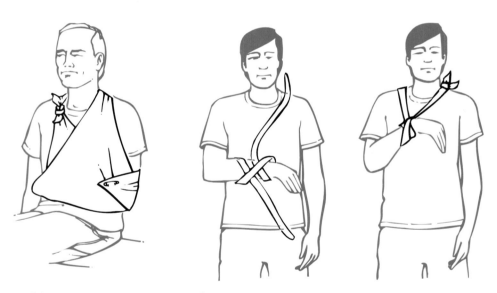

Figure 1.20   **Figure 1.21**

Triangular sling

This keeps the hand well raised and, with a pad under the arm, is used to treat a fracture of the collar bone (Figure 1.22). Place the casualty's forearm across his chest so that his fingers point towards the shoulder and the centre of the palm rests on the breast bone. Lay an open bandage on the forearm with one end (C) over the hand and the point well beyond the elbow (A). Steady the limb and tuck the base of the bandage well under the hand and forearm so that the lower end (B) may be brought under the bent elbow and then upwards across the back to the uninjured shoulder, where it is tied to end (C) in the hollow above the collar bone. The point of the bandage (A) is then tucked well in, between the forearm and bandage in front, and the fold thus formed is turned backwards over the lower part of the upper arm and pinned.

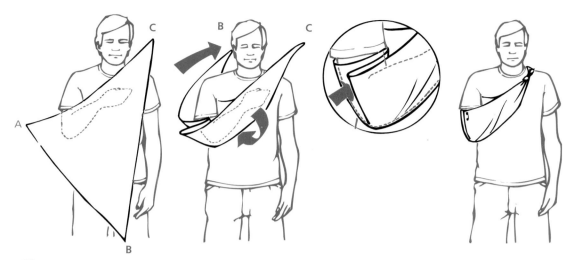

Figure 1.22

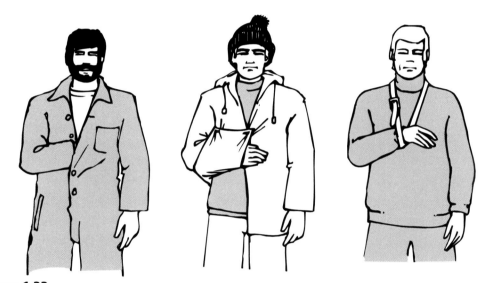

Figure 1.23

Improvised slings and supports

The affected hand or arm can be supported, when no sling is readily available, by simple methods, some of which are illustrated in Figure 1.23.

Splints

Sets of splints of various lengths are included in ships' stores. When properly applied to a limb, they relieve pain by immobilising the fracture and prevent further damage to the surrounding muscles, blood vessels and nerves. The sharp ends of the bone are prevented from piercing the skin and turning a closed fracture into an open fracture with its attendant dangers.

When choosing a splint it should be long enough almost to reach the joint below and the joint above the site of the fracture. The only exception to this rule is the splint used in fractures of the thigh bone. This should be long enough to stretch from the ankle to the armpit.

All splints must be fixed to the limb in at least four places – above and below the site of the fracture and at both ends. Although wooden splints are generally used in first aid, substitutes can be used in emergency situations. These can be in the form of suitably sized pieces of wood or metal, folded cardboard, newspapers or magazines, or pieces of stick or broom handles fastened together to give the necessary width.

Whatever is used, the splint must be padded so that there is a layer of soft material about 1½ cm thick between the splint and the skin. Unpadded splints will cause pain and possible damage to the skin.

Inflatable splints are a useful method for temporarily immobilising limb fractures but are unsuitable for fractures which are more than a short distance above the knee or elbow as they cannot provide sufficient immobilisation in these places. The splint is applied to the limb and inflated by mouth. Other methods of inflation can make the splint too tight and thus slow down or stop the circulation. Inflatable splints can be applied over wound dressings.

The splints are made of clear plastic and any bleeding from a wound can easily be seen. Needless to say, all sharp objects and sharp edges must be kept well clear of the plastic to avoid a puncture.

Inflatable splints may be used to transport a patient about the ship or during moving to hospital. They should not be left in place for more than a few hours. Other means of immobilising the fracture should be used after that period.

Remember that the sound leg is a very good splint to which an injured leg can be secured pending more elaborate measures, and, similarly, the arms can be immobilised against the trunk. If the patient is to be moved by Neil Robertson stretcher, no additional splints may be necessary during first aid.

First aid satchels or boxes

These should contain at least the items required by MSN 1726 for the 'first aid kit'. One should be kept close to the ship's medical store for swift transfer to the site of an accident. If you have more than one, the other(s) should be placed away from the medical store so that if the store is destroyed by fire you have an easily reached first aid kit. These kits should be checked frequently and re-stocked as required.

Severe bleeding

- lay the casualty down;

- press where the blood comes from, using a clean handkerchief, dressing or cloth;

- press with your hand or fist on the wound if nothing else is available. If possible wear disposable gloves.

- if the arms or legs are wounded, lift them up to a near vertical position as this will help to stop the bleeding (Figure 1.24);

- tie a dressing firmly round the wound to maintain the pressure;

- if blood continues to come through the dressing, apply another bandage on the top of the first one. Bandage more firmly.

- keep the injured part as still as possible and the casualty at rest because movement disturbs (and destroys) the blood clot;

- after bleeding has been controlled, rest the limb as shown in Figure 1.24;

- this treatment applies equally to bleeding from an amputation site. Here pressure should be applied over and around the end of the stump.

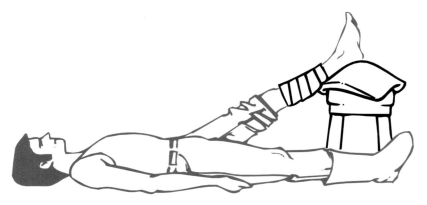

Figure 1.24

Unconscious casualty

The immediate threat to life may be:

- breathing obstructed by the tongue falling back and blocking the throat;

- stopped heart.

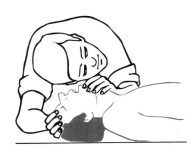

Figure 1.25

Check for breathing at once – Look/Listen/Feel

- look for movements of the chest and abdomen;

- feel for air on your cheek

- listen for breathing with your ear over the mouth and nose (Figure 1.25);

- note the colour of face and lips – normal or blue/grey tinge?

If breathing:

- place the casualty in the unconscious or recovery position (Figure 1.26);

NOTE: no pillows should be used under the head;

- pull up the leg and the arm on the side to which the head is facing, pull up the chin;

- stretch other arm out as pictured

For subsequent treatment of an unconscious patient see Chapter 3.

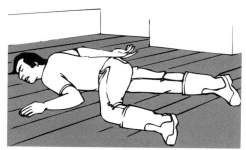

The unconscious position

Figure 1.26

Not breathing:

- With the casualty lying flat on his back, open the airway by making sure that the head is tilted back whilst lifting the chin upwards and forwards (Figure 1.27), which will move the tongue forward and clear the airway.

- Open the mouth and mop out any obvious obstructions such as blood, vomit or secretions. If dentures are worn only remove them if they are broken or displaced. Use your fingers, a handkerchief or a clean piece of cloth.

These actions may relieve the obstruction to breathing. The casualty may gasp and start to breathe naturally. If so, place in the unconscious position.

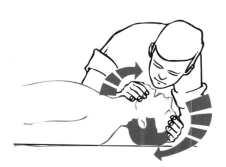

Figure 1.27

Still not breathing:

Begin artificial respiration at once – seconds count.

- Open the airway by making sure that the head is tilted back whilst lifting the chin upwards and forwards.

- work from the side in a convenient position;

- pinch the casualty's nose with your index finger and thumb. After taking a full breath, seal you lips about the patient's mouth and blow into his mouth until you see the chest rise. This should take about 2 seconds for full inflation. (Figure 1.28)

- give two effective inflations quickly, then note if the colour of the face and lips is improving.

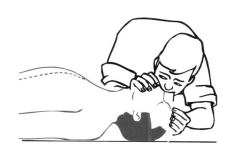

Figure 1.28

If there is improvement:

■ continue the artificial respiration, maintaining a rate of about a dozen inflations each minute. It may help your timing to count to five, slowly, between inflations;

■ see section above on 'If breathing'.

If there is no improvement:

■ listen for heart sounds (Figure 1.29);

■ feel the pulse at the neck (Figure 1.29);

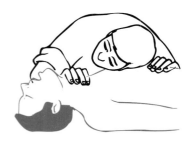

Figure 1.29

If no heart beat is felt, the heart has stopped. A trained first-aider must begin chest compression at once. Unless circulation is restored, the brain will be without oxygen and the person will be dead in four to six minutes:

■ the casualty must be lying on his back on a hard surface, e.g. deck, otherwise the compression will be lost;

■ place your hands together as shown in Figure 1.30;

■ press (¹/₂ second duration, 100 times a minute) firmly and rapidly on the middle of the lower half of the breast bone sufficient to produce a downward movement of about 4 cm (Figure 1.31);

■ artificial respiration (Figure 1.30) must also be carried out when giving heart compression since breathing stops when the heart stops. It can be given by one person, alternately compressing 15 times and then filling the lungs with air twice or, ideally, by two people – one giving heart compression and the other giving artificial respiration, at a ratio of 5 chest compressions to 1 lung inflation;

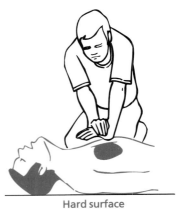

Hard surface

Figure 1.30

■ if the heart starts to beat the colour of the face and lips will improve and the eye pupils will get smaller;

■ listen again for heart sounds and feel for a neck pulse. If they are heard, stop heart compression but continue with artificial respiration until natural breathing is restored.

When you are satisfied that the heart is beating and unassisted breathing is restored, transfer the casualty by stretcher, in the unconscious position, to the ship's hospital or a cabin for further treatment. See Chapter 3 for continued nursing care.

Unfortunately these measures are not always successful. Failure to restart the heart after cardiac arrest is common even in the best environment, such as a fully equipped hospital. It may be necessary to decide to stop artificial respiration and chest compression. If in doubt SEEK RADIO MEDICAL ADVICE.

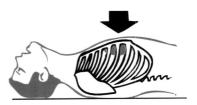

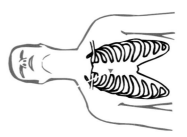

Figure 1.31

Burns and scalds

Clothing on fire

- by far the best way to put out a fire on a person is to use a dry powder fire extinguisher at once;

- if a dry powder extinguisher is not available, then lay the person down and smother the flames by wrapping him in any available material (not made of man-made fibre), or throw buckets of water over him, or use a hose;

- make sure all smouldering clothing is extinguished.

NOTE: The powder from a fire extinguisher will not cause much, if any, eye damage. Most people shut their eyes tightly if sprayed with powder. Any powder which gets in the eye should be washed out immediately after the fire has been extinguished and while cooling is being undertaken.

Heat burns and scalds

- all heat burns should be cooled as quickly as possible with running cold water (sea or fresh) for at least ten minutes, or by immersing in cold water and keeping the injured part in motion; cooling of extensive burns (>15%) should be avoided as hypothermia will result.

- if it is not possible to cool the burn on the spot, the casualty should be taken to where cooling can be carried out;

- try to remove clothing gently but do not tear off any which adheres to the skin;

- then cover the burned areas with a dry, non-fluffy, dressing which is larger than the burns and bandage in place;

- further treatment as in Chapter 4.

Electrical burns and electrocution

- make sure you do not become the next casualty when approaching any person who is in contact with electricity:

- if possible, switch off the current;

- otherwise, insulate yourself. Remove your watch and rings, wear rubber boots or stand on an insulating mat, thick DRY newspaper or wood;

- alternatively, pull the casualty from the source of supply with an insulated flex or push him away with a strong non-conductor, such as a piece of DRY wood;

- check immediately for breathing and heartbeat:

  - if not breathing, give artificial respiration;

  - if heart is stopped, give chest compression and artificial respiration;

- send for help;

- when the casualty is breathing, cool any burned areas and apply a clean, dry, non-fluffy covering to the burned area.

Chemical splashes

- remove contaminated clothing. Drench with water to wash the chemical away;

- carry on washing for at least ten minutes. If you are in any doubt that the chemical has been completely cleared from the skin, repeat the washing for a further ten minutes;

- give priority to washing the eyes if affected, as they are particularly vulnerable to chemical splashes. If only one eye is affected, incline the head to that side to prevent the chemical from running across into the other eye.

Suffocation (Asphyxia)

Suffocation is usually caused by gases or smoke:

- remember that dangerous gases may have no smell to warn you of their presence;
- do not enter enclosed spaces without the proper precautions;
- do not forget the risks of fire and/or explosion when dealing with inflammable gases or vapours;
- get the casualty into the fresh air;
- give artificial respiration if not breathing;
- chest compression may be required if the heart stops;
- when breathing is restored, place in the unconscious position;
- oxygen may be administered later if carried on board.

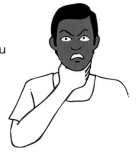

Figure 1.32

Strangulation

- Immediately remove the cause;
- treat as for suffocation above;
- give protective supervision if there is any reason to suspect that the injury was self-inflicted.

Choking

Choking is usually caused by a large lump of food which sticks at the back of the throat and obstructs breathing. The person then becomes unconscious very quickly and will die in 4 to 6 minutes unless the obstruction is removed.

Choking can be mistaken for a heart attack. A person who is choking:

- may have been seen to be eating;
- cannot speak or breathe;
- will turn blue and lose consciousness quickly because of lack of oxygen;
- can signal his distress (he cannot speak) by grasping his neck between fingers and thumb. This is known as the 'Heimlich sign' and, if understood by all personnel, should reduce the risks involved in choking (Figure 1.32).

Up to five firm slaps on the back, between the shoulder blades, may dislodge the obstruction. If not:

If the casualty is conscious, stand behind him, place your closed fist against the place in the upper abdomen where the ribs divide and grasp your fist with the other hand. Press suddenly and sharply into the casualty's abdomen with *a hard quick* upward thrust, five times if necessary. If unsuccessful continue in cycles of five back blows to five abdominal thrusts. (Figures 1.33 and 1.34).

If the casualty is unconscious, place him face upwards, keeping the chin well up and the neck bent backwards. Kneel astride him, place one hand over the other with the heel of the lower hand at the place where the ribs divide. Press suddenly and sharply into the abdomen with a hard, quick upwards thrust. Repeat several times if necessary (Figure 1.35). When the food is dislodged remove it from the mouth and place the casualty in the unconscious position.

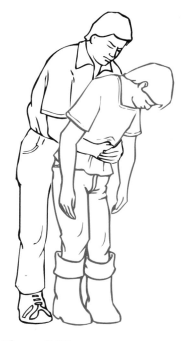

Figure 1.33

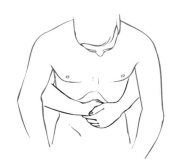

Figure 1.34

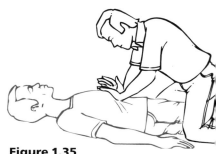

Figure 1.35

Epileptic fits – convulsions

The fit may vary from a momentary loss of consciousness (petit mal) in which the patient may sway but does not actually fall, to a major attack (grand mal) as follows: the patient suddenly loses consciousness and falls to the ground, possibly with a cry; he remains rigid for some seconds, during which he stops breathing and the face becomes flushed; the convulsion then starts with irregular, jerky movements of the limbs, rolling of the eyes, gnashing of the teeth, with perhaps some frothing at the mouth. He may lose control and pass urine or faeces. After a variable time, but usually in a few minutes, the convulsion ceases and he falls into what appears to be a deep sleep.

Treatment

- prevent the patient from hurting himself in the convulsive stage;

- never restrain him forcibly, as this may cause injury, but remove hard objects and surround him by pillows, clothing or other soft material;

- after the fit is over, check for injuries. Assuming the patient is uninjured, let him sleep it off. He may be rather confused and dazed when he comes round. Reassure him and do not leave him until you are sure he is aware of his surroundings and knows what he is doing.

In the event of the patient having several fits, one after the other, it may be necessary to give him an anti-epileptic drug such as Diazepam. SEEK URGENT RADIO MEDICAL ADVICE.

Shock and circulatory collapse

Shock occurs when the body's circulatory system is unable to distribute oxygen enriched blood to all parts of the body. If untreated, the body's vital organs (brain, heart, lungs, kidneys) can fail, leading to collapse, unconsciousness and eventually death.

Causes

The commonest cause is loss of body fluid from the circulation. It can result, either from external or internal bleeding, (e.g. as occurs in fractures of the thigh), the formation of large blisters and the weeping of fluid from large burns and from damaged blood vessels in crush injuries. Shock can also be found in severe heart attacks, and in certain diseases characterised by excessive vomiting and diarrhoea.

The first-aider should always be on the look-out for this condition as it can develop even while the casualty is under close observation and it may be missed. Fear, pain and exposure to cold make shock worse.

Symptoms and signs

The patient:

- will usually lie still, taking little notice of his surroundings

- will complain of feeling faint, cold and thirsty. He may shiver;

- his lips and the edges of the ears may be blue;

- his skin will be pale, cold and clammy;

- his pulse will be rapid and weak;

- his respiration will be rapid and shallow and, as shock deepens, he will give frequent sighs;

- he may start to vomit;

- if untreated, he may lapse into unconsciousness and later die.

Treatment

The primary aim is to treat whatever condition is causing the shock;

- lay the patient flat and, if injuries permit, elevate the feet and legs so that blood flows to the heart and brain (see note below on exceptions to this rule);
- do not move him unless in a position of danger;
- stop any blood loss. Cover burns and scalds. Immobilise fractures.
- loosen any tight clothing which restricts breathing movement;
- keep warm but do not overheat.
- deal with any pain. Morphine may be given as necessary
- give small sips of water if there is no suspicion of abdominal injury but NEVER give fluids to an unconscious casualty. A badly burned or scalded person may require much more fluid;
- move to a place of safety as gently as possible. Rough handling will increase the pain and the shock.

Exceptions to the lay flat rule:

- if there is an injury to the face, mouth or jaw with a lot of bleeding, place in the unconscious position with the head turned with the damaged side underneath and, if possible, with a head-down tilt. This will prevent blood running down into the throat and lungs;
- if there is a penetrating wound of the chest, or if breathing is difficult, prop up to assist breathing;
- if unconsciousness occurs, put into the unconscious position with as little disturbance as possible to the injured part.

Bleeding

External bleeding

Bleeding from small blood vessels occurs when there is a minor cut or abrasion of the skin. Blood oozes from the wound; it usually stops by itself or when a dressing is applied. It is generally of no consequence.

In large and deep wounds, the blood wells up in a steady stream. The volume of blood loss depends on the number of blood vessels damaged and, although it may appear alarming, it is not usually dangerous, unless allowed to continue.

When large arteries are damaged, bright red blood will spurt from the wound in time with the heart beats. This bleeding is usually profuse and the patient's life will be endangered. This is a rare situation.

In all cases of external bleeding, follow the three cardinal rules:

- lay the patient down;
- lift up the affected part if possible;
- press firmly where the blood comes from. Use a dressing or a clean cloth or handkerchief but, if none should be available, use the bare hand or fingers. When possible disposable gloves should be worn to protect yourself.

  This procedure will stop the flow of blood.

When bleeding has been controlled, apply a standard dressing to the wound and bandage firmly and widely in position. There may be a slight staining of blood through the dressing, which is of little consequence, but if blood soaks quickly through the pad it is a sign that the bleeding has not been properly controlled. If this happens, do not disturb the dressing, but put another standard dressing on top and bandage more firmly. This will usually stop the bleeding. Very occasionally, a third dressing may be required.

Do not disturb the dressings until you are prepared to undertake definitive treatment. The bleeding stops because of the formation of a clot. If you remove the dressing, the clot will break and bleeding will start again.

Special types of external bleeding

From an open fracture

The bleeding comes mainly from around the break and not from the bone.

- do not attempt to elevate the part, this will cause further pain and damage;

- apply a dressing, sterile if possible, padding around the wound. Firm bandaging will apply the necessary pressure to the tissue around the exposed bone ends.

From a tooth socket:

- The socket may bleed after the extraction of a tooth. This kind of bleeding is seldom serious. At least two-thirds of the 'blood' which is spat out will be saliva, so the blood loss is unlikely to be great;

- if the gum margins are splayed out, squeeze them gently together to close up the tooth socket;

- fold a piece of gauze tightly and place it in the socket so that it is standing proud of the level of the remaining teeth;

- the casualty should close his mouth, biting firmly on the gauze in the tooth socket. The pressure should be maintained for 20 minutes. If the socket is still bleeding on removing the gauze pad, the procedure should be repeated as often as is necessary (Figure 1.36).

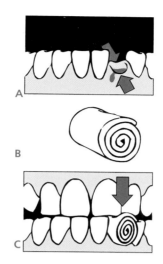

Figure 1.36

From the ear passage:

This is usually caused by a head injury or by blast:

- place a large pad over the ear and bandage it in position;

- keep the affected ear downwards;

- if the casualty is unconscious, place in the unconscious position with the affected ear downwards;

- never plug the ear passage with cotton wool or other material.

From the nose:

- the casualty should sit with his head over a basin or bowl while pinching the soft part of his nose firmly for 10 minutes; (Figure 1.37);

- he should then release the pressure slowly;

- if bleeding has not stopped, he should repeat the manoeuvre for a further 10 minutes;

- it might be necessary to do this for a third time;

- if bleeding has not stopped after half-an-hour, it might then be necessary to pack the nose with ribbon gauze. (See Chapter 4)

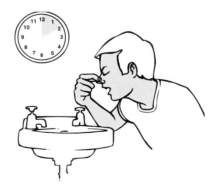

Figure 1.37

From the lips, cheek and tongue:

- press on both sides of the lip, cheek or tongue to stop bleeding;

- use a piece of gauze or a swab on each side to help maintain pressure and stop the fingers slipping (Figure 1.38);

- pressing is usually most easily done by the casualty with direction from another person, or helped by looking in a mirror.

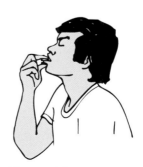

Figure 1.38

Internal bleeding

Internal bleeding may be caused by injury, disease, or by the action of certain poisons. Any severe injury to the body will cause bleeding of varying degree. Bleeding may be limited to the soft tissues, such as muscles, but when a bone breaks there is always bleeding at the fracture site. Minor injury will affect only the superficial tissues and the bleeding may be limited to small amounts which will appear as bruising. Greater force will result, in addition to bruising, in the formation of a collection of blood within the deeper tissues (a haematoma). This causes painful swelling of the affected part and may be difficult to distinguish from a fracture. Whatever the nature of such injuries, the blood loss very rarely endangers life.

In contrast, bleeding from injury to internal organs is always very serious and may quickly endanger life. Such bleeding is always concealed and its presence has to be deduced from the history of the injury, a rising pulse rate and the signs and symptoms of shock which occur rapidly. The abdominal organs are poorly protected by the abdominal wall and they are particularly liable to injury by direct or crushing forces. These internal injuries require expert treatment urgently and every effort must be made to deliver the casualty to medical care. Always get RADIO MEDICAL ADVICE. There is little that can be done aboard because a blood transfusion may be needed.

If internal bleeding is suspected:

- put in bed with a head-down tilt;

- if conscious and in pain or restless, give morphine 10 mg;

- cover with only one blanket;

- record the pulse rate at 10 minute intervals. A falling rate may indicate that the bleeding has stopped (Figure A);

- give fluid per rectum (Chapter 3);

- if the injury is abdominal, allow the patient to suck flakes of ice. With bleeding from other parts of the body, sips of water may be given;

- treat for shock.

Coughing up or vomiting blood

NOTE: remember that bleeding can occur from the back of the nose, a tooth socket, bleeding gums, etc. It is important that this should not be confused with bleeding from the stomach or lungs.

Coughing up of blood

In some lung diseases and cases of injury to the chest, blood may be coughed up. Except in cases of injury this is seldom fatal.

Treatment is the same as for internal bleeding with the exception that the patient should be placed at rest with the head and shoulders raised. It is not usually necessary to give fluid per rectum. For further care see Chapter 4.

See Examination of sputum (Chapter 3).

Vomiting blood

Blood may be vomited if the stomach is injured by a wound of the abdomen or if blood collects in the stomach as a result of a bleeding peptic ulcer. In the latter case the patient may suddenly vomit a quantity of dark brown fluid like coffee grounds. He feels faint and looks pale. If the bleeding and vomiting continue he will suffer increasingly from shock.

Treatment is the same as for internal bleeding. For further treatment of this condition, see Chapter 7. If there is a wound of the abdomen, this should be treated.

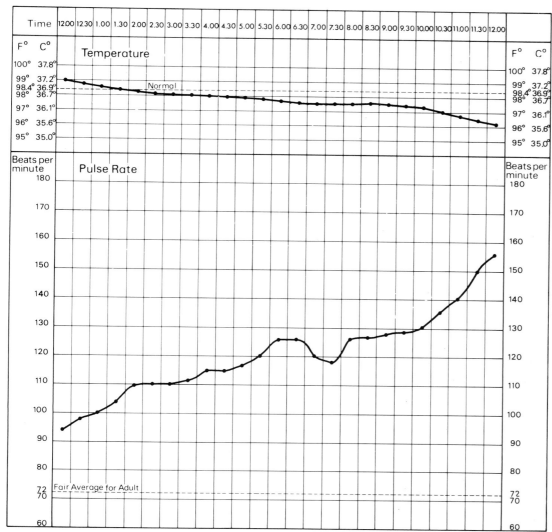

Figure A Haemorrhage – the falling temperature and the rising pulse rate

Wounds

A wound at any site in the body poses three problems:

- control of bleeding;
- prevention of shock
- prevention of infection

 There are some simple rules:

- never wash the wound – except in cases of an animal bite
- never try to remove pieces of metal or glass from a wound unless they are superficial and can be easily lifted out. If pieces can be removed, do it by grasping the material with sterile gauze or use sterile forceps, if available;
- do not pour antiseptic into a wound;
- as soon as possible, cover the wound with a suitable dressing.

Bullet or metal fragment wounds

In this type of injury, look for and treat any exit wound. This is usually larger than the entry wound. Remember that there may be underlying bone fractures and that the bullet or metal fragment may have been deflected from the bone to cause serious internal damage, the only signs of which may be increasing shock.

Chest wounds

A superficial chest wound should be treated as for any wound elsewhere but a penetrating wound (a sucking wound) of the chest must be sealed *immediately*, otherwise air is drawn into the chest cavity and the lungs cannot inflate as the vacuum inside the chest is destroyed. A useful dressing for a sucking wound can be made from a paraffin gauze dressing. Place the paraffin gauze over the wound, smooth the foil on to the chest wall and seal *three edges only* with zinc oxide adhesive plaster. In emergency, a suitable dressing may be improvised from petroleum jelly, gauze and kitchen foil or polythene or, alternatively, a wet dressing may be used to provide an airtight seal. If nothing else is available, use the casualty's own bloodstained clothing to plug the wound temporarily. The aim is to prevent air entering the chest but to allow it to escape if necessary.

The usual rules about stopping bleeding by pressing where the blood comes from also apply. Start a pulse chart soon to check on possible internal bleeding in all chest injuries. The respiratory rate should also be recorded. See also sections on chest injuries.

Conscious casualties should be placed in the half-sitting-up position because breathing is easier in this position.

NOTE: DO NOT GIVE MORPHINE to a patient with this type of wound, even if he is suffering from a lot of pain, as the morphine will increase the breathing difficulties.

Get RADIO MEDICAL ADVICE.

Abdominal wounds

A superficial abdominal wound will require the same treatment as any wound, but for more serious wounds, if the abdominal contents *do not protrude*, cover the wound with a large standard dressing and place the casualty in the half-sitting-up position (Figure 1.39). In this position the wound will not gape open. As the abdominal muscles are slack, the abdominal contents will not bulge through. If the wound runs more or less vertically, it may be best to lay the man flat.

If the abdominal contents *do protrude* through the wound, DO NOT ATTEMPT TO PUT THEM BACK. Cover with a loosely applied large standard dressing or dressings until further treatment can be given. Shock will develop quickly and should be treated as described previously, with the following important exceptions:

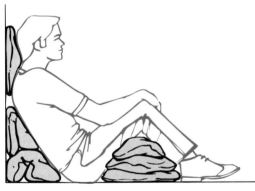

Figure 1.39

- prop up if necessary;
- DO NOT give anything by mouth. If thirsty, the lips should be moistened; nothing more.

    (See also Crush wounds and Stab wounds below).

- Get RADIO MEDICAL ADVICE

Head wounds

The wound itself should be treated in the same way as any other wound. Scalp wounds often bleed briskly. A firm bandage will usually arrest the bleeding, but some ingenuity may be required in applying the bandage so as to keep it firmly on the head and transmit the necessary pressure to the pad. Firm pressure by the fingers over the pad for a few minutes before it is finally fixed in position will help to stop the bleeding.

The possibility of brain damage is of greater importance and two rules should be observed:

- morphine should be given only if conscious and in much pain from more serious injuries elsewhere;
- if unconscious, put in the unconscious position and give the treatment described in Chapter 4.
- Get RADIO MEDICAL ADVICE

Face and jaw wounds

There may be danger of suffocation as a result of blood running into the throat. Lay flat in the unconscious position (Figure 1.26) with the more damaged side underneath. If the casualty is to be removed by stretcher, see that he remains in that position. With severe wounds there may be loss of the power of speech. Give reassurance; speech will probably return to normal when healing has taken place.

Palm of the hand wounds

A deep wound of the palm of the hand may cut the large artery in this area. If this occurs:

- stop the bleeding by pressing where the blood comes from;
- cover the wound with a sterile gauze dressing and ask the patient to grasp firmly on a rolled-up 7.5 cm bandage;
- a hand bandage, firmly applied, will hold the dressing in place and will maintain the pressure necessary to control the bleeding.

Crush injuries

Limbs

After a crush injury, at first there may be very little to see. However, considerable damage may have been done to the muscles and other soft tissues and gross swelling may take place later. Shock, which may be very severe, may also develop.

- treat any wound;
- the affected limb should be immobilised and supported in its most comfortable position;
- treat shock as described but:
  - do not give large amounts of fluid at once as the casualty will vomit;
  - give frequent small amounts of water only.
- GET RADIO MEDICAL ADVICE.

Chest

Crushing of the chest may stop breathing and then artificial respiration will be required.

If ribs have been fractured, treat as described under fractures.

See also section on chest injuries.

Abdomen

Severe crushing of the abdomen may cause rupture of the internal organs and/or internal bleeding. If you suspect that this has occurred, Get RADIO MEDICAL ADVICE. See general advice on abdominal wounds at beginning of this section and stab wounds below.

Stab wounds

Stab wounds are especially dangerous because the underlying structures will have been penetrated and infection will have been carried into the deep tissues.

Chest:

- if the lung has been penetrated, it will collapse giving rise to breathlessness and coughing of bright red frothy blood;
- a sucking wound can be created;
- the heart can be damaged.
- Get RADIO MEDICAL ADVICE
- see also section on chest injuries.

Abdomen

Depending on the position of the wound (see Anatomy Diagrams, Annex II), an organ may be pierced, giving rise to peritonitis and internal bleeding. See general advice at beginning of this section. Get RADIO MEDICAL ADVICE.

Limbs

Muscles, nerves and blood vessels may be cut. Bleeding, both internal and external, will occur. Whatever the site of the stab wound, the immediate treatment is the same:

- stop external bleeding by pressure
- prevent further infection by applying suitable dressings
- treat shock if necessary.

Fractures

A fracture is a broken bone. The bone may be broken into two or more pieces with separation of the fragments or it may have one or more fissured cracks without any separation.

Most fractures are caused by direct force, but force may be transmitted through the body to cause injury indirectly elsewhere. Two classical examples are: a fall on the outstretched hand, causing a fracture of the collar bone; and a fall from a height on to the heels, causing a fracture of the base of the skull.

A much less common type is a stress fracture. The bone becomes weakened in a way comparable to metal fatigue. Sudden, strong muscular effort may snap the bone.

In simple terms, a fracture may be open to infection or closed to infection.

A closed fracture

There is no communication between the fracture and the surface of the body.

An open fracture

There is communication between a skin wound and the fracture. Open fractures are always serious because germs may enter through the wound to cause infection of the broken bone and the surrounding tissues.

NOTE: A skin wound may be present but, unless it is deep enough to reach the broken bone, the fracture is still closed. Open or closed fractures are sometimes *complicated* by damage to important structures such as the brain, lung, blood vessels or nerves.

Principles of treatment

It is not possible to set fractures on board ship. Indeed, many fractures may not require setting and unskilled attempts might prejudice healing. First aid measures should ensure adequate immobilisation. Wherever a fracture case has to be kept on board for more than two or three days, the joints above and below the fracture site should be gently put through a full range of movements, morning and night.

Lasting damage may result if a joint surface is involved in the fracture and in all cases where this is suspected, RADIO MEDICAL ADVICE must be sought.

Antibiotic treatment must always be given as soon as an open fracture is diagnosed or suspected.

Examination

The following signs and symptoms will indicate that the bone is probably broken:

- a heavy blow or other force has been applied to the body or limbs. The casualty or others may have heard the bone break;
- intense pain, especially on pressure or movement at the site;
- swelling. The site may be swollen and/or bruised. This may be due to internal bleeding;
- loss of use. The casualty may be unable or unwilling to use the injured part because of the

pain. He may also experience severe pain if an attempt, even very gently, is made to help him make the movement. Watch his face for signs of pain. Occasionally, if the broken ends of a bone are impacted together, the person may be able to use the part but usually only with a fair amount of pain;

■ distortion. Compare good and bad limbs or sides of the body to see if the part is swollen, bent, twisted or shortened;

■ irregularity. The irregular edges of a broken bone can sometimes be seen in an open fracture. They may be seen or felt under the skin in a closed fracture;

■ *unnatural movement and grating of bone ends.* Neither of these symptoms should be sought deliberately. A limb may feel limp and wobbly and grating may be felt when trying to apply support to the limb. In either of these situations, the bone is certainly broken.

General treatment

■ bleeding should be treated as described;

■ rest the affected part by immobilisation. This prevents further damage, relieves pain and stops further bleeding;

■ all fractures or suspected fractures must be immobilised before making any attempt to move the casualty. This can be done using wooden, improvised or inflatable splints, or by fixing a limb to the body, or – in the case of the legs – by lashing one to the other.

Immobilise a limb in the position in which it is found, if it is comfortable. If it does become necessary to move an injured limb, because of poor circulation or for any other reason, first apply traction by pulling the limb gently and firmly away from the body before attempting to move it (Figure 1.40).

Keep pulling until it has been securely immobilised and then release the traction very slowly. Sudden release can cause pain.

Circulation of the blood in a fractured limb. Check that the circulation to the limb is intact. To do this, press on the nail of the thumb or of the big toe. When circulation is normal the nail becomes white when pressed and pink when released. Continue checking until you are satisfied that all is well. Danger signs are:

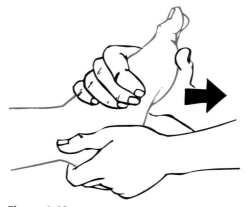

Figure 1.40

■ blueness or whiteness of fingers and toes;

■ coldness of the parts below the fracture;

■ loss of feeling below the injury. Test for this by touching lightly on fingers and toes and asking the casualty if he can feel anything;

■ absence of pulse.

If there is any doubt at all about the circulation, loosen all tight and limb-encircling dressings at once and straighten out the limb, remembering to use traction when doing so. *Check circulation again.* If the limb does not become pink and warm and you cannot detect a pulse, then medical help is urgently necessary if amputation is to be avoided. Get RADIO MEDICAL ADVICE.

■ remember that fractures can cause severe internal bleeding ;

■ always look for and treat for shock;

■ morphine may be necessary to control pain.

Collar bone, shoulder blade and shoulder

Fractures in these areas are often the result either of a fall on the outstretched hand or a fall on to the shoulder. Direct violence to the parts is a less common cause of these fractures.

Place loose padding about the size of a fist into the armpit. Support the arm using a triangular sling (Figure 1.41). Then tie the arm to the body, using a narrow fold bandage. Keep the casualty sitting up as he will probably be most comfortable in this position.

Upper arm

Upper arm fractures are usually caused by direct violence.

Bind the upper arm to the body, using a broad fold bandage. Bend the elbow gently and apply a collar and cuff sling (Figure 1.42). Keep the casualty sitting up so that the weight of the arm can supply traction to the lower fragment.

Alternatively, upper arm fractures may be splinted. Bend the elbow gently. Use three well padded splints. Place one behind the upper arm, one in front and the third from the tip of the shoulder to the elbow. Bandage the splints securely in place. Support the arm with a collar and cuff sling (see also Figure 1.21).

Elbow

Fractures in this area can be especially dangerous because of damage to blood vessels and nerves around the elbow. Check circulation and feeling in the fingers. If the finger tips are white or blue and feeling is absent or altered, the elbow must be straightened at once. Tell the casualty to lie down. Be gentle. Apply traction on the hand and forearm. Bring the arm and forearm slowly and carefully to the casualty's side. Now place plenty of loose padding between the arm and the body and also around the arm. Then bind the forearm to the body by encircling ties. Check the circulation again when you have made the encircling ties. If the circulation is poor, the ties should be loosely secured until the casualty has to be moved (Figure 1.43).

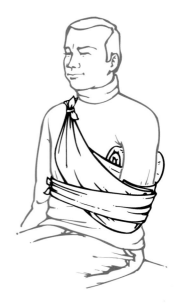

Figure 1.41

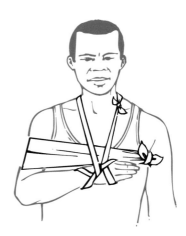

Figure 1.42

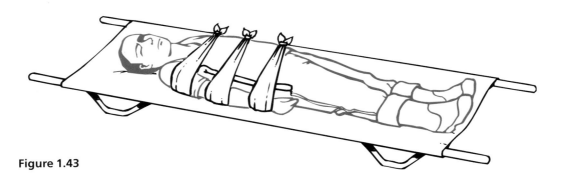

Figure 1.43

Forearm and wrist

Fractures in this area commonly result from a fall on the outstretched hand. Bend the elbow until the forearm is across the body. Then apply an arm sling (Figure 1.20). Remove any finger rings.

Later, apply two well padded splints to the back and front of the forearm and secure firmly, using narrow fold bandages. Support the arm with a broad arm sling. For fractures of the wrist bones, put a broad, well padded splint on the front of the forearm and the palm of the hand. Put plenty of padding on the back of the forearm and hand and secure. Use a broad arm sling for support.

Hand and fingers

Fractures of the hand bones (metacarpals) and the finger bones are a common result of shipboard accidents and expert treatment may be many days away. As fixation in a straight splint is only permissible for a short time, the treatment described in the following paragraphs should be undertaken if the casualty has to be kept on board. Always remove rings immediately.

The hand bones (metacarpals):

- apply a crepe bandage around the hand and wrist firmly enough to support the injured part but not so tight as to prevent movement of the wrist and finger joints;
- check that circulation to the fingers is present;
- elevate the hand by placing the arm in a triangular sling to reduce the swelling;
- encourage the casualty to move the wrist and all the finger joints frequently.

The fingers:

- strap the finger to the adjacent finger, using zinc oxide adhesive plaster (as shown in Figure 1.44);
- be careful that you do not prevent movement of the finger joints. Do not put the plaster directly over the fracture;
- to avoid swelling, elevate the hand by putting the arm in a triangular sling;
- encourage the casualty to move all the finger joints.

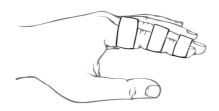

Figure 1.44

Open fracture of the fingers:

- stop the bleeding and apply a dressing to the wound;
- if the dressing prevents strapping to the adjacent finger, use as a splint, a strip of aluminium or other soft metal 2 cm wide and long enough to stretch from the tip of the finger to just below the wrist joint;
- immobilise the finger in the position shown in Figure 1.45. This is done by bending the splint to conform with the joints, using the same finger of the undamaged hand as a pattern, and taking care to ensure that the splint will not dig into the back of the hand or into the wrist;
- pad the splint with two layers of elastic adhesive bandage along its length. Turn the bandage over the ends to protect the skin;
- fix the splint to the finger with zinc oxide plaster cut to suitable widths;
- give standard antibiotic treatment.

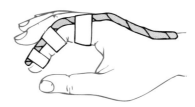

Figure 1.45

Crush injuries to the hand

Severe crushing injuries to the hands may cause multiple open or closed fractures of the metacarpal or finger bones. Other wounds are likely to be present.

- stop the bleeding and apply dressings;

- pain will be severe. Give analgesics (Morphine if necessary);

- if hospital treatment is not available quickly, read the section on definitive treatment of wounds and treat accordingly.

Hip to knee

A broken thigh bone is a potentially serious injury. It causes significant internal bleeding into the muscles of the thigh and, with the associated pain, shock very quickly develops. If it is combined with other serious injuries, the blood loss may be so great as to require blood replacement. Get **RADIO MEDICAL ADVICE**.

- a break of the neck of the thigh bone causes shortening of the injured leg and the casualty will lie with the whole lower limb and foot flopped outwards. There will be severe pain in the region of the hip;

- fractures of the shaft of the thigh bone exhibit the usual signs and symptoms of a fracture. Severe pain is a normal feature.

If you think that the thigh is broken:

- first, pad between the thighs, knees, calves and ankles, using folded blankets or any other suitable soft material;

- bring the good leg to the broken leg. Do this slowly and carefully;

- bring the feet together. If attempting to do this causes pain, apply traction to the injured leg gently and slowly, and then try again;

- tie encircling bandages: around both feet; halfway between the knees and the ankles; just above the knees; and at the upper thighs. Avoid making any ties over the site of the fracture (Figure 1.46);

- the shoe on the affected side can now be removed so that you can check the circulation in the toes – if necessary, loosen any bandages – and then replace the figure-of-eight bandage around the ankles and feet;

- treat for shock and pain – morphine will be needed.

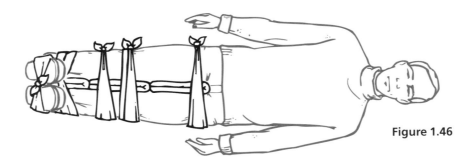

Figure 1.46

Kneecap

This fracture may be caused by direct violence or as a result of a sudden stress on the bone.
    It is commonly a closed fracture. When an open fracture occurs, the wound should be treated before splinting is undertaken and antibiotic treatment should be given.

- place the casualty in a half-sitting-up position and put supports behind his back to maintain this. Raise the leg and hold it in a comfortable position.

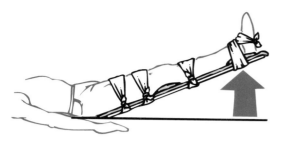

Figure 1.47

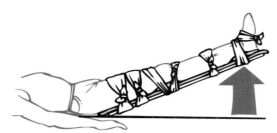

Figure 1.48

- choose a splint long enough to reach from the buttock to beyond the heel, pad it well and apply it along the back of the leg. Put additional padding behind the hollow at the heel so as to lift it off the splint, and also behind the knee;

- secure the splint in place with bandages round the thigh, round the lower leg just below the knee and with a figure-of-eight bandage at the ankle, and elevate the leg on a suitable support (Figure 1.47).

When the casualty is moved to the cabin or to the ship's hospital, he should be kept in a sitting position with the leg elevated.

When medical attention will not be available for some time and it is obvious that there is a wide gap between the fragments of the knee cap, carry out the procedure described above, but put a figure-of-eight bandage round the knee, beginning above the knee cap and finishing over padding applied just below it (Figure 1.48).

This method will draw the fragments together and hold them in place. Check that the circulation is intact.

Knee to foot

Lower limb

These should be treated in the same way as fractures of the thigh. See also below for fractures of both legs.

Ankle

An ankle fracture which is stable and without any deformity can be given adequate but temporary first aid by placing the injured ankle on a number of pillows to keep it at rest (Figure 1.49).

In more serious fractures of the ankle it is usual to find a good deal of deformity and swelling, and splinting may be necessary.

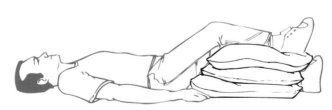

Figure 1.49

- remove the casualty's shoe and sock;

- obtain two splints, long enough to stretch from just below the knee to the sole of the foot. Pad these well to allow for the deformity and swelling, and apply them to both sides of the leg;

- fix them in place with a figure-of-eight bandage to the foot and place other bandages just below the knee and above the ankle;

- check that the circulation is intact.

Heel bone

These fractures usually occur when the casualty has fallen from a height and lands on his heels. As force has been transmitted upwards, there may be more serious fractures elsewhere, e.g. spine and base of the skull, and the patient should be carefully examined to exclude these. Treat as above, for fractures of the ankle.

Bones of the foot

Severe injuries are usually the result of heavy weights being dropped on to unprotected feet or of crushing. Fractures of the toes may occur when they are stubbed against some hard object.

- remove the boot or shoe and the socks carefully;

- treat any wound.

- keep the foot elevated and use pillows to keep it in a comfortable position.

Both legs

As there is no good leg to act as a splint for the other, external splinting will have to be used. There may be considerable blood loss if both legs are broken.

- have well padded splints available. These should reach from the thigh to the ankles on the outside of both the legs for below the knee fractures, and from the armpit to the ankles for above the knee fractures;

- pad between the thighs, knees, calves and ankles;

- bring both feet together as gently as you can, using traction if necessary.

- tie a figure-of-eight bandage round the feet and ankles to keep the feet together;

- apply the padded splints to the outside of both legs;

- tie enough encircling bandages to keep the splints and the legs secured firmly together. Avoid making any ties over the site of any break (Figure 1.50);

- check the circulation in both feet as described for thigh fractures;

- move the casualty in a Neil Robertson stretcher.

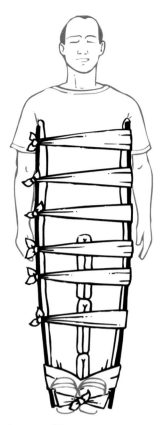

Figure 1.50

Jaw

Normally, fractures of the lower jaw give little trouble.

- the casualty sits with the teeth clenched, often refusing to speak much on account of the pain;

- the spasm of the jaw muscles caused by pain keeps the teeth clenched and jaw immobilised;

- a bandage, tied as in Figure 1.51, will support the lower jaw.

A major hazard arises when both sides of the lower jaw are fractured. In this case, the jaw with the tongue attached on the inside of it, can move backwards and may obstruct the air passage.

- hook a finger, yours or the casualty's, over and behind the lower front teeth and pull the jaw, and with it the tongue, forwards;

- if possible, arrange for the casualty to sit up with his head forwards;

- if he cannot sit up, on account of other injuries, place him in the unconscious position and someone must stay with him, keeping the jaw pulled forward, if necessary, and watching carefully for any sign of obstructed breathing.

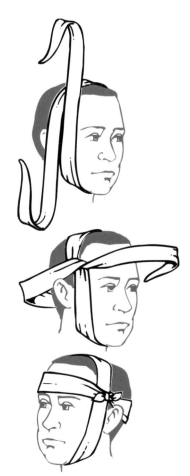

Figure 1.51

Spine

Always suspect a fracture of the spine if a person has fallen a distance of over two metres. Check carefully how the injury happened. Ask if there is pain in the back. Most people with fractures of the spine have pain but a very few DO NOT. If in doubt, treat the injury as a fractured spine.

A FRACTURED SPINE IS POTENTIALLY A VERY SERIOUS INJURY. IF YOU SUSPECT A FRACTURED SPINE, TELL THE CASUALTY TO LIE STILL AND DO NOT ALLOW ANYONE TO MOVE HIM UNTIL FIRST AID TREATMENT HAS BEEN COMPLETED.

Any careless movement of a casualty with a fractured spine could damage or sever the spinal cord, resulting in permanent paralysis and loss of feeling in the legs, and double incontinence for life. He can, however, be safely rolled over onto one side or the other because, if this is done very gently and carefully, there is very little movement of the spine.

First, establish whether the spinal cord has been damaged. To do this:

- ask the casualty if he can feel any tingling of the feet or legs. Tingling usually means that there is some pressure on the spinal cord;

- ask him to move his toes. If he is unable to do this, then paralysis is present and indicates severe damage to the spinal cord;

- run your fingers lightly over the skin of the lower legs and feet. Absence of sensation indicates severe damage to the spinal cord.

If any of these are found, get RADIO MEDICAL ADVICE.

- next, place padding between the legs;

- tie the feet and ankles together with a figure-of-eight bandage and get the casualty lying still and straight. Use gentle traction on the head and on the feet to straighten him out. Do not bend him. Take your time;

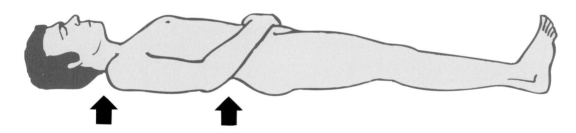

Figure 1.52

- tie a narrow fold bandage around the casualty at the level of his elbows and mid thighs. This method keeps the casualty rigid (Figure 1.53);

- place pads to fill and support the hollows of the spine at the small of the back and at the neck (Figure 1.52);

- he can now lie safely in this position for as long as is necessary. So do not be in a hurry to move him;

- prepare a stiff supporting stretcher ready for the patient. There may be a need to stiffen the Neil Robertson stretcher with broom handles. A canvas stretcher will not do unless it has stiff wooden boards laid transversely over the canvas to provide a rigid support for the back. Two pads must be provided to support and fill the hollows of the spine in the small of the back and behind the neck. The back pad should be larger than the neck pad (Figure 1.52);

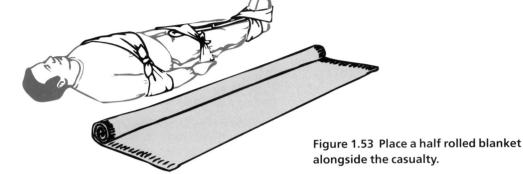

Figure 1.53 Place a half rolled blanket alongside the casualty.

■ when the stretcher has been prepared and is alongside the casualty, the next job is to lift him onto the prepared stretcher as described in Figures 1.53 to 1.58;

NOTE: In Figures 1.54 to 1.58 the encircling bandages shown in Figure 1.53 round the thighs and at the elbows have been omitted for clarity. See also Notes at end of this Section;

■ to lift the casualty, have at least two people grasping each side of the blanket and one person at the head and one at the feet to provide in line support. Those lifting the blanket should be spaced so that more lifting power is available at the body end, which is heavy compared to the legs. A further person is required to push the prepared stretcher under the casualty when he is lifted (Figure 1.57);

■ lift the casualty very slowly and carefully to a height of about half a metre. The height should be just enough to slip the stretcher under the casualty. Be careful, take time, keep the casualty straight (Figure 1.58);

■ slide the stretcher between the legs of the person who is supporting the ankles. Then move the stretcher towards the head end until it is exactly underneath the casualty. Adjust the position of the pads to fit exactly under the curves in the small of the back and neck;

■ lower the casualty very, very slowly on to the stretcher. Maintain support until he is resting firmly on the stretcher (Figure 1.58);

■ the casualty is now ready for removal.

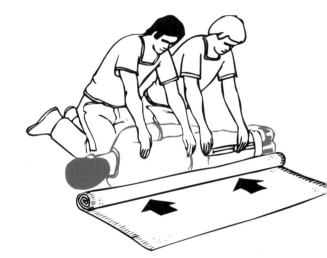

Figure 1.54 Roll the casualty gently onto his side – the attendant closest to his head, or a third attendant, must support the casualty's head.

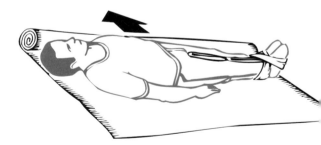

Figure 1.55 Roll the casualty gently over

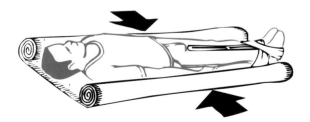

Figure 1.56 Prepare the blanket for lifting the casualty – roll the edges tightly.

When the casualty has been very carefully transported to a mattress on the deck, or other very firm bed, where he may remain undisturbed flat on his back, the most important single point is to keep him as still as possible. He must continue to be supported with pillows, etc., as described later in the text. Every care and attention, and encouragement must be given to help him to remain still, whether or not any paralysis is present. Bags filled with sand should be placed as necessary to prevent the body or limbs rolling. A urine bottle should be constantly available, and a catheter should be used to relieve him if necessary. He should pass any faeces on to cotton wool or other material: he must not be lifted on to a bed pan. His back should be treated, so far as possible, to prevent sores. He must be put ashore at the very earliest possible moment. Get RADIO MEDICAL ADVICE.

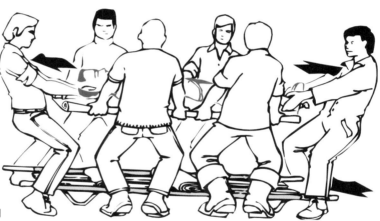

Figure 1.57

NOTES:

(1) As there are a number of people helping and since it is important to take great care in handling the casualty, it may be helpful to have a person read out the particular instruction before each operation is carried out.

(2) At least seven people are required to carry out this manoeuvre. In ships with small crews, there may be insufficient numbers of men available. In this case, do not attempt to move the casualty but carry out the instructions given above on immobilising him and padding the natural curves of the spine. The casualty should then be kept warm, his pain should be treated (see section on analgesics and, if he is on the deck, he should be protected from the elements with suitable waterproof coverings.

Figure 1.58

Neck

Injuries to the neck are often compression fractures of the vertebrae due, for example, to a person standing up suddenly and bumping his head violently, or by something falling on his head. Falls from a height can also produce neck injuries. Treatment is similar to that described above for fractures of the spine, because the neck is the upper part of the spine.

- the casualty should be laid flat, if not already in this position, and should be kept still and straight;

- a semi-rigid neck collar should then be applied gently to stop movement of the neck while an assistant steadies the head. An improvised neck collar can be made quite easily from a newspaper. Fold the newspaper so that the width is about 10 cm at the front. Fold the bottom edge over to produce a slightly narrower back. Then fold this around the neck with the top edge under the chin and the bottom edge over the top of the collar bones;

- tie a bandage, scarf or a necktie over the newspaper to hold it in place. This will keep the neck still (Figure 1.59).

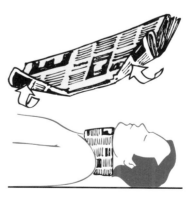
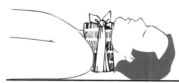

Figure 1.59

Chest

See Fractured ribs.

Pelvis

A fracture of the pelvis will result from direct violence in the pelvic area or from a fall from a height when the casualty has landed on both feet with the legs held stiffly. The main danger of this injury is of damage to the pelvic organs, especially the bladder and the urethra (the pipe which leads from the bladder to the tip of the penis).

- the casualty will complain of pain in the hip, groin and pelvic areas and, perhaps, also of pain in the lower back and buttock areas, made worse by moving or coughing;

- he will be unable to stand, despite there being no injury to the legs;

- he may want to pass urine although he may be unable to do so. If urine is passed, it may be blood-stained.

- there may be signs of internal bleeding;

- the compression test is useful. Press gently on the front of both hip bones in a downward and inward direction so as to compress the pelvis. This will give rise to sharp pain if it is broken. Some movement of the pelvic bones may also be felt if there is a fracture (Figure 1.60), but do not continue pressing in an attempt to elicit this sign, as further damage may be caused.

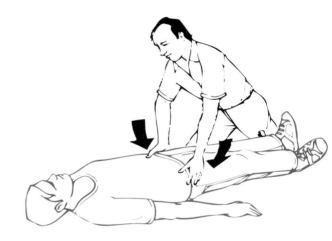

Figure 1.60

If you think that the pelvis may be fractured, tell the casualty:

- not to move;

- not to pass any urine if he can avoid it. If urine is passed, look for staining with blood.

    Remember that:

- if the bladder or urethra is damaged, urine can leak into the tissues;

- bleeding into the surrounding tissues and into the pelvic and lower abdominal cavities may be severe. A pulse chart must be started immediately to check for internal haemorrhage.

- lay the patient in his most comfortable position. This will usually be on his back. If he wants to bend the knees, support them with pillows. Place padding between the legs;

- apply a broad fold bandage round both knees and a figure-of-eight bandage around the ankles;

- move the casualty with great care. Use the same technique as for fracture of the spine.

- keep checking for internal bleeding.

- when moved to a cabin or to the ship's hospital, allow the casualty to lie in whatever position he finds most comfortable;

- morphine may be required to control the pain;

RADIO MEDICAL ADVICE should be obtained.

Dislocations

A dislocation is present when a bone has been displaced from its normal position at a joint (Figure 1.61).

It may be diagnosed:

- when an injury occurs at or near a joint and the joint cannot be used normally;

- movement is limited or impossible;

- there is pain, often quite severe. The pain is made worse by attempts to move the joint;

- the area is misshapen both by the dislocation and by swelling (bleeding) which occurs around the dislocation;

- with the exception of no grating of bone ends, the evidence for a dislocation is very similar to that of a fracture;

- always remember that fractures and dislocations can occur together.

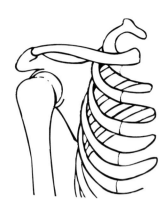

(a) Normal

Treatment

- dislocations can be closed or open. If a wound is present, at or near the dislocation, the wound should be covered, both to stop bleeding and to help to prevent infection; give antibiotic treatment;

- do not attempt to reduce a dislocation. A fracture may also be present and attempted manipulation to reduce the dislocation in these circumstances can make matters worse;

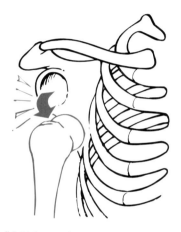

(b) Dislocated

Figure 1.61

- prevent movement in the affected area by suitable immobilisation. The techniques for immobilisation are exactly the same as for fractures of the same area(s).

- look out for impaired circulation and loss of feeling. If these are present, and if you cannot feel a pulse at the wrist or ankle, try to move the limb gently into a position in which circulation can return and keep the limb in this position. Look then for a change of the fingers or toes, from white or blue to pink;

- transport the casualty in the most comfortable position. This is usually sitting up for upper limb injuries and lying down for lower limb injuries;

- for further treatment of dislocations of the shoulder and of the fingers, see Chapter 4.

Head injuries

Head injuries commonly result from blows to the head and from falls, often from a height.

Most preventable serious head injury deaths result from obstructed breathing and from breathing difficulties, not from brain damage. Apart from covering serious head wounds, your attention should be concentrated on the life-saving measures which support normal breathing and which prevent obstructed breathing. This will ensure that the brain gets sufficient oxygen easily. In this way you have a good chance of keeping the casualty alive in order to get him skilled medical aid in a hospital; get RADIO MEDICAL ADVICE.

NOTE: in the case of some head injuries or where a foreign body or a fracture is directly below an open wound, you should NOT control bleeding by direct pressure on top of the wound. In these circumstances a sterile gauze dressing is applied over the wound and a bandage is padded around the wound and over the edge of the dressing, held firmly in place by a bandage.

See Chapter 4 for further information.

Chest injuries

See also Wounds, Crush wounds, Stab wounds.

Fracture of the ribs

This is a common fracture which is usually caused by falling against a hard surface or by a crushing injury. Signs and symptoms are:

- sharp, continuous pain which is increased when breathing in or by coughing;
- shallow breathing to prevent chest movements;
- marked localised tenderness when the injured area is felt gently.

Uncomplicated rib fracture:

- make the casualty sit down in the normal sitting position but, if pain is severe, place him in the half-sitting-up position, leaning over towards the injured side;
- transport him in this position to the ship's hospital or his cabin;
- treat pain;
- do not put strapping around his chest;
- keep him at rest in the position he finds most comfortable, either in bed or sitting in a chair or on the floor (Figures 1.62, 1.63, 1.64).

Severe chest injuries

The ribs form a rigid cage which protects the heart and lungs. Severe force may cause any one or a combination of the following injuries:

- a superficial wound and/or bruising of the chest
- a penetrating (sucking) wound of the chest wall
- multiple rib fractures on one or both sides of the chest, together with injury to the underlying lung and its covering (the pleura);
- a 'stove-in' segment of the chest wall.

The fragments of a fractured rib are usually held in place by the muscles between the ribs. After severe injury, a rib fragment may be driven inwards, causing a tear in the covering of the lung with consequent leaking of blood or air into the chest cavity. The lung on that side will then collapse and/or be compressed, resulting in difficulty in breathing. There may be a blue/grey tinge to the skin of the face and lips, and the casualty may cough up frothy blood-stained sputum.

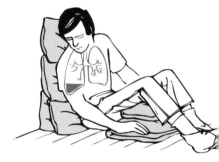

Figure 1.62

Treatment

Get RADIO MEDICAL ADVICE and get the casualty to expert treatment, or expert treatment to the casualty, as soon as possible.

- place in the half-sitting-up position leaning towards the injured side (Figure 1.62). If both sides are injured, keep in the upright half-sitting up position (Figure 1.63);

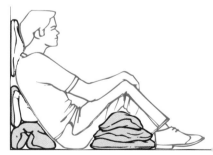

Figure 1.63

- keep the air passage clear. Remove dentures, if worn, and encourage him to spit out any blood, vomit or secretions;
- deal with any sucking wound.
- transport to ship's hospital, or cabin, as soon as possible, but keeping him in the sitting position advised above;
- when in bed, in the correct position, relieve pain but DO NOT GIVE MORPHINE;
- watch for signs of internal bleeding and obstructed breathing.

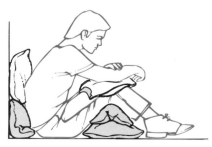

Figure 1.64

Unconscious casualty

Transport and later nurse in bed in the unconscious position, lying on the injured side (not the uninjured side) and with a head-down tilt.

Stove-in chest injury

In a very severe injury, multiple fractures of the ribs may lead to a portion of the chest wall being 'stove-in'. That portion contains adjacent ribs which have been fractured at both ends, thus allowing the portion to have free movement independent from and in the opposite direction to the movement of the rest of the rib cage. This is called paradoxical movement and it is an important sign in diagnosis.

Treatment

- give treatment as for multiple fractures of ribs;
- using the flat hand, either the casualty or the attendant should maintain firm pressure over the stove-in portion of the chest wall;
- a pad of folded cloth should be placed over the damaged area and bandaged firmly in place, using wide crepe bandages to encircle the chest. If breathing movements are hindered by the chest bandage, strips of elastic adhesive bandage, which do not encircle the chest, may be used.
  NOTE: Infections of the lung may appear as a serious complication of any severe chest injury. Whenever a casualty has to be kept on board, always start a course of antibiotic treatment.

Blast injuries

Explosions cause a sudden and violent disturbance of the air; fires can be started and toxic gases produced.

- men may be thrown down and so injured. Further injury may occur from falling wreckage;
- the blast of air itself may strike the body with such violence as to cause severe or fatal internal injuries;
- cases of burns or asphyxia may occur.

  Apart from fractures, wounds, severe bleeding, burns and asphyxia, any combination of the following injuries may be found.

Head

The effect of blast injury to the head is rather like concussion. In some cases there may be paralysis due to spinal cord damage. The patient may be unconscious or he may be extremely dazed. Dazed casualties can be found sitting about, incapable of moving and not caring what is going on. Although apparently to outward appearances uninjured, they do not have the energy, or indeed the will, to move. They will appear confused and disorientated.

- if unconscious, put in the unconscious position immediately. Check for breathing, heart stopped and bleeding;
- if dazed, take them by the hand and lead them to safety. Tell them firmly what they must do. Detail someone to look after them.

Lungs

The blast of air may damage the air sacs and the small blood vessels of the lungs.

- bleeding may take place inside the lungs;
- the patient may be shocked;
- he may have difficulty in breathing. There may be a feeling of tightness in the chest and there may be pain;

- lips, ears and the skin of the face may be blue;
- he may cough up a blood-stained froth;
- take the patient into the fresh air if possible;
- support him in the half-sitting-up position
- loosen tight clothing to allow him to breathe more easily;
- keep him warm and treat for shock;
- encourage him to cough and spit out any secretions produced;
- artificial respiration or assisted respiration may be required if breathing fails or becomes difficult.

PATIENTS WITH CHEST INJURIES MUST **NEVER** BE GIVEN MORPHINE

Abdomen

Abdominal injury to casualties in the sea can happen as a result of underwater explosions but similar injury can be due to explosions on board ship. The force of the explosion damages the internal organs and causes internal bleeding.

The main features of this type of injury are:

- shock;
- abdominal pain;

both of which may become evident some time after the explosion. If these conditions are found, start a pulse chart. Treatment is that for shock and for internal bleeding.

Transportation

Unless there is danger from fire, explosion or toxic substances, do not move a casualty until suspected fractures have been immobilised and bad bleeding has been stopped. Then check out the best route for transport and lift the casualty gently and carry him smoothly. Every jolt means unnecessary pain.

The method of transport will depend on the situation of the casualty and the nature of the injury. Whatever method is used, try to gain the confidence of the person you are carrying by explaining what you are about to do and then carrying out the manoeuvre in an efficient manner.

Ordinary man-handling may be possible, in which case two helpers carry a casualty without forming their hands into a seat, by each using an arm to support the casualty's back and shoulders and each using his spare hand to support the casualty under his thighs.

If conscious, the casualty may help to support himself with his hands on the shoulders of the helpers (Figure 1.65).

The four-handed seat can be used when a heavy person has to be carried. The disadvantage of this type of seat is that the casualty must be able to co-operate and to hold on with both arms around the shoulders of the two men carrying him. It cannot be safely used to negotiate ladders (Figure 1.65).

The hands should be placed as in Figure 1.66.

One advantage of the three-handed seat (Figure 1.67) is that one arm and hand of a helper is left free and can be used

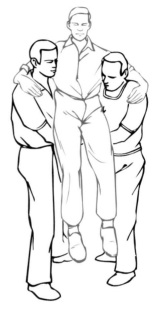

Figure 1.65 Position taken up when man-handled, or a four-arm seat is being used; in the former instance two arms are at the back of the patient and only two are under his thighs.

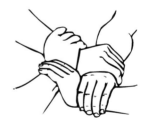

Figure 1.66

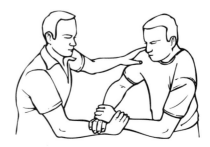

Figure 1.67

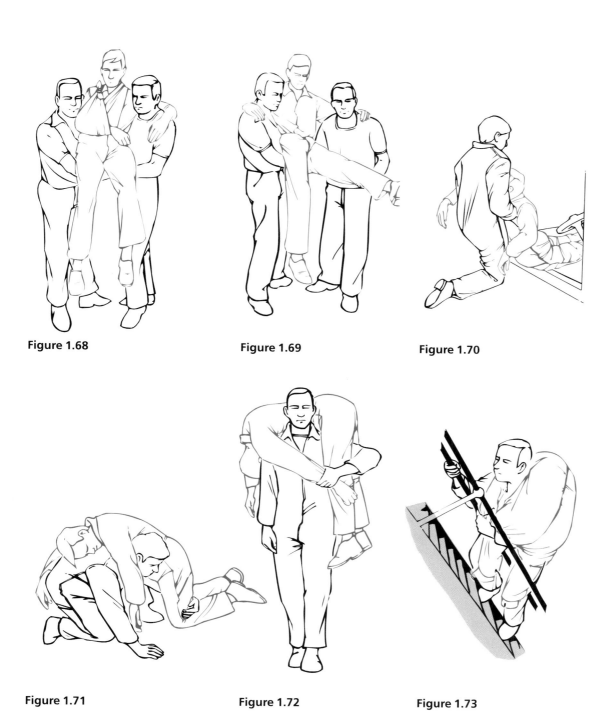

Figure 1.68

Figure 1.69

Figure 1.70

Figure 1.71

Figure 1.72

Figure 1.73

either to support an injured limb or as a backsupport for the casualty. According to the nature of the injury, it is decided which of the two helpers has the free arm (Figures 1.68 and 1.69).

The fireman's lift which should not be used unless the helper is as well built as the casualty is especially useful when you have to move a man by yourself and need the use of your right hand for holding on to a ladder. Roll the patient so that he is lying face downwards, lift him up so that, when you stoop down, you can put your head under his left arm (Figure 1.70). Then put your left arm between his legs and grasp his left hand, letting his body fall over your left shoulder (Figure 1.71).

Steady yourself and then stand upright, at the same time shifting his weight so that he lies well balanced across the back of your shoulders (Figure 1.72). Hold the casualty's arm above the wrist. In this position it is easy to carry the patient up a ladder as one hand is free to grasp the rail (Figure 1.73).

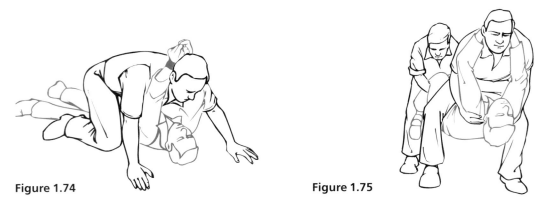

Figure 1.74   **Figure 1.75**

As a last resort, the drag-carry method may have to be used in narrow spaces, particularly where there is wreckage following an explosion and where it may be possible for only one man to reach a trapped casualty and to rescue him. After initial rescue, two men may be able to undertake further movement through a narrow space. The method is demonstrated in Figures 1.74 and 1.75. Ensure that the casualty's wrists, which are tied together, do not interfere with any breathing apparatus the rescuer may be wearing, and safeguard the casualty's head with a bump hat if possible.

Neil Robertson stretcher

This particular type of stretcher is shown in Figure 1.76. It is a simple device for moving a casualty safely from a difficult place where the ordinary stretcher with stiff poles would be useless. Other patterns of rescue stretcher are available but all aim to achieve the same purpose. The casualty is enveloped in a protecting but somewhat flexible case, so that he takes up as little room as possible. The stretcher can be bent slightly in turning sharp corners in narrow passages, as when being hoisted up the ladder ways from engine-rooms, or through the hatches of cargo tanks.

The stretcher is made of stout canvas, stiffened by wooden slats (Figure 1.76). The portion 'A' takes the head and neck, which are steadied by a canvas strap passing over the forehead. Thus, the head of an unconscious patient can be steadied.

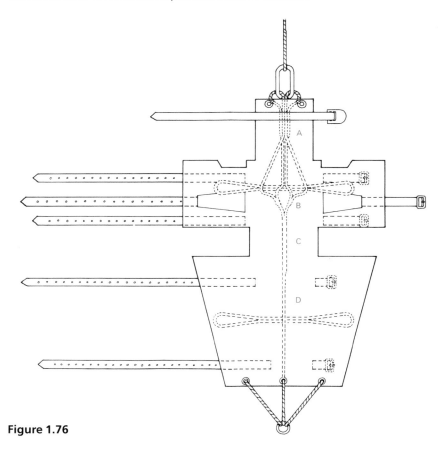

Figure 1.76

The portion 'B' is wrapped round the chest, notches being cut on which the armpits rest. This part has three canvas straps which are used for fastening the stretcher round the chest. The portion 'D' folds round the hips and legs down to the ankles. It is secured by two canvas straps.

A central backbone of stout rope passes along the under surface. This has two beckets passing out from it on either side which can be used as handles, for carrying the patient or for securing tackles when he is slung horizontally.

At the head end, the rope ends in a grommet which takes extra purchase from two brass eyelets let into the canvas. At the foot end of the rope is a galvanised iron ring which is secured to the stretcher by a span going to brass eyelets in the canvas. When more rigidity in the stretcher is required, as in moving those with injuries to the back, a couple of broom handles, slipped through the ropes underneath, will fulfil this purpose admirably.

Some stretchers have a rope about 9 ft long fixed to the galvanised ring at the foot end. This is a steadying rope for use in craft below, or on quay, when the patient is lowered over the side of the ship. When the patient is carried about the ship, this rope can be passed under the various straps to keep it from trailing on the deck or otherwise getting in the way.

The patient should be lifted on to and secured in the stretcher as shown in Figures 1.77 to 1.80.

Cases of fracture of the spine or other back and pelvic injuries should be transferred to the stretcher as directed under spinal injury.

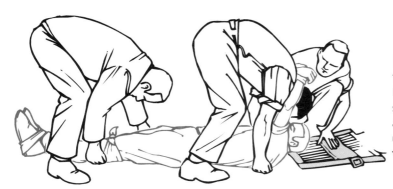

Figure 1.77 Getting ready to lift the casualty sufficiently for the Neil Robertson stretcher to be slid under him. With only three attendants, the wrists of an unconscious patient have to be tied together – but not tightly.

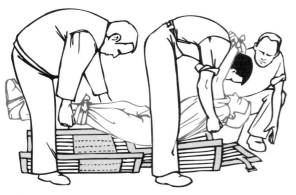

Figure 1.78 Lower the patient slowly – if he is unconscious, support his head.

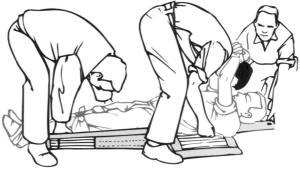

Figure 1.79 Ensure patient's armpits are in the correct place before you finish lowering him.

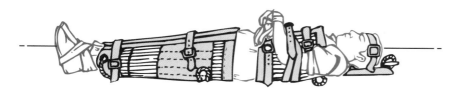

Figure 1.80 Strapped up – the arms can be strapped inside or outside the chest section of the stretcher, depending upon the injuries.

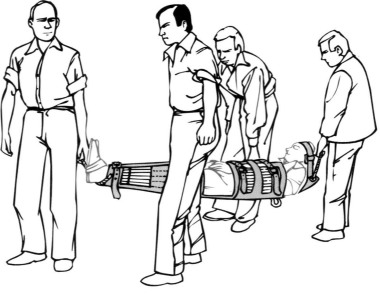

Figure 1.81 Carrying the patient – but keep the head section level with the chest section if the neck may be hurt.

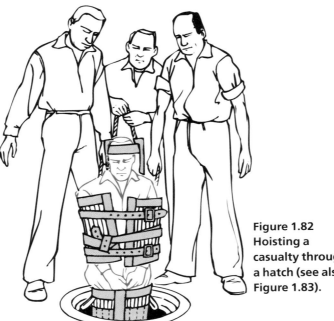

Figure 1.82 Hoisting a casualty through a hatch (see also Figure 1.83).

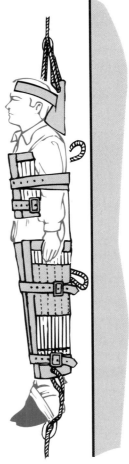

Figure 1.83 Moving a casualty vertically. Note: to steady the stretcher, a rope goes from the foot of the stretcher to a seafarer below.

The patient should be carried by four men, if possible (Figure 1.81). At difficult corners, the stretcher should be lowered at the foot end, and the casualty passed by two of the men to the others. The carry can then be resumed by the four bearers.

When passing the casualty through a narrow hatch, or lifting him up over a height, or lowering him to a boat alongside, put the lifting hook or a rope through the grommet at the head end and a further steadying rope through the galvanised ring at the foot end (Figures 1.82 and 1.83).

Moving an unconscious casualty

If possible, carry an unconscious casualty in the unconscious position and always with a head-down tilt. The tilt is also necessary when carrying a casualty suffering from shock or loss of blood.

Note

More detailed information on the treatment of the effects of specific chemicals is given in the International Maritime Organization's Medical First Aid Guide for use in Accidents involving Dangerous Goods (MFAG) 1994 which your ship may be carrying.

Toxic hazards

Ships carry a number of substances other than cargo which are potentially toxic. For instance, medicines are not generally poisonous but can become so if taken in a manner not prescribed, such as in an overdose. Then there are substances like cleaners, degreasers and disinfectants which can give rise to toxic hazards on their own or through misuse, e.g. emptying a bucket of bleaching solution into a lavatory bowl containing a proprietary caustic cleaner may result in the release of poisonous gas in a confined space. Notes on various specific toxic substances are given at the end of this section. Manufacturer's data sheets also contain specific medical advice.

Toxic substances can harm the body in three ways.

1. They may cause local burns or irritation if they come into contact with skin or eyes.

2. They may be absorbed into the body and cause internal damage or systemic poisoning.

3. They may cause an allergic reaction which could be life threatening.

Toxic substances can enter the body through

- The lungs e.g. fumes or toxic gases.

- The mouth e.g. by swallowing

- The skin and eyes.

The commonest route for a toxin to enter the body onboard a ship is by breathing it in. The toxin may be in the form of a vapour, gas, mist, spray, dust or fume.

Poisons are less commonly swallowed, usually by accident during routine duties, but sometimes deliberately.

The effects of toxins are often sudden and dramatic, but may be subtle, gradual and cumulative. The latter is especially true of inhaled toxins or those absorbed through the skin.

Suspect that every chemical is toxic until you know otherwise. Remember that toxins are poisonous to the rescuer as well as the patient. TAKE ALL POSSIBLE PRECAUTIONS TO PROTECT YOURSELF.

Prompt, safety conscious treatment can avoid many of the complications of poisoning.

Inhaled Poisons

(See Chapter 1 for rescue from an enclosed space.)
Many chemicals produce fumes which can irritate the lungs and cause difficulty in breathing e.g. chlorine. This will alert you to their presence.

Toxic hazards of chemicals including poisoning

Other gases have no odour . This group includes carbon monoxide, carbon dioxide, hydrogen and some refrigerant gases.

Gases such as carbon dioxide and carbon monoxide may also be poisonous, particularly in a confined space, because they replace oxygen in the air and therefore in the blood.

The main symptoms of exposure are :

- difficulty in breathing;

- nausea, headache, dizziness;

- confusion or even unconsciousness in severe cases.

Remember that precautions against fire and explosion may be necessary for some gases.

Treatment

- Remove the casualty at once into the fresh air. Loosen tight clothing and ensure a clear airway. Give oxygen if available.

- Start artificial respiration by the mouth to nose or mouth method if breathing is absent. The use of a Laerdal Pocket Mask (mouth to mask) is recommended for resuscitation in the case of poisoning by solvents, hydrogen cyanide (prussic acid) or petroleum products to avoid poisoning the rescuer. Use oxygen if available.

- Start chest compressions if the heart has stopped.

- In cases of hydrogen cyanide poisoning where breathing and pulse are present, break an ampoule of amyl nitrite into a clean handkerchief or cloth and hold under the patient's nose so that he inhales the vapour.

- **SEEK RADIO MEDICAL ADVICE** as specific treatment may be required.

- Keep the patient at rest in bed for at least 24 hours or until he has recovered.

Complications of inhaled poisons

- Severe difficulty in breathing with frothy sputum (pulmonary oedema).

- Pneumonia and bronchitis.

DO NOT GIVE MORPHINE TO A CASUALTY WHO HAS BEEN GASSED, as this will affect their ability to breathe.

Swallowed Poisons

Astringents

Many substances will cause chemical burns to the mouth, gullet and stomach if swallowed. These include bleaches and other cleaners and disinfectants, acids and alkalis and corrosives as well as petrochemicals.

The main symptoms are blistering of the mouth, lips and tongue and pain in the chest and stomach. The patients breath often smells of the astringent.

DO NOT MAKE THE CASUALTY VOMIT. If the patient is conscious and in pain then he may respond to a glass of milk. Do not give painkillers by mouth. Use suppositories or a painkilling injection if you have any.

Other substances can cause acute abdominal pain and vomiting. These include arsenic, lead, fungi, berries and partly decomposed food. Treat the patient by making them as comfortable as possible, but do not make them vomit.

Drugs and Alcohol

Drugs may cause harmful effects if taken for recreational purposes or as an overdose. An overdose may be taken accidentally or as an attempt at deliberate self harm. Common overdoses include

Sleeping Tablets. These include Diazepam (valium), Temazepam and Nitrazepam. They cause drowsiness and unconsciousness if taken in excess. This may last for 24 hours. The breathing may slow down and become shallow. In severe cases it may stop. A similar picture may be seen with some antidepressants, such as Amitriptyline, or with alcohol.

Simple painkillers such as ***paracetamol*** and ***aspirin*** are often taken as overdoses.

Paracetamol may cause abdominal pain and vomiting initially. Larger overdoses can cause severe liver damage several days later. (Liver damage is rare below 20 tablets)

Aspirin causes vomiting, abdominal pain, ringing in the ears, rapid breathing and semi-consciousness in high doses.

Treatment

Try to discover exactly what was taken (ask the patient, look for empty packets/bottles etc.) but do not waste time doing so in an emergency.

If the casualty is conscious, give one sachet (50g) of oral activated charcoal in 250 mls of fluid, if available. Encourage fluids in conscious cases of aspirin overdose. SEEK RADIO MEDICAL ADVICE.

If the patient is unconscious, then put him in the recovery (unconscious) position and

- Give artificial respiration if breathing has stopped.

- Perform chest compressions if the heart has stopped.

- DO NOT give anything by mouth.

- SEEK URGENT RADIO MEDICAL ADVICE.

Skin Contact

Toxic substances can affect the skin in two ways:

1. direct contact may cause redness and irritation. In severe cases, burns to the skin can occur.

2. Absorption through the intact skin producing general symptoms such as nausea, vomiting, drowsiness, weakness and rarely unconsciousness.

Treatment

- The contaminated clothing and shoes should be removed immediately.

- Wash off the chemical with copious amounts of water for at least 10 minutes. Continue for a further 10 minutes if there is any evidence of chemicals still on the skin.

- If a burn has occurred, see management of burns.

Eye Contact

Many substances, in particular many chemical liquids or fumes of chemicals, will produce redness and irritation if the eyes are accidentally splashed or exposed to the fumes. Treatment should be immediate.

Wash the substance out of the eye with copious amounts of cold fresh water as quickly as possible, keeping the eyelids wide open. This must be done thoroughly for ten minutes. If there is any doubt whether the chemical has been completely removed, repeat the eye wash for a further 10 minutes. If severe pain is experienced, physical restraint to the patient may be necessary in order to be certain of effective treatment. Read about identifying and treating damage to the eye.

For pain, give two paracetamol tablets by mouth every four hours until the pain subsides. If there is very severe pain use Morphine.

General notes

If you are dealing with a suicide attempt, it is your duty to do everything you can to save his life and to guard against further attempts. The patient should not be left without an attendant.

You should save any remains of poison that you may find in a glass, cup, bottle or package. Also collect in a bowl anything that is vomited and seal in a bottle. These may help in identifying the toxic substance and deciding further treatment after the patient has been seen by a doctor or taken ashore.

Notes on specific toxic substances

For treatment see under inhaled poisons, swallowed poisons etc. above.

Disinfectant poisoning

Many types of disinfectants such as carbolic acid, cresol and bleaching solutions are toxic.

Carbolic acid (phenol) and cresols cause a severe rash on contact with the skin in dilute solutions. Strong concentrated solutions will result in painless white burns of the skin. If they are swallowed, burns of the mouth will occur, and the casualty may have severe vomiting, followed by collapse and unconsciousness. Convulsions can occur (see Epileptic fits).

Bleaching solutions (e.g. lavatory cleaners, etc.) are usually solutions of sodium hypochlorite in water. These cause irritation of the skin and are poisonous if swallowed. The patient may complain of burning in the mouth and stomach and feel generally unwell.

On contact with acids, these substances release fumes which are irritating to the lungs causing a cough, a feeling of breathlessness and burning in the mouth. However, these substances are not severely toxic and the symptoms usually subside rapidly.

Solvents, petroleum products and fuel oils

These substances usually cause symptoms after the fumes have been accidentally inhaled. The symptoms are drowsiness, dizziness, nausea and occasionally vomiting. If severe exposure occurs, the patient may become unconscious. If they are swallowed, they usually produce the same symptoms, but nausea and vomiting are worse.

Cyanide

Hydrogen cyanide (prussic acid) gas is used in fumigating ships. Both the solid cyanide and the gas are extremely poisonous, and symptoms and signs may develop very rapidly. They are corrosive either in contact with the skin or after being swallowed, causing external burns, burns in the mouth and intense pain in the abdomen. There will be shortness of breath, anxiety and rapid loss of consciousness. Convulsions can occur. Death may result within a few minutes.

Carbon dioxide (carbonic acid gas)

Suffocation by this odourless gas may occur while dealing with a fire in a hold. The gas is also produced if grain in the hold ferments, and it may be generated by refrigerated cargoes of certain foods; it is also used as a refrigerant. The gas is heavier than air and collects in the lower parts of holds and compartments. When exposed to it, a man has giddiness, difficulty in breathing and headache. Later he may fall down and lose consciousness.

Carbon monoxide

This odourless gas is also produced in hold fires, as a product of an explosion, in the waste gases of petrol and oil driven engines, and when refrigerated meat cargoes decompose. It is lighter than air and very poisonous. In heavy concentration it is inflammable. A patient suffering from the effects of this gas feels giddy, often with muscular weakness. Difficulty in breathing rapidly develops and unconsciousness may come on quickly. In severe cases the lips may be bright red, and the skin of the face and body has a pink colour. Hyperbaric oxygen therapy may be helpful – SEEK ADVICE – consider urgent evacuation.

Refrigerant gases

Ammonia vapour. Breathing ammonia vapour will cause intense irritation, varying from a catching of the breath with smarting and watering of the eyes in low concentrations, up to intense irritation and corrosion of the whole air passages, gasping for breath, collapse and death in the case of highly concentrated vapour.

Carbon dioxide is also present in addition to ammonia. If a person becomes faint or loses consciousness in a refrigerating plant where there is no evidence of escaping ammonia, he is probably suffering from the effects of this gas.

Methyl chloride is a colourless gas, smelling like ether. It may cause drowsiness, mental confusion, coma, nausea, vomiting, convulsions and death. It is also dangerous in low concentration owing to its explosive nature. On no account, should any naked light be exposed in the presence of the vapour; electric motors should be stopped to avoid risk of sparking. A heavy duty electric torch, switched on before approaching the escape, is the only safe light to use.

Trichlorethylene – usually called trilene or 'trike' – is a volatile anaesthetic gas which causes drowsiness, mental confusion, nausea, vomiting and coma. It can also result in death. It is used medically as an anaesthetic because it acts quickly. In the impure form it is used as a dry cleaning agent. Some people are addicted to 'sniffing' it. Exposure may cause palpitations, especially on excitation. Those exposed to it should be kept in a calm environment for at least 6 hours.

Freon is an odourless and harmless gas except in a concentration high enough to deprive a man of sufficient oxygen. The signs of oxygen deficiency are mental confusion, faintness, staggering gait, collapse and unconsciousness.

Poisonous gases from refrigerated cargoes

Certain refrigerated cargoes including fruit, vegetables and cheese, generate carbon dioxide during normal storage. With any failure of refrigerating plant, food cargoes (especially meat) may generate poisonous and inflammable gases. This can be particularly dangerous if the cargo space is flooded. Carbon monoxide, ammonia, hydrogen sulphide and hydrogen may be generated in addition to carbon dioxide. In any great concentration these gases are extremely poisonous and some are explosive. All precautions against fire and explosion must be taken in addition to those against suffocation and poisoning.

Introduction

This section of the Guide is concerned with the care and treatment of bed patients until they recover or are sent to hospital for professional attention.

Good nursing is vital to the ease and speed of recovery from any condition. Attention to detail and comfort may make the lot of the sick or injured person much more tolerable. Cheerful, helpful and intelligent nursing can greatly influence the person's attitude in a positive direction towards his illness or injury.

The nurses

A sick person needs to have confidence in his attendants who should understand his requirements. A nurse should be selected with care and the master or a senior officer should check on the performance of the person chosen.

Sick quarters

Wherever possible a patient sufficiently ill to require nursing should be in the ship's hospital or in a cabin away from others. In this way the patient will benefit from quietness and the risk of spreading any unknown infection will be minimised. The sick quarters should be comfortable and easily cleaned. The room fittings and floors should be cleaned daily.

Adequate ventilation of the sick quarters is of great importance and it is equally important that changes of temperature should be avoided. The ideal temperature for the sick room is between 15.5°C and 18.5°C. If possible, direct sunlight should be admitted to the cabin. If the weather is warm and the portholes will open they should be left open.

Arrival of the patient

It may be necessary to assist the patient to undress and get into bed. A patient with a reduced level of consciousness will have to be undressed. Take off boots or shoes first, then socks, trousers, jacket and shirt in that order.

In the case of severe leg injuries, you may have to remove the trousers by cutting down the seams. In the case of arm injuries, remove the arm from the shirt sleeve on the sound side first, then slip the shirt over the head and lastly withdraw the arm carefully from the sleeve on the injured side.

In cold climates the patient should always wear suitable night wear. In the tropics cotton nightwear is preferable.

Blankets are unnecessary in the tropics but the patient should have some covering, a sheet spread over him.

If your patient has a chest condition accompanied by cough and spitting he should be provided with a receptacle, either a sputum pot or an improvised jar or tin. The receptacle provided should be fitted with a cover. If the sputum pot is not of the disposable variety add a little disinfectant. It should be thoroughly cleaned out twice daily with boiling water and a disinfectant.

CHAPTER 3

General nursing

Your other duties may make it impossible for you to give uninterrupted attention to your patient and a urine bottle should therefore be left within reach of the patient on a chair, stool or locker, and covered with a cloth.

Food, plates, cups, knives, forks and spoons should be removed from the sick quarters immediately after a meal and in no circumstances should they be left there except in infectious cases. In such cases they should be washed up in the cabin and then be stacked neatly away and covered with a cloth.

Visitors

The patient should be protected from long and tiring visits from well-meaning shipmates. Visits to patients who are ill and running a temperature should be restricted to 15 minutes.

Check list

- Ensure that the person is comfortable in bed.

- Check temperature, pulse and respiration twice daily (morning and evening) or more often if not in the normal range (a four-hourly check is usual in any serious illness). Document observations.

- In appropriate cases test a specimen of urine and document.

- Keep a written record of the illness.

- Arrange that soft drinks are easily available unless fluids are to be restricted. No alcohol.

- Specify normal diet or any dietary restrictions.

- Ensure that the person knows to ask for a bottle or a bedpan as needed – some do not unless told.

- Check and record if bowels have moved or not.

- Check fluid-in and fluid-out by asking the person questions about drinking and passing urine. In certain illnesses a fluid chart must be kept.

- Check that the person is eating.

- Re-make the bed at least twice a day or more often if required to keep the person comfortable. Look out for crumbs and creases, both of which can be uncomfortable.

- Try to avoid boredom by suitable reading and hobby material. A radio and/or TV will also help to provide interest for the patient.

- A means of summoning other people, such as a bell, telephone or intercom should be available if the person cannot call out and be heard, or if the person is not so seriously ill as to require somebody to be with him at all times.

- Ensure patient safety.

The body temperature

The body temperature, pulse rate and respiration should be recorded. You should make use of your temperature charts, or if no more charts are available, then your findings should be written down, together with the hour at which they were noted. These readings should be taken twice a day and always at the same hours, and more frequently if the patient is seriously ill.

It will rarely be necessary to record the temperature at more frequent intervals than four-hourly. The only exceptions to this rule are in cases of severe head injury, acute abdominal conditions and hyperpyrexia when more frequent temperature recordings are required.

The body temperature is measured by using a clinical thermometer, except in hypothermia when a low reading thermometer must be used. To take the temperature, first shake down the mercury in a clinical thermometer to about 35°C. Then place the thermometer in the person's mouth, under the tongue. The thermometer should remain in the mouth with the lips closed – no speaking – for at least 1 minute. After 1 minute, read the thermometer, then replace it in the patient's mouth for a further minute. Check the reading and if it reads the same, record the temperature on the chart. Repeat the process if it is different. Then disinfect the thermometer.

Sometimes it will be necessary to take the temperature per rectum, e.g. hypothermia. In that case, first lubricate the thermometer with Vaseline. Then, with the patient lying on his side, push the thermometer gently into the rectum for a distance of 5 cm and leave for 2 minutes before reading it. Do not use the same thermometer as is used in the mouth.

People who are unconscious, restless or possibly drunk should not have their mouth temperatures taken in case they chew the thermometer. These people should have their temperature taken by placing the thermometer in the armpit and holding the arm into the side for 2 minutes before the thermometer is read.

The normal body temperature is 36.9°Celsius (centigrade) and lies in the range 36.3 to 37.2°C. Temperature taken in the armpit is ½°C lower, and in the rectum ½°C higher. In good health, variations in temperature are slight.

Body temperature is raised, and fever is said to be present, in infectious conditions and in a few disorders which affect the heat regulating mechanism in the brain.

Centigrade (Celsius)

Fatal (as a rule)	**Moderate Fever**
43.3	38.3
42.8	37.8
42.2	**Healthy Temperature**
Dangerous Fever	37.2
41.7	36.7
41.1	36.1
High Fever	35.6
40.6	**Hypothermia**
40.0	35.0 and below
39.4	
38.9	

In feverish illnesses the body temperature rises and then falls to normal. At first the person may feel cold and shivery. Then he looks and feels hot, the skin is flushed, dry and warm and the patient becomes thirsty. He may suffer from headache and may be very restless. The temperature may still continue to rise. Finally the temperature falls and the person may sweat profusely, becoming wet through. As this happens, he may need a change of clothing and bedding.

During the cold stage, the person should have one or two warm blankets put around him to keep him warm but too many blankets may help to increase his temperature. As he reaches the hot stage, he should be given cool drinks, not alcohol.

If the temperature rises above 40°C sponging or even a cool bath may be required to prevent further rise of temperature or reduce it. In the sweating stage the clothing and bedding should be changed.

The pulse rate

The pulse rate is the number of heart beats per minute. The pulse is felt at the wrist, or the heart rate is counted by listening to the heartbeat over the nipple on the left side of the chest. The pulse rate varies with age, sex and activity. The pulse rate is increased normally by exercise and excitement; it is decreased by sleep and to a lesser extent by relaxation and some drugs. Pulse rates of 120 and above can be counted more easily by listening over the heart.

Normal resting pulse rate (number of heartbeats per minute)	
Age 2 to 5	About 100
Age 5 to 10	About 90
Adults, male	65 to 80
Adults, female	75 to 85

The pulse rate will usually rise about 10 beats per minute for every 0.5°C over 38°C. In heart disease and shock, a high pulse rate may be found with a normal temperature.

Note and record also whether the pulse beat is regular or irregular, i.e. whether there are the same number of beats in each 15 seconds and whether the strength of each beat is about the same.

If the rhythm is very irregular, count the pulse at the wrist and also count the pulse by listening over the heart. The rates may be different because weak heartbeats will be heard, but the resulting pulse wave may not be strong enough to be felt. Count for a full minute in each case.

The respiration rate

The respiration rate will often give you a clue to the diagnosis of the case.

The rate is the number of times per minute that the patient breathes in. It is counted by watching the number of inspirations per minute. This count should be made without the patient's knowledge by continuing to hold the wrist as if taking the pulse. If the patient is conscious of what you are doing, the rate is liable to be irregular. A good plan is to take the respiration rate immediately after taking the pulse.

The respiration rate varies with age, sex and activity. It is increased normally by exercise, excitement and emotion; it is decreased by sleep and rest.

Normal resting respiration rate (number of breaths per minute)	
Age 2 to 5	28 – 24
5 to Adult	24 – 18
Adult, male	18 – 16
Adult, female	20 – 18

Always count respirations for a full minute, noting any discomfort in breathing in or out.

The pulse rate will usually rise about 4 beats per minute for every rise of 1 respiration per minute. This 4:1 ratio will be altered in chest diseases such as pneumonia or asthma which can cause a great rise in respiration rate.

A Temperature, Pulse and Respiration Chart

Patient's Name 3rd OFFICER M.Y.X. Age 24 years   CABIN

MONTH	NOVEMBER														MONTH
DAY	6th	7th	8th	9th	10th	11th	12th	13th	14th	15th	16th	17th			DAY
DAY OF DISEASE	1	2	3	4	5	6	7	8	9	10	11	12			DAY OF DISEASE

state your diagnosis

TEMPERATURE — °F (107° to 95°) / °C (41° to 35°)

PULSE (180 to 40)

RESPIRATION (55 to 15)

Weight	70.5				68.5										Weight
Faeces	— / —		/ —	— / —	— / —	— / —		/ —		/ —		/		/ —	/ —	— /		Faeces
Urine	2500	3000	4000	3000	2750	2500									Urine
Proteins		POS	NEG	NEG	NEG										Proteins
Sugar		+ +	+	NEG	NEG										Sugar
Ketones		+ + +	+	NEG	NEG										Ketones

See Note

Note   Weight - in kgs : Faeces - number of movements am/pm : Urine - amount in mls
If urine tested record as appropriate , for Protein ; Neg or Pos (not present / present) ; &
for Sugar and for Ketones ; Neg / + / + + / + + +
The remaining rows can be used for other factors significant to the patient's condition

Bed baths

Patients who are confined to bed should be washed all over at least every day. If they are hot, sticky, and feverish, they should be washed at least twice a day. Wash the patient, beginning at the head. If the patient is well enough, he should wash his own face and genital area; otherwise the attendants should do this. Wash and dry one part of the body at a time so that the patient is not uncovered all at once.

When you have finished washing the patient, lightly dust pressure areas and skin creases with talc.

The bed linen should be changed as frequently as necessary, it is much easier using 2 attendants.

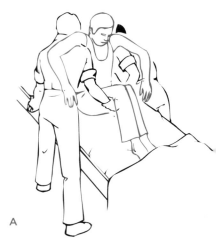

A

Mouth care

Make sure that plenty of drinks are available to prevent dryness and that facilities for brushing teeth and dentures are made available twice a day.

Very ill patients or unconscious patients should have poor fitting dentures removed. The inside of the cheeks, the gums, the teeth and the tongue should be swabbed with dilute glycerine of thymol on a cotton bud, or other suitable material. If the lips are dry, apply Vaseline/petroleum jelly thinly to these areas. This procedure should be repeated as often as is necessary to keep the areas moist.

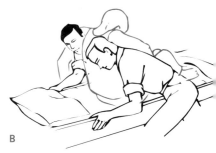

B

Feeding patients in bed

People who are ill or injured may not feel much like eating. They may also have to be encouraged to drink plenty to prevent dehydration. So, always try to find out what the person would like to eat or drink and give him what he wants if you possibly can. Food should also be presented as attractively as possible on a suitable tray. Special diets, when they are prescribed, must be strictly followed. If a weak patient spills food or drink, use towels or sheeting to keep patient and bedding as clean as possible. If they have difficulty in swallowing, soft food only should be given.

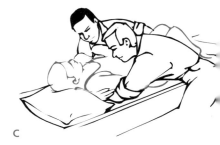

C

Figure 3.1   Moving a patient in bed – always use two helpers, who bend their legs not their backs.

The bed

The bed should be made up and the linen changed at regular intervals. Remember that creases can be most uncomfortable and can cause bedsores. If the patient is gravely ill, incontinent or likely to sweat excessively, use a waterproof sheet covered by a draw sheet across the bottom sheet.

If the patient has a fracture or finds the weight of his bedding to be uncomfortable, you can support the bedding with one or more bed cradles. These can be improvised from a topless wooden box by removing the two shorter (or longer) sides and then inverting it. The cradle goes over the affected part of the patient and the bedding rests on top of the cradle.

Patients who cannot get up can have their bed linen changed by rolling them gently to one side of the bed and untucking the used linen on the unoccupied side. It is then rolled up and placed against the patient. Clean linen is then tucked under the mattress and its outer edge rolled up and placed beside the roll of used linen. The patient can then be very gently rolled over to the clean side of the bed and the job completed. The same technique can be applied, but on an end to end basis, for patients who have to be nursed in a seated position. If the patient is told what you are doing, as you do it, he will know what to expect and will probably co-operate as far as he can. A freshened bed is a comfort to most sick people. Bed making and changing an occupied bed requires two people; it is easier if the bed can be in the centre of the cabin. (Figure 3.1).

Bed sores

Anyone in bed is constantly prone to bed sores (pressure sores) unless preventative action is taken. Unconscious patients and the incontinent are at risk of bed sores. Frequent change of posture, day and night, with, in the case of the incontinent, thorough washing and drying will be required.

Prevention of pressure sores begins by making the person comfortable in bed. Choose a good mattress, keep the sheets taut and smooth. Keep the skin clean and dry. Turning should be done by two or preferably more people. Begin by lifting the person up a little from the bed. Then roll him over slowly and gently.

Figure 3.2 shows the sites on the body where pressure sores may occur. Pillows and other padding can be used to relieve pressure as indicated in the Figure. Wash pressure areas gently and, when dry, dust lightly with talc.

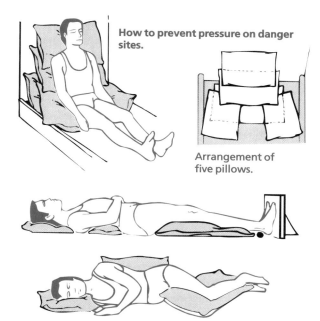

How to prevent pressure on danger sites.

Arrangement of five pillows.

Patient may be further helped by a cushion under the knee joint and one at his feet.

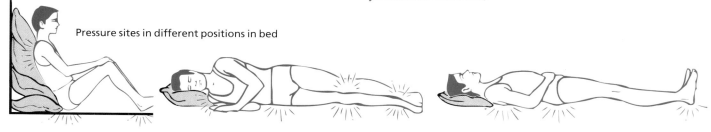

Pressure sites in different positions in bed

Figure 3.2 Pressure sites in bed.

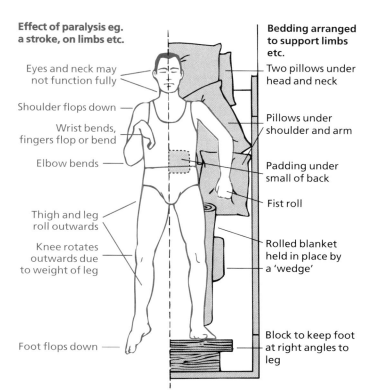

Effect of paralysis eg. a stroke, on limbs etc.

Eyes and neck may not function fully

Shoulder flops down

Wrist bends, fingers flop or bend

Elbow bends

Thigh and leg roll outwards

Knee rotates outwards due to weight of leg

Foot flops down

Bedding arranged to support limbs etc.

Two pillows under head and neck

Pillows under shoulder and arm

Padding under small of back

Fist roll

Rolled blanket held in place by a 'wedge'

Block to keep foot at right angles to leg

Figure 3.3 Paralysed patient.

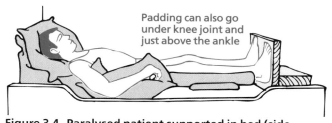

Padding can also go under knee joint and just above the ankle

Figure 3.4 Paralysed patient supported in bed (side view).

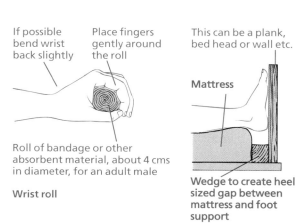

If possible bend wrist back slightly

Place fingers gently around the roll

This can be a plank, bed head or wall etc.

Mattress

Roll of bandage or other absorbent material, about 4 cms in diameter, for an adult male

Wrist roll

Wedge to create heel sized gap between mattress and foot support

Figure 3.5 Two aides for paralysed patients.

Incontinence

Incontinence (urinary and/or faecal) may occur with conscious or unconscious patients. It is acutely embarrassing to conscious patients and they should be re-assured. They must be kept clean. Check the patient frequently.

Collect together all the things which will be necessary to leave the patient in a clean, dry condition, i.e.:

- soap and warm water;
- toilet paper, cotton wool;
- towels;
- talcum powder;
- clean bed linen;
- a change of clothing/pyjamas;
- a plastic bag for soiled tissues;
- a plastic bag for foul linen/clothing.

Clean up with toilet paper. Then wash the soiled areas with cotton wool, soap and water. When the patient has been cleaned, dry him thoroughly by patting. Then dust lightly with talcum powder and remake the bed with clean linen.

If the patient can walk about it may help to assist him into a bath or shower for cleaning up. If a male patient is incontinent of urine place his penis in a urine bottle.

Bodily functions of bed patients

Where the condition of the patient warrants, and if the toilet or a suitable commode is available, it is always better to use these facilities. Privacy is important. The attendant should remain within hearing. Very ill patients may require support or assistance with the bed-pan. Appliances must be emptied immediately and thoroughly cleaned and disinfected. All faeces, urine, vomit, or sputum, should be inspected and a record kept of the amount, colour, consistency, and smell; in some instances it may be necessary to retain samples or to make tests.

Bowel movement in illness

This often worries people. There is no need for the bowels to move every day, nor may it be unhealthy if the bowels do not move for a week and the person feels perfectly well. In illness, food intake is often restricted and, on the basis of less in, less out, bowel motions will not be expected to follow their normal pattern and will probably become less frequent.

Examination of faeces

The bowel habits of patients vary in frequency and character so it is important to establish what is normal for each patient before drawing conclusions from an inspection of the faeces. Constipation should be avoided as this can be very uncomfortable for the patient.

Abnormalities

Common abnormalities to be looked for are blood, pus, slime (mucus), diminished bile pigment content, and worms.
Blood. Black, tarry faeces either formed or fluid but always of offensive odour, indicate bleeding from the stomach or high up in the intestines. The blood has been altered by the digestive process (known as malaena)
Bright red blood suggests an abnormal condition of the lower bowel, rectum or anus.
Haemorrhoids (piles) are the most common cause of this type of bleeding but such cases should be referred to a doctor, when convenient, to exclude more serious causes.
Slimy faeces occur mainly in acute or chronic infections of the large bowel, but irritation of the bowel lining from any cause can also produce excess mucus.

Bile pigment. Pale, putty-coloured faeces caused by a diminished bile content are associated with some liver, pancreas or gall bladder diseases.

Thread worms look like white threads 0.5 to 1 cm in length which can often be seen wriggling about in recently passed faeces.

Round worms resemble earth worms measuring 15 to 20 cm in length and can similarly be seen in recently passed faeces.

Tape worms, the longest of the different varieties can measure 15 metres in length. The body is segmented and flat. Short lengths may break off and be passed in the faeces. The full length is seen only when passed after effective treatment which should be under medical supervision.

Effect of certain diseases

Acute bacillary dysentery. In severe cases up to thirty bowel actions in 24 hours may occur with much slime and blood in the faeces.

Amoebic dysentery. There is often a long history of passing bulky, offensive faeces streaked with blood and mucus.

Cholera. Diarrhoea is frequent and profuse. In severe cases quarts of odourless, watery fluid containing shreds of mucus, the so-called rice water motion, are passed daily.

Typhoid (Enteric). Constipation during the first week may be followed by frequent diarrhoea resembling pea soup.

Testing the urine

In certain illnesses, the urine is found to contain abnormal constituents when the appropriate tests are performed. The tests which are described in this section may help you to differentiate between one illness and another if you are in doubt about the diagnosis.

The urine should always be tested:

- if any person is ill enough to be confined to bed;

- if the symptoms are suggestive of an abdominal complaint;

- if the symptoms are suggestive of disease of the urinary system, e.g. pain on passing urine; or

- if there is some trouble of the genital area.

All tests must be made on an uncontaminated specimen. In males, if there is any discharge from the penis or from behind the foreskin, or in females if there is a vaginal discharge, the genitalia should be washed with soap and water and dried on a paper towel or tissue before passing urine.

Urine glasses or other collecting vessels should be washed with detergent solution or with soap and water and must be rinsed at least three times in fresh water to remove all traces of detergent or of soap. False positive results to the tests will be given if these precautions are not taken.

Examine and test the urine immediately after it has been passed as false results may occur if stale urine is tested.

First examine the appearance of the urine. Hold the urine glass towards a source of light so that the light shines through it. Note the colour and whether the urine is crystal clear, slightly cloudy or definitely hazy (turbid). Note any odour present such as acetone or ammonia. A fishy smell is often found in urinary infections.

Normal urine varies from a pale straw to quite a dark yellow colour. In concentrated urine it becomes brownish in colour. Orange or 'smoky' coloured urine is usually due to blood in small amounts. Greater quantities of blood turn the urine red and cloudy and small clots may be seen. The urine may be the colour of strong tea or even slightly greenish in persons who are jaundiced. Persistent cloudiness is usually due to protein in the urine and can be found in urinary infections.

Test reagents

Simple and reliable Stick tests are available in the medical stores for urine testing – for sugar, ketones, blood and protein, either as separate sticks or a single multi-reagent stick.

The reagent is attached to the plastic stick which is dipped into the urine.

The tests should be done in the following way.

- remove a test strip from its container. Do not touch the test end with your fingers.

- replace the cap of the container at once and screw it on firmly; otherwise the remaining strips will become useless.

- dip the test end into the urine briefly and shake off any excess.

- read off any colour change in the test area by comparing it with the standard colours on the container at the specified times.

- make a note of the date, time and the result of the test in the patient's notes.

NOTE: Urine should be free from blood, sugar and protein. However in some young healthy persons, protein may be found on testing their urine when they are up and about during the day, but it should not occur in a 'first morning' specimen passed after a night in bed. Where protein is found in a young person's urine, the patient should empty his bladder before he goes to bed and a specimen should be passed immediately on rising in the morning. If there is no protein in this specimen, the presence of protein in other specimens taken during the day is of no significance. A similar condition can arise with sugar, but there is no test available on board which can differentiate this from diabetes. If sugar is present in the urine, the patient should be treated as a diabetic until proved otherwise.

Examination of vomited matter

Always inspect any vomited matter, because it may be helpful in arriving at a diagnosis. Note its colour, consistency, odour and approximate amount.

In cases of suspected poisoning, vomited matter should be put in a suitable receptacle, covered with an airtight lid. It should then be labelled and stored in a cool place to be available at any subsequent investigation.

Vomit may contain:

- Partly digested food.

- Bile causing the vomit to be yellow or yellow-green in colour.

- Blood. This may indicate the presence of a gastric ulcer or growth in the stomach, but it may also occur after severe straining from retching, as in seasickness, or as a complication of enlargement of the liver. The blood may be dark in colour, and resemble 'coffee grounds' if it has been retained in the stomach for any length of time. See also 'Note' in Section on sputum below.

- Faecal material. A watery brown fluid with the odour of faeces may be found in advanced cases of intestinal obstruction when there is a reverse flow of the intestinal contents.

Examination of sputum

The quantity and type of any sputum should be noted, and the presence of any blood in it should always be particularly recorded.

- clear and slimy sputum suggests chronic bronchitis.

- thick yellow or green colour suggests acute or chronic respiratory illnes..

- rust colour is due to the presence of small quantities of blood and may occur in pneumonia.

- frothy sputum is characteristic of pulmonary oedema and can be white or pink in colour.

- frothy bright red sputum is associated with lung injury.

NOTE: Remember always in suspected cases of spitting blood (and also of vomiting blood) to inspect carefully the mouth and throat in a good light, and make the patient blow his nose. Coughing and vomiting blood are not common conditions, whereas slight bleeding from the gums and nose is, and an anxious and nervous patient may easily mislead the unwary.

Breathing difficulties

Patients who have difficulty in breathing will be most comfortable half sitting up, either lying back or leaning forward with their forearms and elbows supported on a bed-table with pillows.

Fluid balance

The body has self-regulating mechanisms to maintain a normal balance between fluid in and fluid out.

Fluid in

In a healthy individual, the average daily intake of the fluids from food and drink is about 2.5 litres. In temperate climates it is possible to manage for a short time on as little as 1 litre (just under 2 pints). In hot climates where there is a large fluid loss through sweating, an intake of 6 litres per day may be necessary.

Fluid out

Body fluid is lost through unseen perspiration, the breath, the urine and the faeces. At least 2.5 litres of fluid will be lost a day as follows, in a healthy individual.

	Litres
Unseen perspiration	0.5
Breath	0.4
Urine	1.5
Faeces	0.1
	2.5

To this figure must be added any loss through obvious sweating. This can be high in hot climates.

Measuring fluid imbalance

In any illness where fluid balance is likely to be a problem, eg. where diarrhoea and vomiting are a feature, a fluid chart recording the amount of fluid in and fluid out should be started at once as an aid to you and to the radio medical doctor. The quantity of fluid in and the fluid out should be added up separately every 12 hours and the totals compared. The information in the final column of the record should include as much detail as possible including, where relevant, the duration and the intensity of the fluid loss (e.g. very sweaty for one hour). It will normally be translatable into specific quantities only by a doctor to whom it will be useful.

A normal fluid balance can generally be assumed if the fluid out by way of urine and vomit plus 1 to 1.5 litres equals the fluid in.

Excessive loss of fluid (dehydration)

Dehydration may occur in any patient sweating profusely or suffering from diarrhoea, vomiting, blood loss or burns of areas exceeding about 10% of the body surface. Uncontrolled diabetes can also be a cause of dehydration. Diarrhoea and vomit both have a high fluid content which should be measured or assessed as to the amount and the extent to which it is liquid. Anyone who suffers from either or both will require a high fluid intake to maintain fluid balance. In illnesses where the fluid taken by mouth is vomited back it may be necessary to give fluids per rectum as it may also be for certain unconscious patients.

In these cases a fluid intake and output chart must be used. Signs of dehydration include excessive thirst, high temperature for a long time, dry skin, lack-lustre eyes, dry mouth, lips and tongue, and dark concentrated urine passed infrequently, if in small quantities. Ask a dehydrated patient what he would like to drink and grant him any reasonable, non-alcoholic request. Cool citric fruit juices, sweetened with sugar or glucose, are nourishing.

In conditions, such as heat illnesses, when salt is lost with the sweat, and cholera where profuse diarrhoea occurs and salts are lost from the bowel, salt replacement is necessary. Give re-hydration solution or 1 level teaspoonful of common salt in ½ litre of water, at first in small quantities, repeated frequently.

Giving fluids per rectum

To give fluids per rectum, the patient should lie down on his side with his buttocks raised on two pillows and you should pass a lubricated catheter (26 Charriere or French gauge) through the anus into the rectum for a distance of about 23 cm. The catheter can be lubricated with petroleum jelly (Vaseline). Next, tape the end of the catheter to the skin with the end in a convenient position to attach to a tube and drip set (Figure 3.4). Give 200 ml of water slowly through the tube, taking about 10 to 15 minutes to drip the water in. This amount will usually be retained. Leave the catheter in position and block its end with a spigot, or small cork, or compression clip.

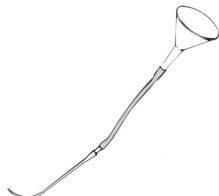

Give the patient a further 200 ml of water every 4 hours. This should give a fluid intake of about 1,200 ml (1 litre) per day. It is worth trying to increase the amount given on each occasion to 250 ml and to give this every 3 to 3½ hours, particularly if the weather is warm and the patient is sweating. However, if any overflow occurs the amount given must be reduced. The rectum will not retain large amounts of fluid and fluid must be retained in order to be absorbed. Occasionally the rectum will not accept fluid readily, especially if it is loaded with faeces. Smaller quantities at more frequent intervals should be tried in these cases. Careful observation will show whether the fluid is being retained and whether or not the patient is being rehydrated. Aim to give at least 1 litre of fluid per day if possible.

Figure 3.6   Make-shift appliance for giving fluids per rectum.

Serious mental illness

Certain guiding principles must be borne in mind when dealing with any patient who, in the opinion of the Master, is of unsound mind.

Every such case should be considered to be, actually or potentially suicidal or homicidal. All possible steps must therefore be taken to have a constant watch kept on the patient.

Should the Master deem it necessary to place the patient under supervision and/or restraint, then the patient should if possible be housed in a single-berth cabin. The cabin should be checked for safety to make sure it contains nothing that the patient might harm himself on, e.g. mirrors, stools or chairs, plastic bags or unprotected light bulbs. Supervision is necessary when water is used in the cabin.

Cutlery should only be allowed under strict supervision and it is advisable to use plastic or paper crockery. No razors, matches or weapons such as knives should be left in the patient's possession. The patient should be encouraged to drink plenty of fluids as there is a real risk of dehydration. The patient should be persuaded to undress and put on clothing that has no pockets. A search can be made for potential weapons or hidden medication. Braces, belts and cords should be removed.

A checklist of all the patient's property should be recorded for future reference, to avoid disputes.

The cabin door must be able to be firmly secured. The disturbed patient, however, may become distressed if he knows he is locked in. Care should be taken to make sure he cannot lock himself in. Any port must be firmly secured and the key removed. It is useful if there is safety glass or window or ventilator in the door, so that the patient can be observed, especially before entering the cabin. It is better for only one person to enter the cabin, but a second person should be nearby in case assistance is required.

The patient should be accompanied by two people if going out on deck. Remember the ship's side is always very near, and if the patient does go over the side the lives of others will be at risk during the rescue attempt.

Many of the patients may have delusions of persecution by their shipmates. The person caring for the patient should be calm, polite and firm, in an attempt to gain the patient's co-operation and trust. Restraint should not be used unless absolutely necessary, as this could aggravate and distress the patient even more. It is worthwhile remembering that a Paraguard or Neil Robertson stretcher can act as a useful restraint when dealing with a seriously disturbed patient.

Unconsciousness

Careful nursing of unconscious people is a demanding, difficult and very important task. The survival and eventual condition of anyone who is unconscious depends greatly on your care, skill and attention.

The 3 MUSTS for Unconscious Patients

■ MUST have a clear airway;

■ MUST be kept in the unconscious position;

■ MUST NEVER be left alone.

Keeping a clear airway is essential and requires the patient to be kept in the unconscious position. A Guedel airway (Figure 3.5) can be used. Any blood, vomit or other secretions from the mouth must be mopped out or removed by the use of a sucker. Unconscious patients must never be left alone in case they move, vomit, have a fit or fall out of their bed.

Airway insertion

An airway (Figure 3.5A) should be inserted if a patient is breathing on his own but is doing so with great difficulty. The function of the airway is to ensure a clear passage between the lips and the back of the throat. Normally use size 4 for adult males, size 1 for small children, and size 3 for others.

First remove any dentures and suck or swab out any blood or vomit which is in the mouth to get a clear airway. Then, with the head fully back, slide the airway gently into the mouth with the outer curve of the airway towards the tongue. This operation will be facilitated if the airway is wetted (Figure 3.5B).

If you notice any attempt by the patient to gag, retch or vomit, it is better not to proceed with the insertion of the airway. If necessary, try again later to insert it.

Continue to slide the airway in until the flange of the airway reaches the lips. Now rotate the airway through 180°C so that the outer curve is upwards to the roof of the mouth (Figure 3.5C).

Bring the jaw upwards and push the airway in until the flange at the end of the airway is outside the teeth (or gums) and inside the lips.

Check that the casualty's breath is coming through the airway. Continue to keep the jaws upwards and the head fully back so that the airway will be held in place by the teeth or gums and by its shape.

As the patient regains consciousness, he will spit out the airway; keep him in the unconscious position and under constant observation until he is fully conscious. If he relapses into unconsciousness it may be necessary to re-insert the airway if his breathing is difficult.

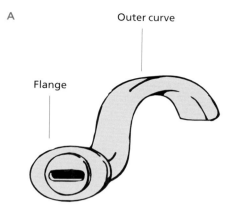

A   Outer curve

Flange

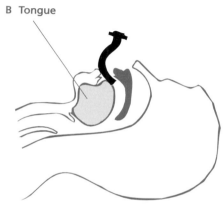

B   Tongue

Head tilted fully back

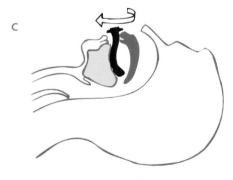

C

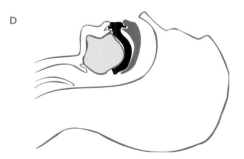

D

Figure 3.7 The Guedel tube airway.

Diagnosis of unconsciousness

As soon as the patient has been put to bed in the unconscious position, assess the circumstances leading to the incident of unconsciousness. Find out all you can from any witness of the occurrence and question close associates on the recent state of health of the patient.

Assess and treat any obvious cause such as a head injury. If patient is unconscious with an injury assume neck is also injured. Otherwise, undress the patient taking care to maintain a clear air passage during the process. Make a general head to toe examination of the patient.

Using the information you have collected and the results of your examination, consult the table and try to identify the cause of the unconsciousness. The following may assist in distinguishing between the main causes.

Fainting

A simple faint will rarely cause difficulty. The patient has usually recovered consciousness within several minutes and he will feel back to normal shortly without any after effects.

Brain concussion

This is usually caused by a direct blow on the head but, sometimes may be caused by a fall from a height even when there has been no direct injury. It could vary in severity from feeling dazed and shaky for a few minutes to, in very severe cases, unconsciousness lasting for hours or even days.

Brain compression

Compression should be suspected if unconsciousness comes on gradually after a head injury, or, if a casualty who has recovered consciousness after a head injury lapses again into unconsciousness.

Epilepsy

The irregular jerking movements of the limbs will have stopped before the casualty has been taken to the ship's hospital. In a single fit these jerking movements will not recur – the patient usually has a history of fits.

Stroke

The presence of paralysis of a limb or limbs on one side of the body should, in the absence of a head injury, point to this cause.

Alcohol abuse

The history obtained from witnesses or close associates will give an indication of the amount of alcohol consumed.

Although a casualty's breath may smell of alcohol, his unconsciousness may not be caused by it. He may for example have sustained a head injury in a fall when drunk.

Diabetic coma

There is usually a history of the casualty feeling unwell for two or three days before the onset of unconsciousness.

The characteristic smell of the breath is very helpful.

The general management of an unconscious patient

Make sure that an unconscious patient cannot injure himself further. Some unconscious and semi-conscious patients can be quite violent, or can move about suddenly, so ensure that they cannot fall onto the floor or hit themselves against any hard edge or surface. A bed with sides will probably be the safest place. Do not put pillows or other padding where the patient might suffocate. Remove any jewellery – rings and earrings in particular.

The person must be turned from one side to the other at least every 3 hours to prevent bedsores, this requires 2 people. Turn the patient gently and roll him smoothly from one side to the other. The head must always be kept back with a chin-up position when actually turning, and at no time must the head be allowed to bend forwards with the chin sagging. This is both to help to keep a clear airway and to prevent neck injuries. If you suspect a broken jaw or that the person has fallen from a height and may have a neck or spine injury, you should be extra specially careful during turning.

Check the breathing and that the Guedel airway is securely in place as soon as you have turned the person.

Make sure that all joints are neither fully straight nor fully bent. Ideally they should all be kept in mid-position. Place pillows under and between the bent knees and between the feet and ankles. Use a bed-cage (a large stiff box will make a good improvised cage) to keep the bedclothes from pressing on the feet and ankles. Check that elbows, wrists and fingers are in a relaxed mid-position after turning. Do not pull, strain or stretch any joint at any time. Make quite sure that the eyelids are closed and that they remain closed at all times, otherwise preventable damage to the eyeball can easily occur. Irrigate the eyes every 2 hours by opening the lids slightly and dripping some saline solution gently into the corner of each eye in such a way that the saline will run across each eye and drain from the other corner. A saline solution can be made by dissolving one level teaspoonful of salt in $1/2$ litre of boiled water which has been allowed to cool.

After 12 hours of unconsciousness further problems will arise. Unconscious people must be given nothing by mouth in case it chokes them. However, after 12 hours of unconsciousness fluid will have to be given, particularly in hot climates and/or if the patient is obviously sweating. Because fluids cannot be given by mouth the fluid should be given per rectum. An input/output chart will be necessary and the instructions given under fluid balance should be followed. The mouth, cheeks, tongue and teeth should be moistened every 3 to 4 hours using a small swab moistened with glycerine of thymol. Carry out mouth care every time the person is turned.

After 48 hours of unconsciousness move each limb joint at least once a day providing other considerations such as fracture do not prevent this. They should be moved very gently in such a way as to put each joint through a full range of movement. Do the job systematically. Begin on the side of the patient which is most accessible. Start with the fingers and thumb, then move the wrist, the elbow and the shoulder. Now move the toes, the foot and the ankle. Then bend the knee and move the hip around. Next, turn the patient, if necessary, with the help of another person, and move the joints on the other side.

Remember that unconscious patients may be very relaxed and floppy – so do not let go of their limbs until you have placed the limb safely back on the bed. Hold the limbs firmly but not tightly and do everything slowly and with the utmost gentleness. Take your time in moving each joint fully before going on to the next.

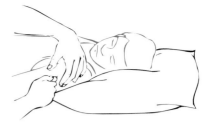

Figure 3.8 Administering a subcutaneous injection.

Injections

Injections are used when rapid absorption is desired, or when the patient cannot or will not swallow a drug, or is vomiting, or the action of the medication would be destroyed by secretions of the stomach or intestine. They can be given under the skin or into a muscle. Before a patient is given an injection he should be asked whether he is allergic to it. If a patient is unconscious you will not be able to ask about allergies.

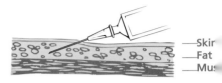

Figure 3.9 Subcutaneous injection - note the very low angle of entry.

Subcutaneous (under the skin)

The site of subcutaneous injections is the fleshy part of the outer arm just below the shoulder. To make the injection, the skin should be grasped between the thumb and forefinger, and the injection is made by inserting the needle 1 cm under the skin surface (Figure 3.7). The maximum effect of the injection usually occurs in about 30 minutes.

Intramuscular (into a muscle)

Medications injected intramuscularly are absorbed more quickly than those given subcutaneously. A maximum effect is obtained in about 15 minutes.

Only two sites are recommended for intramuscular injections. These are the outer side of the middle third of the thigh and the upper outer quarter of the buttock. Great care must be taken to give the injection exactly into the correct site to avoid bone, nerves etc. (Figures 3.8 and 3.9).

If it is impossible to use either of the above sites use the deltoid muscle (upper outer third of the arm) taking care not to hit the bone (Figure 3.10).

Give the injection at right angles to the skin and insert the needle for about 3 centimetres (Figure 3.11).

If you have to give more than one injection, the others must be confined to the areas shown in the Figures but try and alternate between the four sites.

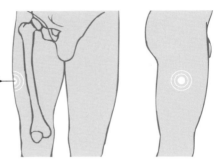

Figure 3.10 Administering an intramuscular injection into the thigh.

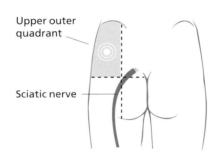

Figure 3.11 Administering an intramuscular injection into the buttock – note: injections into the sciatic nerve can have drastic consequences.

Filling a syringe

Drugs for injection are supplied in either rubber capped vials or in glass ampoules. The name and strength and expiry date of the drug is always marked on the vial. Check this carefully, using a magnifying glass if necessary. If no name is visible or it is indecipherable, that vial should be discarded.

Glass ampoules (Figure 3.14(a)) have a coloured band round the neck at which the top of the ampoule will break off cleanly – use a tissue to break. The rubber cap (Figure 3.14(b)) of the other type of vial is held on by a metal cap. A small tear-off seal may have to be removed before the rubber becomes visible. The tear-off seal should not be removed before the drug is required.

Plastic syringes are supplied either with needles attached or with the needles in separate plastic containers. These pre-sterilised syringes and needles are disposable and must be used once only.

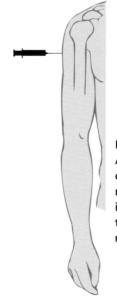

Figure 3.12 Administration of an intramuscular injection into the deltoid muscle.

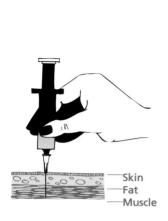

Skin
Fat
Muscle

Figure 3.13 Holding the syringe for an intra-muscular injection. Hold the syringe like a dart. Plunge it into a depth of 2 cms (³/₄ inch).

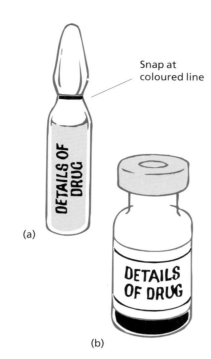

Snap at
coloured line

(a)

DETAILS OF DRUG

DETAILS OF DRUG

(b)

Figure 3.14 Drug vials (a) a glass ampoule, (b) a rubber-capped vial.

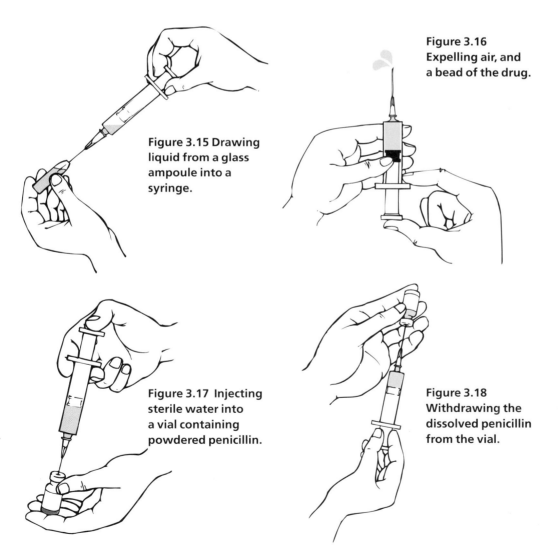

Figure 3.15 Drawing liquid from a glass ampoule into a syringe.

Figure 3.16 Expelling air, and a bead of the drug.

Figure 3.17 Injecting sterile water into a vial containing powdered penicillin.

Figure 3.18 Withdrawing the dissolved penicillin from the vial.

Before giving an injection, prepare:

- The correct drug in its container, either an ampoule or a rubber capped vial.
- A disposable syringe and needle.
- Antiseptic swab.

  Wash your hands thoroughly.

Take the glass ampoule and check that the name, dose and expiry date on the vial is that of the drug which you want to give. Ensure that all the liquid is in the ampoule below the neck by gently tapping the neck region with a finger.

Wrap the ampoule in a swab and gently and firmly break off the top. Make sure that you point the ampoule away from your eyes.

Set the ampoule down and open the syringe following the direction on the package. Remove the syringe and needle, leave the needle cover on until you are ready to use it. If the needle is separate, open the needle case first, leave the needle in the case. Next open the syringe packet and insert the syringe into the needle pressing it down firmly. The needle can then be removed from its sheath. Do not touch the needle shaft at any time. The ampoule is then held in one hand and the syringe and needle in the other. Slightly tilt the ampoule, insert the needle without touching the glass at the opening and draw the liquid into the barrel of the syringe by gently pulling on the plunger. Be careful that you do not push the tip of the needle on to the bottom of the ampoule. This will blunt the needle and make the injection difficult and painful (Figure 3.15).

When the ampoule is empty, withdraw the needle and point it upwards. Tap the barrel of the syringe to ensure that all air comes up to the surface of the liquid, then press the plunger gently to expel the air. A small bead of liquid will appear at the tip of the needle when this has been accomplished. If it is necessary to give less than the full dose, keep on pressing the plunger until the required volume registers on the scale on the barrel (Figure 3.16).

Penicillin in powder

To reconstitute benzylpenicillin 600 mg you will also require a 2 ml ampoule of water for injection.

Prepare a syringe as in the section above, leaving the cover on the needle.

Open an ampoule of the water and, removing the cover from the needle, draw up all the water into the syringe. Replace the cover until you have swabbed the rubber cap of the penicillin vial/bottle with antiseptic swab; then insert the needle through the rubber cap, and depress the plunger to inject the water onto the penicillin (Figure 3.17).

Withdraw the needle, replace the needle cover over it and lay the syringe and needle on the clean towel in a safe place.

Gently shake the vial so that the penicillin is dissolved in the water. Re-swab the rubber cap, allow the spirit to dry, insert the needle just through the rubber cap and invert the vial. The penicillin can now be withdrawn from the vial into the syringe. Then go through the procedure described above to get rid of the air before proceeding with the injection (Figure 3.16).

NOTES:
If you need to give only 300 mg of benzylpencillin, reconstitute 600 mg as above and draw-up 1 ml for immediate use: the balance can be stored for up to 12 hours in the non-freezing section of a refrigerator. (1 ampoule for 1 patient)

Giving the injection

Before giving the injection cleanse the skin with antiseptic swab. Then plunge the needle into the site selected in accordance with the advice given above. Draw back the plunger and look for blood coming into the syringe from a blood vessel. Do not inject if blood comes in, but partially withdraw the needle and reinsert it at a different angle, draw back the plunger and check again for blood.

If no blood appears, give the injection slowly. Then remove the needle and massage the area gently. Safe disposal of needle and syringe is important to avoid sharps injuries to you and others. Do not re-sheath a needles which has been used to give an injection.

Care of the injured

This chapter is about the care and treatment, after first-aid, of a casualty who has been moved to the ship's hospital or to his own cabin, ie. the definitive treatment of injuries sustained onboard.

Cleanliness and sterilising.

To prevent infection in wounds, burns and other conditions, all dressings and instruments should be sterile. Dressings should be supplied pre-packed and sterilised. There are two ways of obtaining sterile instruments:

■ The instruments or equipment can be obtained in pre-packed sterilised containers. Such instruments are for once-only use and are disposable. Disposable equipment is very convenient to use.

■ Instruments, which are not disposable, should be sterilised just before use in a steriliser or by boiling in water for not less than 10 minutes, then allowed to cool.

In using any instrument, the patient, or 'business', end of the instrument must not touch anything before use and only the operator should handle the operator parts of the instrument.

The attendant should similarly guard against infecting the wound:

■ Sleeves should be rolled-up.

■ Hands, wrists and forearms should be thoroughly washed, with soap and running water.

■ Surgical latex (rubber) gloves should be worn to protect both the operator and the patient.

General Care of wounds
Classification of wounds

Wounds vary enormously in extent and depth, depending on how they are caused. They can be classified as follows:

■ Abrasions (Grazes). These are often superficial and if thoroughly cleaned and appropriately dressed usually heal well.

■ Incised wounds. These are caused by sharp implements, such as knives or glass, and may penetrate deeply to and through underlying structures, such as tendons, down to bone. The wound edges are generally healthy and heal well if the edges are carefully opposed.

■ Lacerations. These are caused by blunt injury and involve crushing or tearing of the wound edge. This results in tissue damage or loss, and consequently carries an increased risk of infection.

■ Puncture Wounds. These are not associated with great tissue damage or loss but carry a high risk of infection as organisms or foreign material (e.g. dirt or bits of clothing) may be driven deep into the wound.

■ Bites – human or animal. These are often a combination of puncture and crush and carry an extremely high risk of infection, and will usually require antibiotics.

■ Degloving Wounds. e.g. tissue being torn from a finger by a ring. These injuries involve loss of blood supply to the tissue and require specialist attention.

Wound Healing

There are many factors that can affect how well a wound heals.

Factors that promote healing	Factors that impede healing
Clean incised wound	Ragged crushed wound edges
Fresh wound <6 hours old	Old wound >12 hours old
Uncontaminated	Contamination
No loss of tissue or blood supply	Loss of tissue or blood supply
Scalp/face (good blood supply)	Shin (poor blood supply)

Clean, incised, fresh wounds with no tissue loss and a good blood supply where the edges are held together will heal quickly and relatively painlessly. They will leave a minimal scar.

Wounds where there is a gap between the wound edges, either because of tissue loss or because it is not possible to close the wound completely will heal by growth of new tissue. This process is slow, often associated by some discharge and may be painful. The resultant scar may be unsightly or disabling.

Treatment of Wounds.

Before you start:

■ Ensure the casualty is comfortable and is offered painkillers.

Check for damage to underlying structures. If a wound is on a limb it is essential to check that structures such as major blood vessels, nerves and tendons are intact. It will not be possible to repair them at this stage but such injuries should be documented and attended to at the next port. Injury to a major blood vessel is usually obvious because of bleeding. Apply firm pressure to the bleeding point and GET RADIO MEDICAL ADVICE. DO NOT USE A TOURNIQUET! An area of numbness beyond the injury may indicate nerve injury. Tendon injury will be indicated by inability to move a digit. e.g. extend a finger.

Wash your hands and prepare materials and equipment required to clean, close (stitch if necessary) and dress the wound.

Spread a sterile paper towel over a conveniently located table and lay out the following:

■ A sterile haemostatic clamp(e.g. Spencer Wells forceps).

■ A sterile pair of scissors and a scalpel/scalpel blade.

■ A pair of sterile dissecting forceps.

■ Sufficient sterile gauze swabs to clean and mop the wound.

■ Sterile cleaning fluid, e.g. saline or antiseptic solution/wipes, in a suitable sterile container.

■ Suture materials or steristrips as necessary.

■ A disposable razor if necessary.

■ A suitable dressing.

Ensure you have a container in which to place dirty or soiled dressings to hand.

Remember to wear surgical gloves to prevent (a) contamination of the wound and (b) exposure of yourself to the patient's blood.

Preparation of the wound prior to closure.

If the patient is able, get them to wash the wound and surrounding area under the tap. Use soap on undamaged skin. Next clean the wound then surrounding area thoroughly, with sterile saline or water. If the wound is heavily contaminated with foreign material (grease etc.) then an anti-septic solution, may be used. If necessary use local anaesthetic to infiltrate the wound (see below) prior to gentle scrubbing with a sterile nailbrush.

■ Shave or clip the edges of the wound if necessary in order to see them clearly and to prevent hair being caught in the wound when it is closed. Do not shave eyebrows.

■ Remove any particles of dirt (wood, metal etc.) with the tissue forceps.

■ Trim away any ragged edges or dead tissue with scissors or a scalpel blade, using local anaesthetic if necessary.

Local Anaesthetic

You should decide whether a local anaesthetic (L.A.) will be required. An L.A. should not be necessary for the insertion of 1 or 2 simple stitches; indeed the application of the anaesthetic may in such cases be more painful than the suturing. In more complicated cases it may be desirable to infiltrate lignocaine hydrochloride 1%. Occasionally L.A. is required in order to adequately clean a wound prior to closure. (See MSN 1726 for dose.)

Bleeding.

Exerting firm, sustained pressure to the wound, with a gauze swab, for five minutes or so may control bleeding. If there is pulsatile bleeding, that doesn't stop with pressure, it may be necessary to tie off a small bleeding vessel. If the bleeding vessel can be seen, grasp the end with the pointed tips of the Spencer Wells forceps and make sure the bleeding is controlled. Next take a length of cat-gut and, holding the forceps up, slip the ligature under the forceps and tie it off using a surgeon's knot (see Figure 4.4) so as to encircle the end of the vessel. Now cut the ligature ends short, leaving enough only to ensure that the knot doesn't slip. Then remove the forceps and inspect the wound to ensure the bleeding has ceased. WARNING! If the bleeding is torrential or welling up from deep within the wound, and the bleeding point cannot be identified do not grasp blindly with the forceps as you risk causing further damage. Apply prolonged, firm pressure. If the bleeding is still not controlled, GET RADIO MEDICAL ADVICE.

Wound Closure.

'God heals, we just bring the edges together.'   *A plastic surgeon.*

The purpose of closing a wound is simply to oppose the edges so healing can take place quickly.

Using adhesive skin closures.

(Steristrips)

In the case of superficial lacerations or incised wounds, which nevertheless need closing, it may be possible to hold the edges together using steristrips. These are narrow adhesive strips. Once the wound is prepared for closure the steristrips should be applied as follows:

■ Make sure the wound edges are dry or the steristrips will not stick.

■ Stick the strip to the skin on one side of the wound up to, but not on the wound edge.

■ Pull the strip across the wound so that the edges are brought together.

■ Then stick the strip on the skin on the opposite side of the wound.

Repeat the process along the length of the wound until it is closed (Figure 4.1).

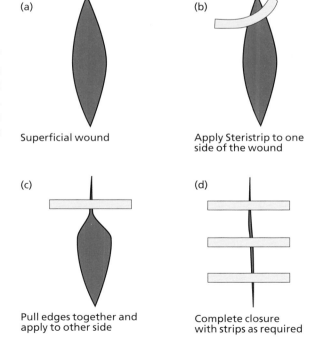

(a) Superficial wound

(b) Apply Steristrip to one side of the wound

(c) Pull edges together and apply to other side

(d) Complete closure with strips as required

Figure 4.1 Butterfly closures holding edges of wound together.

Using Sutures.

Deep and gaping wounds cannot be closed effectively using steristrips alone. For these wounds you will have to consider whether suturing is appropriate.

DO NOT suture if you cannot bring together not only the skin but also the deeper tissue. A 'dead space' will become infected, cause the wound to fall apart, delay recovery and may lead to the loss of the limb or even death (see Figure 4.2c). DO NOT SUTURE A WOUND THAT IS OVER 6 HOURS OLD. WHEN IN DOUBT DO NOT SUTURE.

The circumstances in which a suture should or should not be inserted are shown in Figure 4.2.

When you decide that suturing is appropriate, you will require the items listed above.

Sutures are supplied in sterile dry packs as a length of silk or nylon thread already attached to a surgical, curved, cutting needle. These should not be opened until all is ready for stitching to begin.

Then decide exactly what repair you intend to make. If the cut is linear, for example, how many stitches will you need? If the cut is star-shaped, will one stitch to include the apices of each skin flap be adequate?

Having decided upon the nature of the repair, open the sterile pack and extract the needle with the haemostatic or needle forceps. Hold the needle in the tips of the forceps approximately two- thirds the way down from its point.

Grasp the edge of the wound furthest from you with the toothed forceps, then with a firm sharp stab drive the needle through the whole thickness of the skin at least 0.6 cm from its edge. Then grasp the skin on the immediate opposite side of the wound with the toothed forceps and drive the needle upwards through the whole thickness of the skin so that it emerges at least 0.6 cm from the wound edge (Figure 4.3). Make sure the depth of the suture is the same on both sides of the wound, or you will create a step on the surface . Now cut sufficient thread off the main length to tie a surgeon's knot with sufficient tension exerted (and no more) to bring the cut edges of the skin together. If the wound is deep and clean insert the needle deeply into the underlying tissue so as to draw it and the skin together. Insert further stitches as required at intervals of not less than 1 cm. After tying, cut off the ends of the knots, leaving about 1 cm of thread free to facilitate later removal of the stitches (Figure 4.3). If the cut edges of the skin tend to curve inwards into the wound, correct with toothed forceps (Figures 4.2, 4.3 and 4.5). As soon as the stitching is completed, clean the whole area with sterile saline, and apply a sterile occlusive dressing. Dispose of sharps safely.

If you have a difficult, deep and tense wound to close use a mattress suture (Figure 4.6). A mattress suture ensures that you bring together the edges of the wound not just on the surface but throughout its depth and length.

Deep and gaping wounds that cannot be sutured (Figure 4.2(d))

If the wound is to be allowed to heal without suturing, lightly dress the wound with sterile paraffin gauze. Then place about three layers of sterile gauze over this and make fast with bandages. Re-dress the wound on alternate days until it is healed. If the wound is on a limb, it should be elevated to encourage draining and reduce swelling.

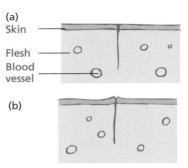

(a)

Skin
Flesh
Blood vessel

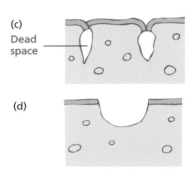

(b)

Wounds A and B can be stitched

(c)
Dead space

(d)

Wounds C and D should not be stitched

Figure 4.2

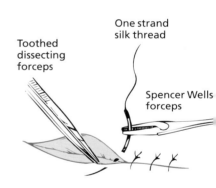

One strand silk thread
Toothed dissecting forceps
Spencer Wells forceps

Figure 4.3 Stitching a wound.

Wound Infection.

A greater or lesser degree of infection of the wound is inevitable after injury. This means that there will be a certain amount of fluid from the damaged and inflamed tissues, which should be allowed to escape. Remember this when inserting stitches; do not put them so close together that it is impossible for pus to discharge if it forms. Also, when inspecting a wound after stitching, look closely to see if there is swelling or tension on a stitch in any part of the wound, indicating the formation of pus within the wound. If there is, remove the stitch and allow free drainage of the wound.

Antibiotics?

Consider whether antibiotic therapy is necessary. Simple sutured wounds and superficial packed wounds should not require antibiotics. In other cases, and especially with deep wounds involving damage to muscles, start the antibiotic treatment. When in doubt, give antibiotics.

Tetanus.

Check whether the casualty has had a tetanus injection within the last 10 years. If not, give 0.5ml tetanus vaccine by intra-muscular injection. This injection should be noted in the casualty's records and you should also ensure that he understands that he has been given a tetanus injection.

Removal of stitches.

Once the wound has healed the stitches can be removed and a simple dressing worn until healing is complete. Remember that some wounds take longer to heal than others. Unless otherwise stated most sutures can be removed after one week.

The removal of stitches is a simple and painless operation if carried out gently. Clean the area with sterile saline. Grasp one of the ends of the stitch with sterile forceps and lift it up, so as to be able to insert the pointed blade of sterile scissors immediately under the knot. Cut the stitch level with the skin and by gently pulling with the forceps withdraw it (Figure 4.8).

Site of Wound	Remove sutures after:
Face	4–6 days
Scalp	5–7 days
Upper limbs	7 days
Lower limbs	8–10 days
Back	10–12 days
Over a joint (e.g. elbow, knee)	12–14 days

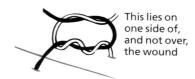

This lies on one side of, and not over, the wound

Figure 4.4 Surgeon's knot.

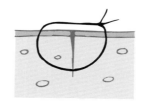

Stitches should be inserted by using curved 'cutting needle' so that each completed stitch is 'round'.

Figure 4.5 Cross section of stitched wound.

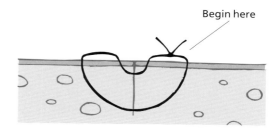

Begin here

Figure 4.6 A Mattress suture.

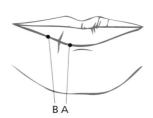

B A

First stitch between A and B on the lip margin

Figure 4.7 Stitched lip.

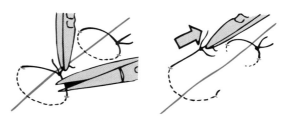

Figure 4.8 Removing a stitch.

Internal injuries

The site of each major internal organ is shown in Annex II. If you suspect any organ is damaged, always start a 10 minute pulse chart so that internal bleeding can be recognised as soon as possible by a rising pulse rate. If the pulse rate is or becomes high (>100 beats per minute) GET RADIO MEDICAL ADVICE.

Restlessness is often a sign of internal bleeding – so all patients who are restless after injury need careful watching.

If the patient is restless because of great pain, and other injuries permit (not head or chest injuries), give morphine. This will control the pain, help to keep the patient calm and quiet, and thus diminish bleeding by rest.

Injury to the abdomen with protrusion of gut.

GET RADIO MEDICAL ADVICE. This injury requires hospital treatment ashore at the earliest moment. Until then, put the patient to bed lying on his back with his knees drawn up to relax the abdomen. No attempt should be made to push intestines back into the abdomen. Exposed intestines (gut) should be covered with a clean, non-fluffy very damp bed sheet. The covering should be kept damp with cooled boiled water and should be held on loosely by a binder. Alternatively the intestines could be loosely wrapped in cling-film. Nothing should be given by mouth. If the patient cannot be taken off the ship within about 12 hours, fluid should be given via the rectal route.

Keep the patient warm, give morphine to keep the patient pain-free at rest and start antibiotics until he can be taken off the ship.

Head injuries

The majority of head injuries are not serious. However, all but the most superficial head injuries are potentially dangerous. Careful examination is therefore essential.

In the first instance, the aim of examination is to distinguish whether the patient has sustained, or is at risk of, a brain injury.

The characteristic sign of brain injury is alteration in the level of consciousness.

Assessment of the Head Injured Patient

History

If the patient is conscious they are usually able to tell you what happened. For patients who are unconscious it is essential to get as much detail of what happened from other crew members, particularly whether the patient's level of consciousness has changed since the injury occurred.

Examination

There are three key indicators of brain injury.

- Level of consciousness,

- pupil size and reaction to light, and

- signs of paralysis down one side of the body.

Level of consciousness (L.O.C.)

After ensuring that the casualty's airway is clear and he is breathing adequately, your first priority is to establish the patient's L.O.C. This can be done simply and quickly using the A.V.P.U. score, detailed below, or the Glasgow Coma Scale (GCS) if you are familiar with it.

1. Is the patient **A**lert (talking sensibly etc.)?
2. If not does he respond to **V**erbal stimuli (i.e. your voice)?
3. If not does he respond to **P**ain (e.g. Firm pressure on a fingernail with a pen)?
4. Or is the patient **U**nresponsive?

This is the most important indication of brain injury, and if the patient's L.O.C. is deteriorating, following a head injury GET RADIO MEDICAL ADVICE, YOUR PATIENT REQUIRES URGENT TRANSFER TO HOSPITAL.

Pupil Response

- Are the pupils equal in size?

- Do they constrict (get smaller) when a light is shone into them?

The pupils should be the same size and constrict quickly and equally when a bright light is shone into them. Some people always have unequal pupils, however, in an unconscious patient, following a significant head injury, a pupil that is widely dilated and unreactive to light probably indicates a serious, life threatening brain injury. GET RADIO MEDICAL ADVICE YOUR PATIENT REQUIRES URGENT TRANSFER TO HOSPITAL.

Signs of Paralysis down one side of the body

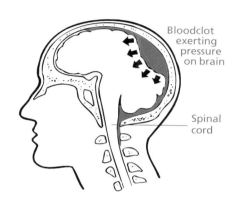

Is the patient moving one side of his body more than the other? You may have to inflict a painful stimulus, like pressure on a fingernail, to get an unconscious patient to move. Unilateral paralysis may indicate that a blood clot is forming in the skull and putting pressure on the brain (Figure 4.9a). Under these circumstances, GET RADIO MEDICAL ADVICE YOUR PATIENT REQUIRES URGENT TRANSFER TO HOSPITAL.

Figure 4.9a Compression of the brain.

Care of the Unconscious Head Injured Patient

It is essential that you do not allow the patient to come to any further harm.

Move the patient to a safe environment, place him in the recovery position and ensure that his airway is clear and he is breathing adequately. If necessary, assisted respiration or artificial respiration should be given. He must be kept constantly under observation in case he should vomit, have fits or become restless and throw himself out of the unconscious position. The observation should be maintained when consciousness returns in case he lapses into coma once again.

Caution! Injuries to the neck are often associated with severe head injuries, so every care should be taken to minimise movement of the neck, and a neck collar, if available, should be fitted to the patient.

Once the patient is in a safe environment, GET RADIO MEDICAL ADVICE and continue to monitor the patients breathing pulse and level of consciousness.

Other Signs of Serious Head Injury

Skull Fractures

A skull fracture indicates that the patient has sustained a significant head injury. In severe injury a depressed fracture may be apparent on careful examination. There is a depression in the skull and sometimes, bony fragments may be present in the wound (Figure 4.9b). Linear fractures of the sides or top of the skull (the vault) are less obvious and normally only diagnosed on x-rays. However, they are occasionally seen or felt at the base of a head wound. Base of skull fractures are the result of indirect force which is transmitted to the base of the skull from a heavy blow to the vault, from blows to the face or jaw or when the casualty falls from a height and lands on his feet. They can be diagnosed by deduction from the history of injury and certain examination findings.

1. CSF (cerebro-spinal fluid) leakage from the ears or nose. This fluid normally circulates around the brain and spinal cord, cushioning them from injury. It appears as bloodstained or sticky clear fluid that trickles from the ear or drips from the nose.

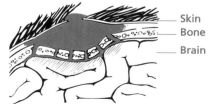

2. 'Panda Eyes' Bleeding from a base of skull fracture ends up appearing around both eyes giving the patient two black eyes.

Figure 4.9b Depressed skull fracture with brain compression.

There is little you can do about the skull fracture itself. If you suspect a depressed fracture, suturing any laceration should control bleeding.

An open wound needs to be covered to prevent infection. However DO NOT poke around in scalp wounds, press over the wound, or try to remove fragments of bone from scalp wounds.

Using scissors, trim the hair around the wound then shave the scalp with a disposable razor so that the edges of the wound can be seen clearly. Carefully clean the wound and surrounding scalp by irrigating the area with sterile saline or boiled, cooled water. Dry the scalp then suture the laceration with silk, and cover this with sterile swabs before bandaging. Hair should not be allowed to enter the wound. Give benzyl penicillin 600 mg intramuscularly, followed by oral antibiotic treatment. If the casualty is unconscious, continue to give benzyl penicillin 600 mg intramuscularly every 6 hours. If allergy develops read the section on allergy and GET RADIO MEDICAL ADVICE.

Fits or Convulsions

Fits may occur after a head injury. If the movements are violent, do not attempt to restrain the casualty by the use of excessive force. It is only necessary to prevent him from causing further injury to himself. If the fit continues for more than a minute give diazepam 5mg rectally. If this dose fails to control the fit, give a further 5mg after 3–4 minutes and GET RADIO MEDICAL ADVICE YOUR PATIENT REQUIRES URGENT TRANSFER TO HOSPITAL.

Headaches

Headaches are common after all types of head injury, even when trivial. However, they usually subside over the days following the injury. A headache becomes concerning if it increases in severity and particularly if it is associated with the onset of drowsiness, confusion or vomiting. Under these circumstances GET RADIO MEDICAL ADVICE.

Vomiting

One or two episodes of vomiting following a head injury is relatively common and not cause for concern. Persistent 'effortless' vomiting, however, may be an indication of increasing pressure within the skull caused by an enlarging blood clot. When associated with increasing headache, drowsiness or confusion, this should be taken seriously and you should GET RADIO MEDICAL ADVICE.

Communication

When communicating with a medical advisor on the ship's radio it is essential that clear, concise information is conveyed. You should report using the format in Chapter 13 including particularly:

- A report of the patient's ABC status. A=Airway Is the patient maintaining a clear airway (Noisy breathing indicates a partially obstructed airway.) A clear airway should be maintained at all times. B=Breathing Is the casualty breathing adequately? What is the respiratory rate (breaths per minute)? C=Circulation What is the pulse rate? Is the pulse full or thready?

- A report of the patient's level of consciousness (A.V.P.U), pupils size and reaction, and signs of paralysis. This should include any change since the injury occurred.

- Details of any other injuries.

Longer term management of serious head injuries.

If a casualty with a serious head injury has to remain on board for more than a few hours, it will be necessary to monitor his condition. You should record as much information as possible to help those to whom the casualty will eventually be transferred and possibly deal with certain complications.

Include in your records:

- Date and time of the accident.

- How the accident happened in detail.

- The casualty's condition when first seen.

- The condition of the casualty subsequently.
- Details of the treatment you have carried out.

The essential observations should be recorded every half-hour while you are preparing to evacuate the casualty. They are, in the order of importance:

- The respiratory rate. A clear airway should be maintained at all times. If the respiratory rate drops below 8 breaths per minute assisted or artificial ventilation should be used.
- The pulse rate.
- The level of consciousness. (A.V.P.U.)
- The state of the pupils. (Size and reaction to light)
- The development of any signs of paralysis.

Concussion and Minor Head injuries

Concussion

Concussion of the brain can occur when a heavy blow is applied to the skull. It occurs because the brain is fairly soft and its function can be subject to widespread disturbance when shock waves pass through its substance. Suspect this condition if the casualty loses consciousness for only a few minutes. It is characterised by a loss of memory for events before or after the injury, headache and sometimes nausea and vomiting. The casualty should be put to bed and allowed to rest for 48 hours. Headache may be troublesome and paracetamol or codeine phosphate may be required. These headaches may continue for many weeks after an accident. The casualty should be warned to report immediately if he notices increasing headaches or drowsiness or if he vomits. He should be sent to see a doctor at the next port.

Bruising

Bruising will occur if a moderate force is applied. Because the head is well supplied with blood, a collection of blood (haematoma) will form in the tissues under the scalp. It may be sharply defined, hard and tense, or it may be a fairly diffuse soggy swelling (Figure 4.10). If the soggy area is large it may indicate an underlying fracture so the patient should be closely monitored. No specific treatment is required. An ice pack held over the area might control the bleeding.

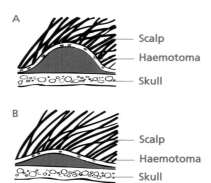

Figure 4.10 Bruising of the head.

Scalp Lacerations

These are common because there is little tissue between the skull and the scalp. The wound will bleed freely and often out of proportion to the size of the wound. Surrounding tissues may be swollen and soggy with the blood that has leaked into them. The scalp edges will be ragged, not clean-cut (Figure 4.11). Control the bleeding by pressure. If necessary, stitch the wound as detailed above. Ensure that you can see the wound clearly by shaving the scalp for distance of 1cm from the wound edge.

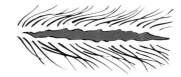

Figure 4.11 Scalp wound.

Pain Relief in Head Injuries

Paracetamol should be used in minor injuries for relief of headaches. 1g orally every 4–6 hours (maximum 4g per 24 hours)

Codeine phosphate may be used if Paracetamol is not effective. 30–60mg orally or intramuscularly every 4–6 hours.

Morphine should not be given unless the head injury is trivial and the casualty has serious and painful major injuries elsewhere.

Eye injuries

The eye(s) can be injured in several ways which include foreign bodies, direct blow as in a fight, lacerations, chemicals and burns. The eye is a very sensitive organ and any injury must be treated seriously.

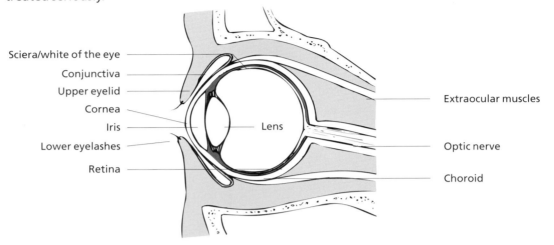

Sciera/white of the eye
Conjunctiva
Upper eyelid
Cornea
Iris
Lower eyelashes
Retina
Lens
Extraocular muscles
Optic nerve
Choroid

Figure 4.12 Diagram of the eye.

Anatomy

The eyes lie partially protected in bony cavities of the skull. They are guarded by the eyelids (upper and lower) which have the faculty of blinking and closure. The white part of the eye is the sclera and the clear transparent central part is the cornea.

The cornea covers the coloured iris which controls the size of the pupil. Behind the pupil, which appears black in colour, is the lens which is not normally visible. The retina is the inner lining of the eyeball and it provides the sight receptors. The conjunctiva is the outer lining, a thin membrane which covers both the inner surfaces of the upper and lower eyelids, and the visible part of the eyeball except for the cornea (Figure 4.12).

Examination

The first stage in treating an eye injury is to record a full account of the injury, what happened and the details of the symptoms. It will then be necessary to carry out a careful examination. It helps if the casualty is lying down, with head supported and held slightly back, during the examination.

Basic requirements are:

- Good illumination (overhead light, lamp, or hand held torch or strong day light);

- Magnifying glass;

- Soft paper tissues;

- Moist cotton wool swabs or moist cotton buds;

- Fluorescein drops (stain);

- Anaesthetic eye drops;

- Basic antibiotic eye ointment. NOTE: any opened tube should only be used for treating one patient for one course of treatment.

First record the general appearance of the tissues around the eye(s), looking for swelling, bruising or obvious abnormality; and then examine the affected eye(s) starting with the sclera, the conjunctiva, which covers both the sclera and the backs of the eyelids, and the cornea. Comparing one eye with the other is helpful and a diagram is the best method of recording the findings.

The sclera can be viewed by gently holding apart the eyelids with the fingers and asking the patient to look in four different directions. Make sure you can see well into each 'corner' of the eyelids. The inside of the lower lid can be inspected by gently pulling down the lower lid with the eyes looking upwards. The upper lid must be rolled back (everted) before the underlying conjunctiva can be inspected. There are two methods of doing this. Both require the casualty to keep looking down towards the feet while the technique is being completed.

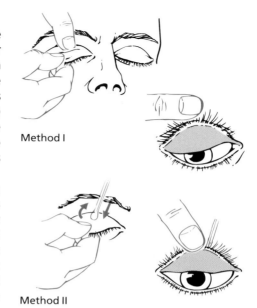

To evert the upper lid, ask the casualty to remain looking downwards then place the index finger of one hand across the upper lid while grasping the eyelashes firmly but gently between the index finger and thumb of the other hand. Pull gently downwards on the eyelashes and then with a downward pressure of the index finger fold the eyelid back over it. The index finger is then withdrawn and the everted lid can be held back by pressing the eyelashes against the bony margin of the socket, under the eyebrow. The underneath surface of the lid can now be examined. The eyelid will return to normal position if the casualty looks upwards and then closes the eyelids together (Figure 4.13 – Method I).

Figure 4.13 Eversion of upper eyelid – two methods.

The alternative methods use a cotton bud laid on or across the upper lid, instead of a finger. The same procedure is followed, with the casualty looking downward and the eyelid being folded upwards over the cotton bud, which is then withdrawn. These procedures ensure that the whole area of conjunctiva is inspected for damage or foreign bodies (Figure 4.13).

The cornea and surrounding area should next be inspected and it helps to slant the light across the surface to show up any abnormality. The magnifying glass is beneficial for this examination. The cornea should be clear and any area of cloudiness or opacity, or the presence of foreign bodies should be noted. The surrounding sclera may be reddish in colour which can signify corneal irritation. Any obvious loose foreign body should be removed at this stage (see below).

Staining the eye with fluorescein will highlight any area of corneal or conjunctival damage. The fluorescein drops should be instilled with the lower lid everted with the casualty looking upwards. Wipe any excess dye off the eyelids. Any area of corneal or conjunctival damage will attract the dye and be stained green. Any such area should be clearly shown on the diagram in the casualty's notes.

The more common injuries affecting the eyes and the treatments are described in the following paragraphs. Treatment for the relief of pain should be appropriate to the degree of discomfort being experienced.

Blows on or adjacent to the eye (black eye)

These blows may result either in the complete or partial detachment of the retina or in bleeding into the eyeball. If, after an injury, there is any marked deterioration in sight the casualty should be put to bed and seen by a doctor as soon as possible. Get RADIO MEDICAL ADVICE. Even if there is no discernible deterioration of sight the casualty should be advised to visit a doctor at the next port.

Corneal abrasions

A scratch or abrasion on the cornea can be caused, for example, by a foreign body under the eyelids or by a fingernail touching the eye. Pain is felt immediately and the casualty thinks there is some-thing in the eye. Corneal abrasions can be identified by staining the eye with fluorescein. Antibiotic eye ointment should be placed along the inside of the lower lid, and blinking the eyelids will smear the ointment across the eye. An eye pad held in place by loose strapping should be applied for 24 hours. Next day re-examine the eye, using the fluorescein stain. If there is no sign of staining after careful examination, the treatment can be stopped. If the cornea still stains, repeat the treatment every 24 hours until the staining ceases or the casualty visits a doctor.

Loose foreign bodies

These can often be removed from under the lids or over the conjunctiva without the use of anaesthetic eye drops. Use moistened cotton wool on a stick or a moistened cotton bud. Be very gentle. After you have removed the foreign body or foreign bodies, stain the eye with fluorescein and mark any areas of staining on an eye diagram. If there is any staining, treat as for corneal abrasion.

However, the eyes of some persons are so sensitive that it is impossible to examine the eye thoroughly or remove a foreign body unless anaesthetic eye drops have been used. These drops may cause slight smarting for several minutes after being put into the eye. Wait for this effect to wear off before examining the eye or attempting to remove a foreign body by the method described above. Remember that the surface of the eye will be insensitive so you must be very gentle. After the foreign body has been removed treat as for corneal abrasion.

A foreign body may occasionally adhere to the surface of the eye and an attempt to pick it up using a cotton bud will fail. The anaesthetic eye drops should then be used before one attempt is made to remove the foreign body using a nylon eye loop. The greatest care must be taken not to injure the eye and should the attempt fail it must not be repeated. Afterwards, whether successful or not, treat as for corneal abrasion.

Foreign bodies embedded in, or completely inside, the eye

When very small pieces of metal, grit etc. become embedded in the cornea or the sclera, it may be very difficult to see either the wound or the object, even with the help of fluorescein, and the patient may not have felt any pain when the accident occurred. However, you should suspect such an accident if questioning the patient reveals that he has been hammering, chipping, milling, boring or striking metal with a tool, or standing near someone who was doing so, or has rubbed his eyes after getting dirt in them.

If you believe an injury of this kind has occurred, or you are in any doubt about it, treat the eye as for corneal abrasion. However, the application of antibiotic eye ointment should be repeated often enough to keep the eye comfortable but not less frequently than every six hours. The casualty should see an eye specialist as soon as possible. Do not attempt to remove the foreign body yourself.

Wounds of the eyelids and eyeball

Get RADIO MEDICAL ADVICE AT ONCE, if the eyeball is cut and if the eye leaks fluid or jelly. In the meanwhile close the eyelids or approximate them as best you can. Cover the eyelid with one or two layers of paraffin gauze to keep the eyelid shut. Then place an eye pad over this. Stick the eye pad in place with strips of adhesive tape or sticking plaster. Give the standard antibiotic treatment.

Chemical burns

If this has not already been done, wash the chemical out of the eye with copious amounts of water for as long as is necessary to ensure that no chemical remains in the eye. This period is rarely less than 10 minutes.

Then stain the eye with fluorescein. If there is marked staining of the eye, antibiotic eye ointment should be applied copiously to prevent the lids sticking to the eyeball. Apply the ointment every 4 hours, and cover the eye with paraffin gauze and an eye pad. The casualty should be seen by a doctor as soon as possible.

Less severe damage should be treated by 4–hourly applications of antibiotic eye ointment with an eye cover of paraffin gauze and a pad. Re-examine the eye each day, using fluorescein. Treatment should be continued for 24 hours after the eye is not stained by fluorescein and is white.

Arc eyes ('Welder's Flash')

The ultra-violet (UV) in an electric arc can cause 'sunburn' of the surface of unprotected eyes. In arc eyes, both eyes feel gritty within 24 hours and look red. Bright light hurts the eyes. The eyes should be carefully searched for foreign bodies and be stained with fluorescein. If one eye only is affected it is probably not an arc eye. It may be due to an embedded corneal foreign body or an area of corneal damage which will show on staining with fluorescein.

Bathing the eyes with cold water and cold compresses applied to the lids will give some relief of symptoms. Dark glasses help the discomfort caused by light. If the eyes feel very gritty, apply antibiotic ointment to the eyes every 4 hours. The condition will usually clear up spontaneously within about 48 hours if no further exposure to UV occurs. Further exposure to welding should be avoided and dark glasses should be worn in bright sunlight until the eyes are fully recovered.

Ear injuries

Foreign bodies

Sand, an insect, or some other small object in the ear may cause irritation, discomfort or pain. If it is clearly visible, it may be possible to remove it using tweezers. If this cannot be achieved easily NO other efforts should be made to extract it by any means. You may pierce the ear drum if you try to remove objects which are not visible or which are stuck in the ear passage; also you might push the object further in.

If nothing is visible, flood the ear passage with tepid groundnut (arachis), olive or sunflower oil which may float the object out or bring it out when the casualty drains his ear by lying over on the affected side. If these measures are unsuccessful send the casualty to a doctor at the first available opportunity.

Injuries to the internal ear

If the ear drum has been perforated as the result of a skull fracture there may be a flow of cerebro-spinal fluid and this should not be stopped by inserting anything into the ear. The casualty should be placed on his injured side, with his shoulders and head propped up; this will allow the fluid to drain freely. For other injuries, put a dressing over the ear and apply a bandage. Do not put cotton wool in the ear passage. In all cases, get **RADIO MEDICAL ADVICE.**

Nose injuries

Foreign bodies
Sometimes, when a foreign body is stuck in one nostril, the casualty can blow it out by compressing the other nostril and blowing down the blocked one. Otherwise, if the object can be seen and is loose it may be removed by using forceps. Unless this is clearly feasible no attempt should be made to remove the object and the casualty must be seen by a doctor.

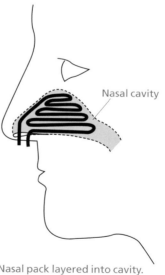

Nasal cavity

Injuries inside the Nose

If bleeding cannot be controlled by the method described in Chapter 1 then it may be necessary to pack the nose. This is done by lubricating ribbon gauze thoroughly with petroleum jelly (Vaseline) and inserting it in the nostril with the aid of forceps (Figure 4.14). Put in sufficient gauze to fill the nostril without stretching it unduly. Leave the gauze in place for 48 hours, and then gently pull it out.

A fracture of the nose cannot be dealt with on board ship and the only problem will be to stop any persistent bleeding. Any distortion of the nose will have to be corrected in hospital.

Nasal pack layered into cavity.
NOTE: floor of nose is horizontal.
Do not pack

Figure 4.14

Mouth and dental injuries

Cuts inside the mouth and a broken jaw

When there has been a severe blow to a jaw, especially if the jaw is broken, there may be complications caused by broken dentures, by the loss of teeth and by wounds to gums, the lips, the tongue and the inside and outside of the mouth. For external wounds to the cheek and lips treatment is as for any skin wound.

For wounds inside the mouth the casualty should first rinse his mouth well with antiseptic mouthwash which should remove any loose fragments. You should not try to extract pieces of tooth from the gum. If the casualty is in pain read the section on analgesics.

Treatment for a lost tooth is given in Chapter 1, and for other teeth in Chapter 7.

No attempt should be made to stitch deep wounds of the cheek and tongue. Serious bleeding should be controlled by pressure.

If a jaw is or may be broken the upper and lower jaws should be held together by a bandage with, as far as possible, the upper and lower teeth fitting together as they normally do. If the patient has dentures which still fit adequately he should wear them; they will help to act as a splint.

If the wounds on the face or inside the mouth are other than very slight give antibiotic treatment. If the casualty is unable to take tablets by mouth give benzyl penicillin 300 mg intramuscularly every six hours for five days.

Burns and scalds

The treatment of burns and scalds caused by dry or wet heat respectively is the same.

Classification

Skin has an outer layer (epidermis) and a deep layer (dermis). The latter contains the sweat glands, hair follicles and nerves relaying sensation and pain to the skin.

FIRST DEGREE BURNS affect only the outer skin layer, causing redness, mild swelling, tenderness and pain.

SECOND DEGREE BURNS extend into the deeper skin layer (dermis):

- Superficial second degree burns cause deep reddening, blister formation, considerable swelling, and weeping of fluid.

- Deep second degree burns may not be easy to distinguish from third degree burns immediately after the injury. Pain may be severe because of damage to the nerve endings.

THIRD DEGREE BURNS involve the whole thickness of skin, and may extend to the underlying fat, muscle and bone. The skin may be charred, black or dark brown, leathery or white according to the cause of the burn. Pain may be absent due to destruction of the nerve endings.

Fluid loss

The fluid lost in burns is the colourless liquid part of the blood (plasma). The degree of fluid loss may be determined more by the area of the burn than by its depth. The greater the plasma loss, the more severe the degree of shock. Further, due to loss of plasma, the remaining blood is 'thicker', and more difficult to pump round the body, throwing extra strain on the heart.

Area of burn – the rule of nines

A recognised method of calculating the surface area of the body is the 'rule of nines' (Figure 4.15). In children (not babies) the percentage for the head should be doubled and 1% taken off the other areas.

Treatment

Try to remove to hospital within 6 hours or otherwise seek RADIO MEDICAL ADVICE in the case of:

- third degree burns, especially those which encircle chest or limbs;
- babies;
- burns of face and genitalia, and large burns around joints;
- burns of over 18% of the body surface in adults or 10% in children or older persons (Figure 4.15).

Until removed to hospital put the patient to bed and seek to restore the fluid balance by encouraging the patient to drink as much as possible. Put rehydration powder into the drink according to the instructions; (if not available dissolve 1 teaspoonful of salt in $^{1}/_{2}$ litre of water). If vomiting occurs and persists, fluid per rectum may be necessary. Relieve pain and start antibiotic treatment. Remove rings, jewelry or constricting items of clothing. Anxiety may be relieved by giving diazepam 5 mg, repeated every 4 hours. Cling film makes a good temporary dressing for large burns.

Less serious cases can be treated aboard ship. First assemble:

- a plentiful supply of soap, warm boiled water and gauze pads;

- at least two sets of sterile scissors and forceps; sufficient paraffin gauze burn and wound dressing to cover and overlap the cleansed burned areas;

- sterile gauze and sterile cotton wool to go on top of the dressings as padding;

- suitable sterile bandages;

- face mask for each attendant

Wash your hands and forearms thoroughly and put on a face mask. Remove the first-aid dressing to expose either a single burned area (in multiple burns) or a portion of a single burn e.g. a hand and forearm, or a quarter of the back. The aim is to limit the areas of burned skin exposed at any one time to lessen both the risk of infection and the seepage of fluid. Clean the skin around the edges of the burn with soap, water and pads. Clean away from the burn in every direction. DO NOT use cotton wool or other linty material for cleaning as it is likely to leave bits in the burn.

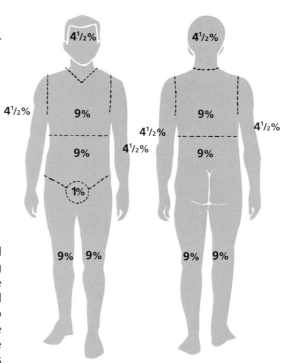

Figure 4.15 Rule of nines – to determine the extent of burns.

Leave blisters intact but clip off all the dead skin if blisters have burst. Flood the area with clean warm boiled water from a clean receptacle to remove debris. Soak a pad in warm boiled water to dab gently at any remaining dirt or foreign matter in the burned area. Be gentle as this will inevitably cause pain.

Next cover the burn with the paraffin gauze dressing, overlapping the burn or scald by 50–100 mm, according to its size. To absorb any fluid leaking from the burn apply a covering of absorbent material, e.g. a layer of sterile gauze, covered with a layer of sterile cotton wool. This is held in place by a suitable bandage.

Thoroughly wash your hands and arms before proceeding to deal as above with the remainder of a large burn or another burn in the case of multiple burns. In serious cases, start antibiotic treatment.

Dressings should be left undisturbed for a week unless the dressing becomes smelly or very dirty, or the temperature is raised. Re-dress such areas as above. Supercicial second degree burns will usually heal in a week to ten days without scarring. Deeper second degree should heal with little scarring in about three weeks.

Special burns

Severe *sunburn* with blistering should be treated as a second degree burn according to the area of the body involved. In mild cases, (first degree burns) keep the patient out of the sun and apply calamine lotion or zinc ointment to the painful areas.

Scalds and burns of mouth and throat. Wash out with water and give ice to suck.

Respiratory burns are caused by the inhalation of hot gases and air particles, and smoke. Expect such a burn when you find burns around the mouth, nose, face, hair and neck. Heat from a flash fire may also cause a burn-related swelling of the top of the throat, even though there is no sign of burns on the face.

A patient with a mild injury to the respiratory passage may have only a cough, hoarseness, or a sore throat. In more severe cases the patient may suffer from marked shortness of breath, persistent coughing, wheezing and hoarseness. In very severe cases the respiratory passages may be blocked by a swollen throat and the lungs may partially collapse.

If the patient has difficulty in breathing and is unconscious insert a Guedel airway. In any event, get **RADIO MEDICAL ADVICE IMMEDIATELY.**

Dislocations

The commonest dislocations are of the shoulder and the finger joints. Try to deal with (i.e. reduce) these dislocations if a doctor cannot see the casualty within about six hours.
All other dislocations should be left for treatment by a doctor. Until this is possible, place the patient in a comfortable position and relieve pain.

NOTE: In some cases a dislocation may be accompanied by a fracture of the same or a related part, so be careful.

Dislocated shoulder

The shoulder will be painful and cannot be moved by the patient. Undress the patient to the waist and note the outline of the good shoulder and compare it with the affected side. Usually in a shoulder dislocation the outward curve of the muscle just below the shoulder is replaced by an inward dent, and the distance from the tip of the shoulder to the elbow is longer on the injured side. This is because the head of the arm-bone usually dislocates inwards and downwards. If you think that the shoulder is dislocated, give the casualty 15 mg of morphine intramuscularly. When the pain is relieved (in about 15 to 20 minutes), the casualty should lie face downwards on a bunk, couch or table, the height of which should be sufficient for the arm to hang down without touching the deck. As the casualty lies down on the bed, hold his dislocated arm until you have placed a small pillow or big pad under the affected shoulder. Then lower the arm slowly until it is hanging straight down the side of the bunk and leave it to hang freely. The patient should remain in this position for about 1 hour, letting the weight of the arm overcome the muscle spasm caused by the dislocation. At the end of this period, if the dislocation is reduced, the patient should roll onto his good side and then use the injured arm by bending the elbow and then touching the good shoulder with the fingers. Afterwards he should be helped to sit up and the arm should be kept in a collar and cuff sling until the shoulder is fairly comfortable. This might take up to 48 hours. When the sling is removed, the patient should exercise the joint slowly and carefully. A check x-ray should be taken at the next port. If the above treatment does not reduce the dislocation, get RADIO MEDICAL ADVICE.

Dislocated finger

Finger dislocations can usually be reduced by pulling firmly on the finger. It is often a good idea to begin by binding the patient's elbow to a right-angle. Pull firmly on the finger for about one minute while a helper is pulling in the opposite direction at the elbow. Keeping the ends of the bones apart by pulling, gently ease the joint back into its normal position. The affected finger should be immobilised by strapping to an adjacent finger. After 24 hours, the strapping should be removed and the patient should exercise the finger slowly and carefully. A check x-ray should be taken at the next port.

Sprains and strains

These injuries are usually the result of twisting, turning or tripping. Pain is usually felt at once, and later swelling at the site of injury will occur due to bleeding.
There is no sure clinical method of excluding fracture associated with sprains and strains except by x-ray. When there is doubt, it is therefore safer to assume the possibility of fracture and to treat accordingly.

Whether the injury is seen immediately or later when much swelling may have occurred, put the casualty in his bunk and elevate the injured part, if this is possible. Cold water compresses kept in place by a crepe bandage should be applied. An ice-pack wrapped in a damp cloth may also help to reduce swelling. Avoid prolonged use of ice as skin damage can occur.

Rest and elevation may be necessary for two to three days (or sometimes longer according to the severity of the injury). Continue support with a crepe bandage. Pain relief may be necessary.

If an associated fracture is not present, gentle movement of the injured part should be encouraged. Sprains and strains do much better with early movement than with too long a period of rest. The casualty can usually judge when he can use the injured part for full or restricted duties.

If not fully recovered, get an x-ray at the first port of call.

Causes and prevention of disease

Causes of disease

This chapter deals with common-sense measures and some necessary precautions which should be taken to preserve the health of those aboard ship and to prevent the spread of disease where it has occurred. Of the many causes of disease, infection by living organisms is the commonest and an understanding of their mode of spread is necessary if healthy living and working conditions are to be maintained.

Microbes (germs) can be classified in broad terms as viruses, bacteria, and fungi. They are widely disseminated throughout nature and although most of them are not harmful to mankind certain organisms may invade the body and produce particular diseases. They gain entry to the body, usually through the nose or mouth or the broken skin. Infection can take place directly from person to person or it may be conveyed indirectly in air, water or food or by a parasite carrier (such as an insect).

The viruses of influenza, that of the common cold and much more rarely Legionnaires disease are examples of air-borne infection which is spread when the sufferer coughs or sneezes.

Typhoid fever is an example of a water-borne bacterial infection. The excreta of infected persons contaminate water supplies. Hence the necessity for safeguarding the water supply for washing as well as for drinking at all times.

Examples of two well-known bacterial diseases brought about by personal contact are syphilis and gonorrhoea.

A number of diseases are conveyed by carriers. The plague germ is conveyed by the bites of fleas living on the rat. Typhus is conveyed in similar manner by lice. Malaria and yellow fever organisms inhabit the salivary glands of the mosquito and are injected into the blood when the mosquito bites. Flies, because of their behaviour, are very prone to convey disease germs from filth to food.

Ringworm is an example of a disease caused by a fungus through contact.

Potable water

This covers water used for drinking, cooking, the washing of cooking and eating utensils, and water used for general cleaning and bathing. Additional advice is given in Merchant Shipping Notices M.1214 and M1401.

Fresh water should be free from causes of infection and be bright, clear and virtually colourless. It should be aerated, that is, it should bubble when shaken, otherwise it has an insipid taste.

The Merchant Shipping Crew Accommodation Regulations 1997 and Merchant Shipping Crew Accomodation (Fishing Vessels) Regulations 1975 require all fresh water produced on board ship to be disinfected automatically. Electro-silver ionisation systems are acceptable for this requirement.

Fresh water storage tanks

These water tanks are coated internally with an anti-corrosive material which will not contaminate the water. It is recommended that the tanks should be emptied annually, or more frequently if contamination is suspected, for inspection and maintenance after which they should be thoroughly scrubbed and flushed out, and the whole water system disinfected by chlorine (see below). Anyone entering any potable or washing water tanks should wear clean clothing and footwear, and should not be suffering from skin infections, diarrhoea or any communicable disease.

Disinfection of the fresh water tanks and distribution system by super-chlorination

It is recommended that the storage tanks and the whole of the fresh water system should be disinfected at intervals of not more than twelve months even if the quality of the water that has been used to fill them is not suspect.

The chlorine compounds that may be used for disinfecting are chlorinated lime, high-test hypo-chlorite or commercially prepared sodium hypo-chlorite solution.

NOTE. Before being diluted by the water in the potable water system these compounds:

- are dangerous to eyes and skin – see IMO Medical First Aid Guide;

- deteriorate on exposure to air – they should, therefore, be purchased in small containers which should be sealed tightly after use;

- should be kept in a cool, dry and dark place, but where they can be easily seen and removed when needed or there is a likelihood of fire;

- Calcium Hypochlorite – is liable to spontaneous combustion if not stored as above, or if in contact with animal, vegetable, plastic or other inorganic material;

- Chlorinated Lime – is liable to facilitate fires.

See also the International Maritime Dangerous Goods Code.

Determine the volume of water necessary to fill the tanks and distribution system completely and the amount of chlorine compound required. The latter can be calculated from the manufacturer's instructions or from the table or formula shown below.

Amount of chlorine compound required for a 50–ppm (50-mg/litre solution)

Capacity of system (including tanks and piping)	Amount of chlorine compound required			
	Chlorinated lime 25%	High-test calcium hypochlorite 70%	Sodium Hypochlorite solution	
			5%	10%
for each:	Kg	Kg	litre	litres
1,000 litres	0.2	0.08	1	0.5
5,000 litres	1	0.4	5	2.5
10 tonnes	2.0	0.8	10.0	5.0

NOTE.

1. Before using the above chlorine compounds check that the percentages are as in table above – if not adjust the quantity you use accordingly.

2. When chlorine compounds or solutions other than those mentioned in the table are used the dosages should be:

for powders:
$$\frac{70 \times \text{dosage in 70\% column}}{\text{percentage of chlorine in compound}}$$

for liquids:
$$\frac{5 \times \text{dosage in 5\% column}}{\text{percentage of chlorine in liquid}}$$

Chlorinated lime

Place the required amount of chlorine compound in one or more clean, dry buckets (or drums). Add a small amount of water to each bucket and mix the lime into a thick paste. Dilute the paste by adding warm water gradually, and stirring constantly, until there are about six litres of solution in each bucket. Allow the solution to stand for 30 minutes, so that the undissolved particles may settle to the bottom. Decant the clear liquid (the chlorine solution) and, if necessary, filter it through muslin or cheese-cloth prior to putting it into the tank

Chloride of lime may be sold as:

Chloride of Lime (Stablochlor) Chlorinated Lime Calx Chlorinata	British
Calx Chlorinata	U.S.A.
Chlorure de Chaux Sel de Javelle	French
Chlorkalk Calcaria Chlorata	German
Calx Chlorata	Danish, Norwegian and Swedish
Cloruro di Calce	Italian
Hipoclorito Calcico Clorurado	Spanish
Hipoclorito de Calcio	Mexican
Cal Chlorada	Portuguese

High-test calcium hypochlorite

Place the required amount of the compound in one or more clean, dry metal buckets (or drums). Add fresh water and stir until the powder is dissolved (disregard any slight turbidity).

Sodium hypochlorite solution

No preparation is required.

Procedure

Introduce the chlorine solution into nearly empty fresh water tanks and immediately fill them to overflowing with fresh water. The turbulence of the incoming water will ensure adequate mixing.

Open the taps and outlets of the fresh water distribution system nearest the storage tanks, and allow the water to flow until you can smell chlorinated water. Then close those taps and outlets, and, working outwards from the tanks, open and close successively the other taps and outlets until they have all been flushed with chlorinated water. Care should be taken to ensure that the pressure tank is filled with chlorinated water.

In flushing the system a certain amount of the chlorinated water will have been drawn from the storage tanks. They should be refilled to overflowing, and chlorine solution should be added to make up the concentration in the tanks to 50 ppm (50 mg/litre), ie if you have drained off 380 litres of water you will need to add, for example, an additional 75 grams of chlorinated lime 25% solution.

The chlorinated water should be allowed to remain in the storage tanks and the distribution system preferably for twelve hours but not less than four hours. After the contact period the tanks and distribution system should be drained and flushed with potable water until the water no longer has an objectionable taste of chlorine.

Hoses

Hoses, where carried on board for the purposes of transferring water from shore mains supply or water barges, should be used solely for this purpose. They should also be suitably marked and, after use, should be drained and capped at both ends. The hoses should be stowed away from the deck in a place free from contamination.

Disinfection of hoses should be carried out as a routine measure every 6 months – or whenever any contamination is suspected – with a chlorine solution of 100 ppm (100 mg/litre). This should be allowed to stand in the completely filled hose for a period of at least one hour.

A 100 ppm strength solution can be obtained by doubling the quantities of chlorine shown in the formula for the 50 ppm hyper-chlorine solution used for disinfecting ships' water tanks which is shown in the above table.

Taking water on board

Before taking on water check that the delivery cocks on the shore and the receiving point on the ship are properly cleaned. Examine the hose to ensure that it is clean, in good working order, and free from leaks (germs can get in through leaks in the hose). Ensure that the ends of the hose do not drag across the deck.

If you are taking water for potable purposes from a source which is new to you or about which you have doubts, you should ask the British Consul or your agents for advice as to whether the water is likely to contain germs or harmful minerals such as lead. Remember that a bright, clear, sparkling water may easily contain either deadly organisms such as cholera, or harmful minerals such as lead. It is unlikely that fresh water taken on board will contain sufficient (if any) chlorine to ensure complete safety.

It is recommended therefore that the chlorination of water outlined in the following paragraph be carried out in all vessels, including those equipped with distillation units and/or ultra violet sterilizers.

Routine treatment of fresh water by chlorine

All fresh water taken from shore or water barge for drinking or washing should be chlorinated on loading to ensure a residual free chlorine content of 0.2 ppm at all outlets throughout the ship's freshwater distribution system. As free chlorine in a ship's water system is progressively lost in passing through the system it will, in practice, be necessary to chlorinate the water held in the storage tanks to a higher concentration than 0.2 ppm. Finding the best actual level of initial concentration may be a matter of experiment as much will depend on the size of the tank or the distribution system.

If chlorine test facilities are available, samples of treated water should be taken at tap and shower outlets at [weekly/monthly] intervals, preferably using outlets that would otherwise not be used (e.g. in unoccupied cabins) in order to reduce the presence of standing water in the system. The result of these tests should be used to adjust the concentration of chlorine in the system to obtain a minimum of 0.2 ppm at the outlets.

It should be remembered however that if drinking water supplies pass through charcoal filters close to the outlets, there will be no free chlorine at these points.

It is recommended that, initially a concentration of 0.5 ppm in the storage tanks is aimed for and this may be achieved by using an automatic chlorination unit in the ship's deck filling line or by the traditional manual method using the manufacturer's instructions for the chlorine compound in use or by calculating the quantities required by use of the following table or formula:

Amount of chlorine compound required for a 0.5 ppm chlorine solution

	Amount of chlorine compound required			
	Chlorinated lime 25%	High-test calcium hypochlorite 70%	Sodium Hypochlorite solution	
			5%	10%
for each:	g	g	ml	ml
1,000 litres	2	0.8	10	5
10 tonnes	20	8	100	50

Water making plant

All water made from seawater by low pressure evaporators or reverse osmosis plant requires to be treated by means of an automatic chlorination unit adjusted to give the required concentration on delivery to the storage tanks, or by an elctro-silver ionisation system.

Ultra violet sterilizer units should only be used as a supplement to chlorination.

Maintenance of distribution system

The various elements of the freshwater system which might include sand filters, evaporators, reverse osmosis plant, softeners etc., should be inspected, cleaned, flushed out, back washed, recharged or items replaced where appropriate, in accordance with the maker's instructions and it is recommended that a Freshwater System Maintenance Log be kept itemising each principle unit in the system.

Food

A balanced diet is essential for the maintenance of good health and should contain the correct proportions of protein, carbohydrate, fats, vitamins and essential minerals such as iron. It should be varied in accordance with the needs of the consumers and the climate in which they are working. Protein is derived from such foods as meat, fish and beans; carbohydrates from cereals and bread; and vitamins and essential minerals from all of these and from fruit and vegetables.

It is also essential to avoid contamination in the food preparation area. Raw food, especially meat, should be kept separate from cooked products. Separate utensils and cutting boards etc. must be kept for each and stored separately. The food handler must wash between handling different foods and especially after handling raw meat and poultry; cooked food should be manipulated by tools and utensils and not by the hands; and work surfaces and equipment must be cleaned thoroughly and disinfected efficiently. Cleaning equipment must also be disinfected adequately.

Vegetables

Fresh vegetables, such as lettuce, radish, carrot, beetroot, celery and spinach should never be eaten, cooked or raw, without first being thoroughly washed in clean running water.

In many countries such crops are fertilised with human excreta and are, therefore, potentially dangerous as a source of transmission of intestinal disease such as typhoid, dysentery and intestinal parasites.

Wherever practicable, boil vegetables before serving. Where the origin of any vegetable to be eaten raw is not known, it should be soaked for two minutes in a solution of 3.5 g of stabilised chloride of lime to 5 gallons of water followed by at least two thorough rinsings in potable water.

Fruit

Fruit, such as oranges, bananas, grapefruit, that must be peeled before eating is generally safe. Fruit, such as apples, tomatoes, grapes, dates, that is not generally peeled, is a frequent source of diarrhoea. Before eating they should be treated in the way recommended for raw vegetables.

Canned foods

Each tin should be carefully examined before being opened. Never accept or use tins which are rusty, dented, damaged or blown.

Bacteria in food

Bacteria require moisture and warmth for growth. The most favourable temperature for growth is normal body heat, although most will thrive at temperature between 15°C and 45°C. Bacteria can multiply very fast in favourable conditions.

Unpreserved foods should therefore be stored in a refrigerator or freezer. When perishable bulk food packs are opened for use, any unused portion should be resealed and returned to the refrigerator or freezer as quickly as possible (before defrosting has occurred, if frozen).

When removed from the cold for cooking, food should be thoroughly thawed, carefully prepared, and heated to a minimum temperature of 63°C. It should be served and eaten at once, or kept above the minimum cooking temperature if there is to be any delay in serving. Inadequate defrosting before cooking food, particularly meat and poultry, may mean that the centre does not reach the minimum temperature to destroy bacteria (i.e. is only partially cooked). This is a common source of food poisoning. Frozen meat and poultry which have thawed out should not be refrozen before being thoroughly cooked.

All cooked unconsumed food should be cooled rapidly and stored in a refrigerator for up to 48 hours or in a freezer if it is to be kept for a longer period. Any food to be reheated must be heated thoroughly to the temperature necessary to kill bacterial contamination. Under no circumstances should meat products or rice be reheated more than once.

Further guidance is available in Marine Guidance Note 61 (M+F).

In any outbreak or suspected outbreak of food poisoning or illness with diarrhoea on board, the following steps should always be taken:

■ try to identify the food(s) which have caused the outbreak. Make sure that no further consumption of these foods is possible by discarding them. Keep a sample if near port so that laboratory identification is possible.

■ inspect all food handlers for general cleanliness and for the points listed. Forbid anyone who does not meet these standards to handle food. You may thus remove the cause of the outbreak.

■ inspect all food storage and preparation areas and make sure that good food hygiene practices are being followed (next section).

■ if near port, keep samples of diarrhoea or vomit (in sealed containers inside a plastic bag in a cold place, away from catering facilities) so that laboratory identification of the cause may be possible.

■ treat all affected persons and prevent them spreading the disease.

Catering staff: personal hygiene

It is of prime importance that catering staff should maintain a high standard of personal hygiene. Only by insistence that these standards are maintained will outbreaks of diarrhoea and of food poisoning be avoided.

The staff should be supplied with, and should wear, clean clothing when handling food. There should be ample supplies of soap, towels, nail brushes and hot water available for washing hands, and it is important that thorough washing of the hands follows a visit to the toilet.

Food handlers should be free from communicable diseases. Anyone suffering from a septic skin condition should be removed from duty until the condition is cured. A person who has had an attack of typhoid fever or of dysentery, and who may have become a carrier of the disease, or who has suffered from an unexplained or unusual illness, should not be allowed to prepare or handle food or utensils until cleared for such duty by a doctor.

Food handlers should be made aware of their responsibilities for the health of others and should be educated and trained in good food hygiene practices.

General cleanliness on board ship

Cleanliness, both of the person and the environment, is essential at all times on board ship. Frequent monitoring by the master and senior officers will help to keep the crew aware of the necessity to maintain scrupulous cleanliness and will detect infestations.

Cloths for cleaning working surfaces and tables are a common source of infection. They should regularly be either boiled or soaked in disinfectant (e.g. hypochlorite solution) or replaced. It is strongly recommended that disposable cloths are used to minimise the risk of contamination.

Insecticides

Insecticides should conform to the specification in MSN1726. They should be used only in accordance with the manufacturer's instructions and the recommendations in M1534. If going to tropical areas check that you have sufficient appropriate insecticides to deal with mosquitoes.

Insecticides are usually carried in two forms:

- a liquid insecticide intended for the destruction of flying insects such as flies and mosquitoes, and also non-flying insects such as cockroaches, bugs and ants;

- an insecticide powder intended for use on the body, personal clothing, bedding, blankets and such like, for the destruction of bugs, fleas and body lice.

In addition there are insecticides in tablet form which have to be heated by, for example, a low wattage electric lamp. These are used particularly for killing tropical mosquitoes.

It is important to appreciate the difference in practice between the control of flying insects and non-flying insects:

Flying insects are controlled by spraying the insecticide into the affected space. The spray diffuses rapidly and will kill the insects in flight. Do not attempt to hit individual insects as this only wastes the insecticide.

Crawling insects such as cockroaches usually hide and breed in cracks and crevices and in the spaces behind lockers and cooking stoves. The area around their hiding places should be thoroughly and liberally sprayed so that they come into contact with the insecticide as they emerge to feed. As this spraying cannot kill the insects' eggs, it must be repeated at regular fortnightly intervals to kill the young insects as they hatch.

Bugs may be present in the sheathing, wainscoting, wooden bunks, etc. The surfaces should be sprayed thoroughly to ensure the rapid destruction of the bugs as they run over the sprayed area.

The best way to deal with an infestation of bugs in bedding, mattresses, etc. is by means of a thorough dusting with insecticide powder. The bugs will eventually come into contact with the powder and be killed.

Disinfection

A disinfectant is a substance used for cleaning instruments, materials, lavatory pans, bed pans, etc. The instructions on the container should be followed.

An antiseptic has a similar anti-bacterial action, but is generally more suitable for application to human tissues.

A deodorant dilutes or obscures odours only and has no disinfecting properties.

Disinfestation is the destruction of rats, mice and insects of all kinds which may or may not carry disease to humans.

Sterilisation

In ships this term means the destruction of germs by the use of boiling water or steam. It is a very simple and effective way of rendering free from germs articles of all kinds. Articles to be sterilised must be boiled for 10 minutes, at least. Boiling cannot, of course, be used to sterilise certain fabrics which are damaged by boiling, such as those containing wool. A disinfectant solution must be used for these.

Disinfection at end of illness

This term means the disinfection of a room after it has been occupied by an infectious patient.

First remove all bedding, blankets and movable articles of furniture. The bedding and blankets should be disinfected. The furniture should be left on deck, preferably in the sun, after having been thoroughly scrubbed. After emptying the cabin, give the whole surface, including the bulkheads, deck, ceiling and all internal and external surfaces of cupboards and such like, a thorough washing down. The principal object is to clean the cabin surfaces, lockers, etc., and thereby to remove any dust and dirt that may have accumulated and which may contain germs of the disease. On completion of this procedure the room can safely be occupied.

A more thorough procedure is necessary in the case of serious infectious illnesses, such as plague, cholera, typhus, or typhoid fever. At sea, dispose of all bedding, mattresses, etc., and, after a thorough cleansing of the cabin, close it down and do not use it until authorised to do so by the Medical Officer of the next port of call. He may consider it desirable to carry out a further disinfection by other means. He should also be asked to disinfect ashore all the patient's personal clothing and belongings, remembering that the patient will require his effects, either during his subsequent stay in hospital or after his discharge from hospital.

Isolation

The isolation of an ill patient will prevent the spread of disease to other persons on board. It is convenient to categorise isolation into two types:

- strict;

- standard.

Details of the type of isolation necessary are given in Chapter 6 at the beginning of each section dealing with a particular illness.

Strict isolation

The patient is confined to the ship's hospital or to a cabin set aside for his sole use in a quiet part of the ship and which has been stripped of all unnecessary furnishings and carpets to facilitate cleaning and disinfection.

He must be seen only by the person who nurses him.

If disposable eating and drinking utensils are available, these should be used and later destroyed. Should ship's dishes and cutlery have to be used, they should be washed and sterilised after use and kept in the cabin or hospital. They should never be washed up with utensils used by other members of the crew.

All used bed linen and towels should be sterilised by boiling or by disinfection. Faeces and urine should be passed into bedpans or urine bottles and at sea disposed of in a flushing WC set aside for the purpose. The attendants should wear disposable gloves when handling these items and care should be taken not to splash the contents about. The pans and bottles should be sterilised after use. In port, faeces and urine should not be flushed away but should be disinfected and disposed of after consultation with the Port Health Authority. It is important to dispose of any used syringes and needles in the correct way. Place the needle and syringe into a 'sharps' box (safety container designed for disposing of contaminated sharp items which could accidentally injure and thus infect another individual). The containers should be kept in the isolation room until arrival in port when they should be handed to the Port Health Authority for disposal. The attendant's gloves should be bagged, sealed and disposed of in the same way.

NOTE: The attendant should wash his hands each time the gloves are removed.

Standard isolation

The patient is isolated in the ship's hospital or in a cabin set aside for his use. There is no need to observe the stringent rules for strict isolation. Whilst the patient is ill, visitors should be discouraged. When he shows signs of recovery, this ban can be lifted but visitors should be instructed to stay only for short periods. Whilst he is convalescing visiting should be encouraged to relieve boredom.

In certain cases it will be necessary to deal with urine and faeces in accordance with the procedure for strict isolation, e.g. enteric fever.

Ventilation

Adequate ventilation and a free flow of air to the crew accommodation and food stores is important for the health of all on board ship. This is often arranged by means of a recirculating air-conditioning system. With such a system, it is obviously undesirable that the air from a room occupied by an infectious person should be recirculated. Purpose-built ships' hospitals therefore have separate ventilation systems. However, when a person with an infectious disease has to occupy a cabin, all possible steps should be taken to prevent contaminated air from re-circulating. For example, a porthole or external door not subject to an inflow of air should wherever possible be opened to exhaust the contaminated air.

Port health clearance

Measures for the prevention and control of the spread of epidemic diseases by international transport are governed by a code of rules which have been drawn up and agreed by practically all the maritime countries of the world (International Health Regulations 1969 – Third Annotated Edition). The Regulations are applied in most countries by Port Health Officers.

A Maritime Declaration of Health should be completed before arrival at the first port of call in a new country. This, however, only relates to Yellow fever, Pulmonary plague and Cholera.

It is advisable to seek advice and to give information by radio, preferably within 4–12 hours of the estimated time of arrival at the port, in any of the circumstances described below.

1. The occurrence on board during the voyage of:

- death other than by accident;

- illnesses where the person concerned had:

- a temperature of 38°C or greater, which was accompanied by a rash or a glandular swelling or jaundice, or which persisted for more than 48 hours;

- diarrhoea severe enough to interfere with work or normal activities.

2. The presence on board of:

- a person suffering from an infectious disease or who has symptoms which may indicate the presence of an infectious disease;

- any animal or captive bird of any species including rodents and poultry, noting any mortality or illness among such animals or birds.

3. Any other circumstances which are likely to cause the spread of infectious disease.

Preventing heat illness

In very hot conditions the minimum of light clothing should be worn to allow the largest possible surface for free evaporation of sweat. If there is much direct heat from the sun (radiant heat), light white cotton clothing will reflect the heat and keep the body temperature below danger limits. Fair-skinned people should remember that they burn more easily and should take precautions.

Perspiration is the body's best heat control mechanism but the sweat consists mainly of salt and water which must be replaced. The salt is best taken with food and supplemented by salt-containing drinks to prevent heat cramp. At least 4 litres of fluid is required per day in conditions of moderate heat. If working in high temperatures, the requirement may rise to 6–7 litres.

When the ambient temperature is above 32°C in very humid climates, or above 43°C in dry air, there will be a risk of heat illness, especially when work has to be carried out. This applies particularly to work in engine-rooms and other enclosed spaces.

Air temperature, movement of air, humidity and radiant heat all combine to cause heat exhaustion. A number of ships, especially those operating in hot climates, will carry an hygrometer. This comprises two thermometers, one wet-bulb and one dry-bulb. The readings of the two thermometers can be used to determine a 'composite temperature' which will give an indication of the amount of work that can be undertaken per hour in given circumstances.

The 'composite temperature' is calculated by adding the wet-bulb temperature x 0.7 to the dry- bulb temperature x 0.3 measured in °C. The resulting 'composite temperature' can be used to establish the work/rest ratio as follows:

*Composite temperature °C			Work/rest ratio
Light Work	Moderate Work	Heavy Work	
30	27	25	Continuous work
30.5	28	26	75% work/25% rest per hour
31.5	29.5	28	50% work/50% rest per hour
32	31	30	25% work/75% rest per hour

*Add 1° to the composite temperature if there is some radiant heat

*Add 2° to the composite temperature if there is intense radiant heat

If the composite temperature is above the values in the table, extreme caution should be exercised in allowing work at all because there will be a risk of heat-stroke. In emergency conditions where the work must be done, short spells of work (say 10 minutes) may be permitted but the person must be allowed to cool off completely before being allowed back into the hot environment.

Exposure

Sunburn, frostbite, heat illness and hypothermia may occur in the course of routine duty, and must be guarded against. Sunburn, although often only a minor discomfort, can be dangerous. A person drowsy after drinking alcohol who decides to sleep in the sun may very well wake up suffering from serious burns. Special care should also be taken against frostbite and hypothermia (lowering of the body temperature). Hypothermia will most frequently be present in men who have fallen overboard. Normal body temperature cannot be maintained in water at temperatures below 20°C. Discarding clothing and swimming movements accelerate heat loss. Treatment of heat illnesses and exposure problems are dealt with in Chapters 7 and 11.

Lifting heavy weights

Backache, sciatica, lumbago and slipped disc are frequently caused by incorrect lifting or by attempting to lift heavy weights. If the legs are not bent and the object is lifted by straightening a bent back, there will always be a risk of damage to the spinal column. Leg and thigh muscles are the most powerful in the body and they should be used when lifting, the torso and head being kept straight to avoid bending stresses. Crew should be properly instructed in the correct technique for lifting and carrying heavy weights. They should not be allowed to attempt to raise excessively heavy objects (see Code of Safe Working Practices for Merchant Seamen).

Exercise and boredom

Very few seafarers aboard ship exercise hard enough to cause them to become breathless or to increase the rate of their heart-beat. Ideally 20 minutes of aerobic exercise (exercise that raises the heart rate and makes breathing faster) should be taken twice a week, to help maintain cardio-vascular fitness. Such regular exercise will also help maintain muscle tone, strength and mobility. Individuals unused to regular exercise should start training programs gently and seek advice if in doubt about initial levels. If it hurts, don't do it.

On long, tedious voyages there will be boredom and lack of interest which will also be detrimental to health and well being. Awareness of the danger is the best protection.

Communicable diseases are those that are transmissible from one person, or animal, to another. The disease may be spread directly, via another species (vector) or via the environment. Illness will arise when the infectious agent invades the host, or sometimes as a result of toxins produced by bacteria in food.

The spread of disease through a population is determined by environmental and social conditions which favour the infectious agent, and the relative immunity of the population. An outbreak of infection could endanger the operation and safety of the ship. An understanding of the disease and the measures necessary for its containment and management is therefore important.

Infectious agents and examples of diseases

The organisms that cause disease vary in size from viruses, which are too small to be seen by a light microscope to intestinal worms which may be over a metre long. The groups of infectious agents are listed with examples of diseases they cause.

Bacteria
Pneumonia, tuberculosis, enteric fever, gonorrhoea

Viruses
Measles, varicella, influenza, colds, rabies

Fungi
Ringworm, tinea pedis (athlete's foot)

Protozoa
Malaria, giardia

Metazoa
Tapeworm, filariasis, onchcerciasis (river blindness), hookworm

Prions
Kuru, Creutzfeld-Jacob disease, Bovine spongiform encephalopathy (BSE)

Modes of transmission

Direct transmission

■ Direct contact with the infected person as in touching, kissing or sexual intercourse

■ Droplet spread through coughing sneezing, talking or explosive diarrhoea

■ Faecal-oral spread when infected faeces is transferred to the mouth of a non infected person, usually by hand.

Indirect transmission

■ Indirect transmission of infectious organisms involves vehicles and vectors which carry disease agents from the source to the host.

Infectious agents

Modes of transmission

Definitions and terms used

Symptoms and signs

General management and treatment

Anthrax

Cellulitis

Chickenpox (Varicella)

Cholera

Dengue fever

Diphtheria

Enteric fever (typhoid and para-typhoid fevers)

German measles (Rubella)

Glandular fever

Hepatitis (viral)

Influenza

Malaria

Measles

Meningitis

Mumps

Plague

Poliomyelitis

Rabies

Scarlet fever

Tetanus

Tuberculosis

Typhus fever

Whooping cough (Pertussis)

Yellow fever

Sexually transmitted diseases including HIV (AIDS)

NOTE. Other communicable diseases such as Lassa Fever do not fall within the competence of this book. When in doubt notify the Port Health Officer.

Communicable diseases

Vehicles are inanimate or non-living means of transmission of infectious organisms. They include:

- Water. If polluted, specifically by contaminated sewage. Water is the vehicle for such enteric (intestinal) diseases as typhoid, cholera, and amoebic and bacillary dysentery.

- Milk is the vehicle for diseases of cattle transmissible to man, including bovine tuberculosis, brucellosis. Milk also serves as a growth medium for some agents of bacterial diseases such as campylobacter, a common cause of diarrhoea.

- Food is the vehicle for salmonella infections (which include enteric fever), amoebic dysentery, and other diarrhoeal diseases, and poisoning. Any food can act as a vehicle for infection especially if it is raw or inadequately cooked, or improperly refrigerated after cooking, as well as having been in contact with an infected source. The source may be another infected food, hands, water or air.

- Air is the vehicle for the common cold, pneumonia, tuberculosis. influenza, whooping cough. measles. and chickenpox. Discharges from the mouth. nose, throat, or lungs take the form of droplets which remain suspended in the air, from which they may be inhaled.

- Soil can be the vehicle for tetanus, anthrax, hookworm. and some wound infections.

- Fomites. This term includes all inanimate objects, other than water, milk, food, air, and soil, that might play a role in the transmission of disease. Fomites include bedding, clothing and the surfaces of objects.

  Vectors are animate or living vehicles which transmit infections in the following ways:

- Mechanical transfer. The contaminated mouth-parts or feet of some insect vectors mechanically transfer the infectious organisms to a bite-wound or to food. For example, flies may transmit bacillary dysentery, typhoid, or other intestinal infections by walking over the infected faeces and later leaving the disease-producing germs on food.

- Intestinal harbourage. Certain insects harbour pathogenic (disease causing) organisms in their intestinal tracts. The organisms are passed in the faeces or are regurgitated by the vector, and the bite-wounds or food are contaminated. (e.g. plague, typhus.)

- Biological transmission. This term refers to multiplication of the infectious agent during its stay in the body of the vector. The vector takes in the organism along with a blood meal but is not able to transmit infection until after a definite period, during which the pathogen changes. The parasite that causes malaria is an example of an organism that completes the sexual stages of its life cycle within its vector, the mosquito. The virus of yellow fever also multiplies in the bodies of mosquitoes.

Terms used in connection with communicable diseases

A *carrier* is a person who has the infection, either without becoming ill himself or following recovery from it.

A *contact* is a person who may have been in contact with an infected person.

The *incubation period* is the interval of time that elapses between a person being infected with any communicable disease and the appearance of the features of that disease. This period is very variable and depends upon the infectious agent and the inoculum (the amount of the infectious agent).

The *isolation period* signifies the time during which a patient suffering from an infectious disease should be isolated from others.

The *period of communicability* is the time during which a patient who may be incubating an infectious disease following contact can communicate the disease to others.

The *quarantine period* means the time during which port authorities may require a ship to be isolated from contact with the shore. Quarantine of this kind is seldom carried out except when serious epidemic diseases, such as, for instance. plague. cholera, or yellow fever are present or have recently occurred on board.

Symptoms and signs

In reality it is often very difficult to make an accurate diagnosis of an infectious disease without laboratory investigations. It may be possible if there are very specific features such as a rash (varicella) or cluster of suggestive features (regular fever, enlarged spleen and history of mosquito bites in an endemic area). Because of the difficulty in making an accurate diagnosis on board ship you may have to give a variety of treatments each directed at different infectious agents.

Onset

Almost all communicable diseases begin with the patient feeling unwell and perhaps a rise in temperature. This period may be very short, lasting only a few hours (meningococcal sepsis), or more prolonged (hepatitis). In some diseases the onset is mild and there is not much general disturbance of health, whereas in others it is severe and prostrating. During the onset it is rarely possible to make a diagnosis.

The rash

The diagnosis of some communicable diseases is made easier by the presence of a characteristic rash. In certain diseases (e.g. scarlet fever) the rash is spread evenly over the body, in others it is limited to definite areas. When examining an individual suspected to be suffering from a communicable disease, it is of great importance to strip him completely in order to get a full picture of any rash and its distribution.

General rules for the management of communicable diseases

Isolation

The principles of isolation are described in Chapter 3 and Chapter 5. If you have a suspicion that the disease with which you are dealing is infectious it is advisable to invoke isolation precautions as soon as possible.

Treatment

An essential element in treatment is maintaining the patient's well being. This is achieved through good general nursing and it is important to ensure that the patient does not become dehydrated.

Advice on specific medical treatment for infectious diseases which are likely to respond to specific drugs is given under the sections on treatment for the individual diseases. You may also be advised to administer drugs to prevent secondary infection occurring.

See Chapter on General Nursing and on how to reduce a high fever.

Diet

Diet will very much depend on the type of disease and severity of fever. Serious fever is invariably accompanied by loss of appetite and this will automatically tend to restrict diet to beverages such as water flavoured with lemon juice and a little sugar or weak tea with a little milk and perhaps sugar.

Essential basic rules

- Isolate. If anyone suffers from a temperature without obvious cause it is best to isolate him until a diagnosis has been made.

- Strip the patient and make a thorough examination looking for any signs of a rash in order to try to establish the diagnosis.

- Put him to bed, and appoint someone to look after and nurse the patient.

- Give non-alcoholic fluids in the first instance.

- If his temperature exceeds 39.4C make arrangements for tepid sponging.

- Arrange for the use of a bed pan and urine bottle if the patient shows any sign of prostration or if his temperature is high.

- If the patient is seriously ill and if in any doubt as to the diagnosis seek RADIO MEDICAL ADVICE, failing which you should consider the need for making for port.

- Treat symptoms as they arise.

Do not attempt to get the patient up during convalescence if he is feeble, but keep him in bed until the next port is reached.

When approaching port, send a radio message giving details of the case to enable the Port Health Authority to make arrangements for the isolation of the case and any contacts on arrival and Disinfection.

Immunisation and travel advice

It is important that up to date advice on immunisation and the prevalent diseases should be obtained before arrival in a foreign port. This is most easily available from the following publications:

Health Information for Overseas Travel, produced by the UK Department of Health, and *International Travel and Health*, WHO, Geneva

Anthrax

French: *Charbon*   German: *Milzbrand*   Italian: *Carbonchio*   Spanish: *Carbon*
Incubation Period: 2 to 7 days, usually 2
Period of communicability: No evidence of transmission from person to person
Isolation Period: No evidence of transmission from person to person
Quarantine Period: None.

Anthrax is an uncommon but serious communicable disease which may occur in man and animals. It occurs in man either as an infection of the skin (malignant pustule), or as an attack on the lungs or intestines, or as a widely spread infection throughout the body by means of the blood circulation.

Anthrax is, in man, usually contracted by handling infected animals, skins, hides, or furs. It can also be conveyed by the consumption of infected or insufficiently cooked meat, or by the inhalation of dust containing the organism.

Symptoms and signs

In most cases anthrax is accompanied by severe symptoms such as fever and prostration. When it appears as a skin infection, it begins as a red itching pimple which soon changes into a blister and within the next 36 hours progresses into a large boil with a sloughing centre surrounded by a ring of pimples. Alternatively it may take the form of a painless widespread swelling of the skin which shortly breaks down to form pus in the area.

The gastro-intestinal form of anthrax resembles food poisoning with diarrhoea and bloody faeces. The lung form develops into a rapidly fatal pneumonia.

Treatment

Should a case of anthrax occur at sea, which is unlikely unless as a result of handling animals, hides, skins, etc., all dressings or other material that come into contact with the discharge must be burnt or disposed of by disinfection.

Instruments must be used to handle dressings as far as possible, and the instruments must subsequently be sterilised by vigorous boiling for not less than 30 minutes, since the spores of the anthrax germ are difficult to kill.

Treatment is not easy on board and the patient should be put ashore as soon as possible. In the meantime treatment is with Penicillin

No attempt at surgical treatment (incision or lancing of the sore) should be made as it does no good. Cover the sore with a dressing.

Seek advice from a Port Health Authority about the treatment of cargo.

Cellulitis (Erysipelas)

French: Erysipèle   German: Erysipel   Italian: Erisipela   Spanish: Erisipela
*Incubation Period:*1 to 7 days
Period of communicability: None
Isolation Period: None
Quarantine Period: None

This disease is an acute inflammatory condition of the skin caused by a germ entering the body through a scratch or abrasion. Cellulitis occurs anywhere, but most commonly on the legs, arms and face.

The onset is sudden with shivering, and a general feeling of malaise. The temperature rises rapidly and may reach about 40°C. The affected area becomes acutely inflamed and red on the first or second day of the infection and the inflammation spreads rapidly outwards with a well-marked, raised, and advancing edge. As the disease advances the portions of the skin first attacked become less inflamed and exhibit a yellowish appearance. Blisters may appear on the inflamed area which can be very painful.

General treatment

The patient must be kept in bed during the acute stage.

Specific treatment

Give the patient benzyl penicillin 600 mg followed by oral antibiotic treatment. Paracetamol can be given to ease the pain.

Chickenpox (Varicella)

French: *Varicelle*   German: *Windpocken*   Italian: *Varicella*   Spanish: *Varicela*
Incubation Period: 14 to 21 days, usually 14
Period of communicability: Up to 5 days before the onset of the rash and 5 days after the first crop of vesicles
Isolation Period: Until the vesicles become dry
Quarantine Period: None

This highly infectious disease starts with fever and feeling unwell. Within a day or two the rash appears on the trunk but soon spreads to the face and elsewhere, even sometimes to the throat and palate.

The rash starts as red pimples which quickly change into small blisters (vesicles) filled with clear fluid which may become slightly coloured and sticky during the second day. Within a day or two the blisters burst or shrivel up and become covered with a brownish scab. Successive crops of spots appear for up to five days. Although usually a mild disease, sometimes the rash is more severe and very rarely pneumonia may occur.

Treatment

A member of the crew who has had chickenpox, and therefore has immunity, could make a suitable nurse. If all of the crew have had chickenpox in the past then there is no need to isolate the patient. The patient need not be confined to bed unless he is unwell. He should be told not to scratch, especially not to scratch his face otherwise pock marks may remain for life. Calamine lotion, if available, dabbed onto the spots may ease the itching.

Cholera

French: *Choléra*   German: *Cholera*   Italian: *Coléra*   Spanish: *Cólera*
Incubation Period: 1 to 5 days, usually 2–3 days
Period of communicability: Usually for a few days after recovery
Isolation Period: Until diarrhoea has settled
Quarantine Period: 5 days

Cholera is a severe bacterial infection of the bowel producing profuse watery diarrhoea, muscular cramps, vomiting and rapid collapse. Infection occurs principally through drinking infected water and sometimes through eating contaminated uncooked vegetables, fruit, shell fish or ice cream. It generally occurs in areas where sanitation is poor and where untreated sewage has contaminated drinking water. Other bacterial and viral causes of diarrhoea can sometimes produce a similar clinical picture and may be just as severe.

Symptoms and signs

Most cases are mild and will not be differentiated from any other form of diarrhoea. In a severe case the onset is abrupt, the vomiting and diarrhoea extreme with the faeces at first yellowish and later pale and watery, containing little white shreds of mucus resembling rice grains. The temperature is below normal, and the pulse rapid and feeble.

The frequent copious watery faeces rapidly produce dehydration. Vomiting is profuse, first of food but soon changing to a thin fluid similar to the water passed by the bowel. Cramps of an agonising character attack the limbs and abdomen, and the patient rapidly passes into a state of collapse.

As the result of the loss of fluid, the cheeks fall in, the eyes become shrunken and the skin loses its normal springiness and will not quickly return to its normal shape when pinched.

The body becomes cold and covered with a clammy sweat, the urine is scanty, the breathing rapid and shallow, and the voice is sunk to a whisper. The patient is now restless, with muscle cramps induced by loss of salt, and feebly complaining of intense thirst.

This stage may rapidly terminate in death or equally rapidly turn to convalescence. In the latter case the cessation of vomiting and purging and the return of some warmth to the skin will herald convalescence.

Treatment

If there is a suspected case of cholera on board RADIO MEDICAL ADVICE ON MANAGEMENT SHOULD BE OBTAINED PROMPTLY.

The patient should be isolated and put to bed at once. Every effort should be made to replace fluid and salt loss. Therefore, keep a fluid balance chart. The patient should be told that his life depends on drinking enough and he should be encouraged and if necessary almost forced to drink as much as possible until all signs of dehydration disappear (until his urine output is back to normal). Thereafter he should drink about 300 ml after each stool until the diarrhoea stops. It is best to drink oral rehydration solution (ORS), if this is not available, make up a solution from 20 gm of sugar with a pinch of salt and a pinch of sodium bicarbonate and juice from an orange in 500 ml sterile water.

Give Doxycycline 200 mg first dose then 100 mg once daily. If vomiting, give an anti-emetic tablet or injection before each dose. The patient must be kept in bed until seen by a doctor.

Caution

Cholera is a disease which is transmitted from person to person. If cholera is suspected, the ship's water supply must be thoroughly treated to make sure that it is safe. The disposal of infected faeces and vomit must be controlled carefully since they are highly infectious. The hygiene precautions of all attendants must be of an order to prevent them also becoming infected and all food preparation on board must be reviewed.

Dengue fever

French: Dengue
Italian: Dengue; Febbra dei sette giorni
German: Denguefieber; Siebentagefieber
Spanish: Fiebre dengue
Incubation Period: 3 to 14 days, usually 7 to 10 days.
Period of communicability: No person to person transmission. Infective for mosquitoes for about 5 days from just before the end of the febrile period.
Isolation Period: None
Quarantine Period: None

This is an acute fever of about 7 days' duration conveyed by a mosquito. It is sometimes called break-bone fever. It is an unpleasant, painful disease which is rarely fatal. A severe form of the disease, dengue haemorrhagic fever, can occur in children. Features of the disease are its sudden onset with a high fever, severe headache and aching behind the eyeballs, and intense pain in the joints and muscles, especially in the small of the back. The face may swell up and the eyes suffuse but no rash appears at this stage. Occasionally an itchy rash resembling that of measles but bright red in colour appears on the fourth or fifth day of the illness. It starts on the hands and feet from which it spreads to other parts of the body, but remains most dense on the limbs. After the rash fades, the skin dries and the surface flakes.

   After about the fourth day the fever subsides, but it may recur some three days later before subsiding again by the tenth day.

General treatment

There is no specific treatment, but paracetamol will relieve some of the pain, and calamine lotion, if available, may ease the itching of the rash. Control is by removal of Aedes mosquitoes.

Diphtheria

French: Diphtérie   *German:* Diphterie   *Italian:* Difterite   *Spanish:* Difteria
Incubation Period: 2 to 5 days
Period of communicability: Usually less than 2 weeks, shorter if the patient receives antibiotics
Isolation Period: 2 weeks
Quarantine Period: None

Diphtheria is an acute infectious disease characterised by the formation of a membrane in the throat and nose. The onset is gradual and starts with a sore throat and fever accompanied by shivering. The throat symptoms increase, swallowing being painful and difficult, and whitish-grey patches of membrane become visible on the back of the throat, the tonsils and the palate. The patches look like wash leather and bleed on being touched. The neck glands swell, and the breath is foul. The fever may last for two weeks with severe prostration. Bacterial toxins may cause fatal heart failure and muscle paralysis.

General treatment

Immediate isolation is essential as diphtheria is very infectious, the infection being spread by aerosols.

Specific treatment

Specific treatment is diphtheria anti-toxin which should be given at the earliest possible opportunity if the patient can get to medical attention. Antibiotic treatment should be given to all cases to limit the spread of infection but it will not neutralise toxin which has already been produced.

Enteric fever – typhoid

French: *Fièvre typhoide*
Italian: *Febbre tifoidea*
German: *Typhus abdominalis*
Spanish: *Fiebre tifoidea*
Incubation Period: 1 to 3 weeks, depending on size of infecting dose
Period of communicability: Usually less than 2 weeks. Prolonged carriage of salmonella typhi may occur in some of those not treated.
Isolation Period: Variable.
Quarantine Period: None

The term enteric fever covers typhoid and para-typhoid fevers. Enteric fever is contracted by drinking water or eating food that has been contaminated with typhoid germs. Seafarers are advised to be very careful where they eat and drink when ashore. Immunisation gives reasonable protection against typhoid but not para-typhoid.

In general the para-typhoids are milder and tend to have a shorter course.

The disease may have a wide variety of symptoms depending on the severity of the attack. Nevertheless, typhoid fever, however mild, is a disease which must be treated seriously, not only because of its possible effect upon the patient, but also to prevent it spreading to others who may not have been immunised. Strict attention must be given to hygiene and cleanliness and all clothing and soiled linen must be disinfected.

During the first week the patient feels off-colour and apathetic, he may have a persistent headache, poor appetite, and sometimes nose bleeding. There is some abdominal discomfort and usually constipation. These symptoms increase until he is forced to go to bed. At this stage his temperature begins to rise in steps reaching about 39–40°C in the evenings. For about two weeks it never drops back to normal even in the mornings.

Any person who is found with a persistent temperature of this kind should always be suspected of having typhoid, especially if his pulse rate remains basically normal. In 10 to 20% of cases, from about the seventh day, characteristic rose-pink spots may appear on the lower chest, abdomen and back, which if pressed with the finger will disappear and return when pressure is released. Each spot lasts about 3–4 days and they continue to appear in crops until the end of the second week or longer. Search for them in a good light, especially in dark-skinned races. During the second week, mental apathy, confusion and delirium may occur. In the more favourable cases the patient will commence recovery but in the worst cases his condition will continue to deteriorate and may terminate in deep coma and death. Even where the patient appears to be recovering, he may suffer a relapse. There are a variety of complications but the most dangerous are haemorrhage from, or perforation of, the bowel. Where the faeces are found to contain blood at any stage of the disease the patient must be kept as immobile as possible and put on a milk and water diet. If the bowel is perforated, peritonitis will set in.

General treatment

Anyone suspected of having typhoid or para-typhoid fever should be kept in bed in strict isolation until seen by a doctor. The patient's urine and faeces are highly infectious, as may be his vomit. These should all be disposed of. The attendants and others coming into the room should wash their hands thoroughly after handling the bedpan or washing the patient, and before leaving the room.

The patient should be encouraged to drink as much as possible and a fluid input/output chart should be maintained. He can eat as much as he wants, but it is best if the food is light.

Specific treatment

If you suspect somebody has enteric fever get RADIO MEDICAL ADVICE. Give ciprofloxacin 500 mg every 12 hours for one week. On this treatment the fever and all symptoms should respond within 4–5 days.

All cases should be seen by a doctor at the first opportunity. The case notes including details of the amount of medicine given should be sent with the patient.

German measles – rubella

French: *Rubéole*   German: *Röteln*   Italian: *Rosolia*   Spanish: *Rubéola*
Incubation Period: 14 to 23 days, usually 17
Period of communicability: For about 1 week before to at least 4 days after the onset of the rash
Isolation Period: Until 7 days from the appearance of the rash
Quarantine Period: None

German measles is a highly infectious, though mild disease. It has features similar to those of mild attacks of ordinary measles or of scarlet fever. For the differences in symptoms and signs see the table.

Usually the first sign of the disease is a rash of spots, though sometimes there will be headache, stiffness and soreness of the muscles, and some slight fever preceding or accompanying the rash. The rash is absent in half the cases and lasts from 5 to 6 days.

The glands towards the back of the neck are swollen and can easily be felt. This is an important distinguishing sign. This swelling will precede the rash by up to 10 days.

General treatment

Give the patient paracetamol, and calamine lotion, if available, for the rash.

Specific treatment

NOTE: Particular care should be taken to isolate patients with German measles from pregnant women: Any pregnant woman on board should see a doctor ashore as soon as possible so that her immunity to rubella can be confirmed. If a patient has seen his wife in the last week he should be asked whether his wife might be pregnant. If so, his wife should be advised to see her doctor.

Glandular fever – infectious mononucleosis

French: *Fièvre glandulaire; Mononucleose infectieuse*
German: *Drusenfieber; Infektiose Mononukleose*
Italian: *Febbre ghiandolare (Mononucleosi infettiva)*
Spanish: *Fiebre glandular (Mononucleosis infecciosa)*
Incubation Period: 4 to 6 weeks
Period of communicability: Prolonged, excretion of virus may persist for a year or more
Isolation Period: None
Quarantine Period: None

This malady is an acute infection which is most likely to affect the young members of the crew. Convalescence may take up to two or three months.

The disease starts with a gradual increase in temperature and a sore throat; a white covering often develops later over the tonsils. At this stage it is likely to be diagnosed as tonsillitis and treated as such. However it tends not to respond to such treatment and, during this time, a generalised enlargement of glands occurs. The glands of the neck, armpit and groins start to swell, and become tender; those in the neck to a considerable extent. The patient may have difficulty in eating or swallowing. His temperature may go very high and he may sweat profusely. Occasionally there is jaundice between the fifth and fourteenth day. Commonly there is a blotchy skin rash on the upper trunk and arms at the end of the first week. Vague abdominal pain is sometimes a feature. A diagnosis of diphtheria may be considered due to the appearance of the tonsils, but the generalised glandular enlargement is typical of glandular fever.

General treatment

Paracetamol should be given to relieve pain and to moderate the temperature. Any antibiotics which have been prescribed to treat the tonsillitis should be discontinued.

There is no specific treatment. If complications arise get RADIO MEDICAL ADVICE.

Hepatitis (viral)

French: *Hépatite : Hepatitis*   German: *Hepatitis*   Italian: *Epatite*   Spanish: *Hepatitis*
Incubation Period: 15 to 50 days for hepatitis A, 60 to 90 days for hepatitis B (may be much longer)
Period of communicability: None after jaundice has appeared in hepatitis A, can be indefinite for hepatitis B
Isolation Period: During first week of illness
Quarantine Period: None

This is an acute infection of the liver caused by viruses. There are two main causes of acute hepatitis: hepatitis A and hepatitis B. Two other viruses may cause hepatitis (C and E), but these are uncommon. The most likely cause will be hepatitis A and this is spread by the faecal-oral route (as is hepatitis E). Hepatitis B is spread sexually or by contaminated blood or needles. There is no way of differentiating one type of viral hepatitis from another. The urine and faeces will show the typical changes associated with jaundice.

Treatment

There is no specific treatment. The patient should be put to bed and nursed in isolation. Plenty of sweetened fluids should be given until the appetite returns. When the appetite returns a fat-free diet should be given. No alcohol should be allowed. All cases must be seen by a doctor at the next port.

Influenza

French: *Grippe; Influenza*   German: *Epidemische Influenza; Grippe*
Italian: *Influenza*   Spanish: *Influenza; Grippe*
Incubation Period: 1 to 5 days
Period of communicability: 3 to 5 days (7 in children) from the onset of illness
Isolation Period: Often impractical because of the delay in diagnosis. In an outbreak it would be advisable to keep all affected individuals together and away from those who are well
Quarantine Period: none

This is an acute infectious disease caused by a germ inhaled through the nose or mouth. It often occurs in epidemics. The onset is sudden and the symptoms are, at first, the same as those of the common cold. Later the patient feels much worse with fits of shivering, and severe aching of the limbs and back. Depression, shortness of breath, palpitations, and headaches, are common.

Influenza may vary in severity. Commonly a sharp unpleasant feverish attack is followed by a prompt fall in temperature and a short convalescence. Pneumonia is a possible complication.

General treatment

The patient should be subject to standard isolation. He should be watched for signs of pneumonia such as pains in the chest, rapid breathing and a bluish tinge to the lips. He should be given plenty to drink and a light and nutritious diet if he can manage it.

Specific treatment

There is no specific treatment for the uncomplicated case, but the patient should be given paracetamol as needed.

Malaria

French: *Paludisme*   German: *Malaria*   Italian: *Malaria* Spanish: *Paludismo*
Incubation Period: 12 days or more, depending on the type of malaria
Period of communicability: The patient will remain infectious for mosquitoes until they have been completely treated
Isolation Period: None if in mosquito-proof accommodation
Quarantine Period: None

Malaria is a recurrent fever caused by protozoa introduced into the blood stream by the bite of the Anopheles mosquito. The malaria-carrying mosquito is most prevalent in districts where there is surface water on which it lays its eggs. It is a dangerous tropical disease which causes fever, debility and, sometimes, coma and death.

Malarial areas

Ports between latitudes 25°N and 25°S on the coasts of Africa (including Malagassy), Asia, and Central and South America should be regarded as infected or potentially infected with malaria. Enquiries should be made prior to departure to allow appropriate prophylaxis to be arranged and treatment drugs obtained. Before arrival in port further enquiries should be made as to the current malaria situation and prophylaxis issued to the crew if necessary.

Prevention of malaria

The risks of attacks of malaria can be very greatly reduced if proper precautions are taken and the disease can be cured if proper treatment is given. Despite this, cases have occurred in ships where several members of the crew have been attacked by malaria during a single voyage with severe and even fatal results.

The precautions are:

■ avoidance of mosquito bites;

■ prevention of infection.

Avoidance of mosquito bites

The best way to prevent malarial infection is to take measures to avoid being bitten. The advent of air conditioned ships has made many traditional preventive measures obsolete. However, when within two miles of a malarial shore it remains important that:

■ doors are kept closed at all times after dusk;

■ any mosquitoes which enter compartments are killed using insecticide spray;

■ persons going on deck or ashore after dusk wear long sleeved shirts and trousers to avoid exposing their arms and legs;

■ no pools of stagnant water are allowed to develop on deck or in life boats, where mosquitoes might breed.

In ships which are not air conditioned other traditional measures to protect against mosquitoes should be implemented. These include:

■ placing fine wire mesh over portholes, sky lights, ventilators and other openings;

■ screening lights to avoid attracting mosquitoes;

■ fixing mosquito nets over beds where accommodation spaces cannot be made mosquito proof.

Prevention of infection

The fewer the bites, the smaller is the risk of infection but even when the greatest care is exercised it will seldom be possible entirely to prevent mosquito bites either on shore or in the ship. For this reason in all cases when a ship is bound for a malarial port, Masters (in addition to taking all possible measures to prevent mosquito bites) should control infection by giving treatment systematically to all the ship's crew.

Preventive treatment (prophylaxis) does not always prevent a person from contracting malarial infection, but it will reduce the chance of disease.

All persons, therefore, should be warned that they have been exposed to the chance of malaria infection and that, if they fall ill at a later date, they should inform their doctor without delay that the fever from which they are then suffering may be due to malaria contracted abroad.

The most appropriate prophylaxis will vary with the location as there are different types of malaria in various parts of the world. There is also increasing resistance to anti-malarials which will affect their effectiveness. Up to date information should be obtained before departure if possible or from the local health authorities.

General guidelines

Start taking the prophylaxis before arrival at a malarial area in accordance with specific instructions and depending on the region. (Usually 1-3 weeks before departure).This will allow the tolerance and side-effects (if any) of the prophylactic drug to be assessed. Prophylaxis should be continued for 4 weeks after leaving the malarial area so as to ensure all stages of the parasite have been killed.

No drugs for the treatment of malaria are specified in the MSN 1726 as the advice varies with destination and the pattern of disease in any given malarial area at the time.

For information, the UK's present guidelines recommend 3 different regimes depending on destination:

- Proguanil 200 mg once daily and chloroquine 300 mg weekly

- Mefloquine 250 mg once weekly

- Maloprim (a combined tablet of dapsone and pyrimethamine) 1 tablet weekly and chloroquine 300 mg weekly

    Other regimes may be used in areas of high level resistance

Treatment of malaria

Features of the illness

Malaria cannot be diagnosed with certainty without laboratory assistance. If the person has been in a potentially malarial area within the last few months and has a fever they should be assumed to have malaria. The characteristic patterns of fever associated with malaria (fever every 2 to 3 days) may not be obvious. The illness may progress rapidly without many features other than fever and sweating. There will often be a severe headache. If there is any doubt about whether to treat or not get RADIO MEDICAL ADVICE.

General treatment for mild or severe malaria

The patient should be put to bed in a cool place and his temperature, pulse and respiration taken four hourly. If body temperature rises to 40°C or over, cooling should be carried out. The temperature should be taken and recorded at 15 minute intervals until it has been normal for some time. Thereafter the four-hourly recording should be resumed until the attack has definitely passed.

Specific treatment for mild or severe malaria

Anti-malarial drugs are not specified in MSN 1726 as treatment depends on the area and patterns of resistance. If anti-malarials are to be carried seek appropriate advice on which to obtain/use.

The following examples of current regimes are given for information:

- Quinine 600 mg every 8 hours for 7 days followed by Fansidar (see below) 3 tablets as a single dose

    or

- Mefloquine 500 mg (2 tablets) for 2 doses 8 hours apart

Chloroquine is not used for treatment except for proven single infections with vivax and other benign malarias because of drug resistance. If quinine, Fansidar or mefloquine are not available then chloroquine 300 mg 8 hourly for three doses then 300 mg daily for 2 days should be used.

If the patient is unable to take medicine by mouth or is vomiting then quinine 600 mg should be given by intramuscular injection every 8 hours. As soon as the patient is able to swallow it should be given by mouth. Quinine may produce ringing in the ears or dizziness, but this should not normally be a reason to stop treatment.

NOTE: All patients who have been treated for malaria or suspected malaria must see a doctor at the next port because further medical treatment may be necessary.

Measles

French: *Rougeole*   German: *Masern*   Italian: *Morbillo*   Spanish: *Sarampion*

Incubation Period: 7 to 18 days usually 10 until onset of fever, 14 days until rash
Period of communicability: about 10 days, minimally infectious after the second day of the rash
Isolation Period: 4 days after onset of rash
Quarantine Period: None

Measles does not often occur in adults. See also the sections on German measles and scarlet fever and the table of differences of symptoms.

The disease starts like a cold in the head, with sneezing, a running nose and eyes, headache, cough and a slight fever 37.5°C–39°C. During the next two days the catarrh extends to the throat causing hoarseness and a cough. A careful examination of the mouth during this period may reveal minute white or bluish white spots the size of a pin's head on the inner side of the cheeks, or the tongue and inner side of the lips. These are known a 'Koplik spots' and are not found in German measles and scarlet fever.

The rash appears on the fourth day when the temperature increases to 39–40°C. Pale rose-coloured spots first appear on the face and spread down to cover the rest of the body. The spots run together to form a mottled blotched appearance. The rash deepens in colour as it gets older. In four or five days the rash begins to fade, starting where it first appeared. The skin may peel.

The main danger of measles is that the patient may get bronchitis, pneumonia or middle ear infection.

General treatment

This highly infectious disease is conveyed to others when the patient coughs or sneezes. There is no specific treatment, but the patient may have paracetamol. Calamine lotion, if available, may be applied to soothe the rash.

Meningococcal disease (meningitis and septicaemia)

French: *Méningite cérébro-spinal épidémique*
German: *Epidemische Meningitis Cerebro-spinal*
Italian: *Meningite cerebro-spinal epidemica*
Spanish: *Meningitis cerebro-spinal epidemica*

Incubation Period: 2 to 10 days, usually 3 to 4
Period of communicability: Generally not communicable whilst the patient is on antibiotics
Isolation Period: For 24 hours after the start of antibiotics
Quarantine Period: None

Infection caused by the meningococcus (a bacterium) can cause either meningitis, with inflammation of the membranes surrounding the brain and spinal cord, or a septicaemia characterised by a generalised rash that does not fade on pressure. Unless treated promptly and effectively, the outcome is nearly always fatal. It occurs in epidemics which may affect closed communities such as a ship. The infection enters by the nose and mouth.

Meningitis starts suddenly with fever, considerable headache and vomiting. Within the first day the temperature increases rapidly to 39°C or more and the headache becomes agonising.

Vomiting increases and there is general backache with pain and stiffness in the neck. Intolerance of light (photophobia) is usually present. The patient may be intensely irritable and resent all interference, or may even be delirious.

As the meningitis develops the patient adopts a characteristic posture in bed, lying on the side with his back to the light, knees drawn up and neck bent backwards. Unconsciousness with incontinence may develop.

The septicaemia caused by the meningococcus also starts suddenly with a flu like illness. A rash develops quickly, starting with pin prick like spots which will not blanche when pressed. This rash may progress to form large dark red areas.

Individual cases may vary in the speed of onset, the severity of the illness and the clinical features which are present.

If meningitis is suspected get RADIO MEDICAL ADVICE and it will help the doctor if the results of the two following tests are available:

The neck bending test

Ask the patient to attempt to put his chin on his chest. In meningitis the patient will be unable to do so because forward neck movement will be greatly restricted by muscle contraction. Try to increase the range of forward movement by pushing gently on the back of his head. The neck muscles will contract even more to prevent the movement and the headache and backache will be increased.

The knee straightening test
– Figure 6.1

A. Bend one leg until the heel is close to the buttock.

B. Move the bent leg to lie over the abdomen.

C. Keeping the thigh as in (B) try to straighten the lower leg.

In meningitis it will be impossible to straighten the knee beyond a right angle and attempts to force movement will increase the backache.

General treatment

The patient should be nursed in a quiet, well-ventilated room with shaded lights in strict isolation. He should be accompanied at all times by an attendant who should wear a face mask to cover his nose and mouth. Tepid sponging may be necessary and pressure points should be treated. Usually there is no appetite but he should be encouraged to drink plenty of fluid. Ice packs may help to relieve the headache.

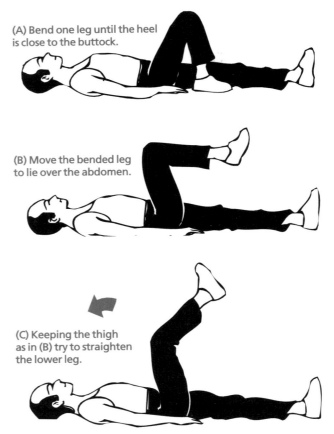

(A) Bend one leg until the heel is close to the buttock.

(B) Move the bended leg to lie over the abdomen.

(C) Keeping the thigh as in (B) try to straighten the lower leg.

Figure 6.1 The knee straightening test.

Specific treatment

Give benzyl penicillin 3 g intramuscularly at once, and get RADIO MEDICAL ADVICE as to the amount and frequency of subsequent injections of benzyl penicillin. Until such advice is received, give benzyl penicillin 2.4 g at six hourly intervals.

The headache should be treated with codeine. The patient should come under the care of a doctor as soon as possible.

Mumps

French: *Oreillons*
Italian: *Malaria Orecchioni*

German: *Mumps – Ziegenpeter*
Spanish: *Orejones*

Incubation Period: 12 to 26 days, usually 18
Period of communicability: 7 days before glandular swelling and up to 9 days after
Isolation Period: 9 days after swelling started
Quarantine Period: None

Mumps is a viral disease which causes the swelling of the salivary glands in front of the ears and around the angle of the jaw. The swelling usually affects both sides of the face though it may only affect one side and it may make the mouth difficult to open. The onset is usually sudden and may be accompanied by a slight fever. The swelling gradually diminishes and should disappear entirely in about 3 weeks.

About 20% of men with mumps get orchitis which is the swelling of one or both testicles; when this occurs it usually happens around the tenth day. Whilst very painful, orchitis does not usually result in infertility and never in impotence.

General treatment

The patient should be put in standard isolation for 9 days and stay in bed for 4 to 5 days or until the fever is no longer present. He can be given paracetamol to relieve the symptoms, but there is no specific treatment.

If he develops swollen painful testicles (orchitis) he should stay in bed. He should support the scrotum on a pad or small pillow. The testicles should also be supported if the patient gets up for any reason.

Plague

French: *Peste*   German: *Pest*   Italian: *Peste*   Spanish: *Peste*

Incubation Period: 2 to 6 days
Period of communicability: As long as infected fleas are present. Person to person spread is uncommon except with plague pneumonia.
Isolation Period: For 3 days after the start of antibiotic treatment
Quarantine Period: 6 days

Plague is a serious bacterial disease transmitted to man by infected rat fleas. It may present in three ways

Bubonic in which buboes (swollen lymph nodes) are the most obvious feature. The nodes are painful and may ooze pus.

Pneumonic in which pneumonia is the main feature. The type of plague is very infectious as the sputum contains the plague bacterium.

Septicaemic which is rapidly fatal.

The attack begins suddenly with severe malaise, shivering, pains in the back and sometimes vomiting. The patient becomes prostrated and is confused. His temperature reaches about 38°C C and the pulse is rapid. After about 2 days the buboes may develop, most commonly in the groins. The buboes may soften into abscesses.

General treatment

The patient should be cared for by an attendant who should wear a face mask to cover his nose and mouth The patient should be isolated and taken as soon as possible to a port where he can be treated. He should rest in bed, be encouraged to drink as much fluid as possible and have a very light diet. If the abscesses burst they should be dressed with a simple dressing, but they must not be lanced. Soiled linen and bed clothes should be boiled for 10 minutes or destroyed.

Specific treatment

Give Doxycycline 100 mg once daily for at least 5 days. The patient should remain on complete bed rest during convalescence.

Prevention

Plague should be notified to the local health authorities at the next port of call. The quarters of the patient and the crew should be treated with insecticide powder and dust to ensure the destruction of fleas.

Warning

Dead rats should be picked up with tongs, placed in a plastic bag, which should be sealed with string, weighted and thrown overboard; if the ship is in port, the dead rats should be disposed of in the manner required by the port medical health authority.

Poliomyelitis – infantile paralysis

French: *Poliomyélite*
Italian: *Poliomielite*
German: *Poliomyelitis*
Spanish: *Poliomielitis*

Incubation Period: 3–21 days, commonly 7–14 days
Period of communicability: Cases are most infectious during the first few days before and after the onset of symptoms
Isolation Period: Not more than 7 days
Quarantine Period None

Poliomyelitis is an acute viral disease that occurs mostly in children. It is a disease almost entirely preventable by immunisation.

The severity ranges from non-apparent infection to non-specific febrile illness, meningitis, paralytic disease and death. Symptoms of the mild disease include fever, malaise, headache, nausea and vomiting. If the disease progresses, severe muscle pain and stiffness of the neck and back, with or without paralysis will occur. The most commonly affected parts are the legs and arms, shoulders, diaphragm and chest muscles. The development of paralysis is generally complete within two days and then recovery begins. The recovery may be complete or leave some degree of paralysis

Affected muscles are usually painful and tender if touched. They are always limp and movements of the affected parts are either weakened or lost by the wasting which appears very soon after paralysis.

Paralysis of the respiratory muscles may cause breathlessness and blueness of the lips.

General treatment

There is no specific treatment but much can be achieved by good nursing. The patient should have complete rest in bed. Pain should be treated with paracetamol and/or codeine.

If a limb has been affected it should be supported by pillows in such a way that the paralysed muscles cannot be stretched. The joints above and below the paralysis should be put through a full range of movement morning and evening to prevent stiffness.

In all cases, as soon as paralysis appears, RADIO MEDICAL ADVICE must be sought. If the respiratory muscles are affected, breathing difficulty may ensue. Urgent steps must be taken to get the patient to skilled hospital treatment as soon as possible.

Rabies – hydrophobia

French: *La rage*   German: *Tollwut*   Italian: *Rabbia*   Spanish: *Rabia*

Incubation Period: in humans the incubation period is usually 2 to 12 weeks, shortest for patients bitten about the head and those with extensive bites
Communicability: Rabies is rarely, if ever, spread from human to human. Nevertheless for the duration of the illness contamination with saliva should be avoided by wearing gloves when nursing the patient
Isolation Period: Duration of the illness
Quarantine Period:

Rabies is an acute infectious viral disease that is almost always fatal. When a rabid mammal bites humans or other animals, its saliva transmits the infection into the wound, from where it spreads to the central nervous system. Rabies is primarily an infection of wild animals such as skunks, coyotes, foxes, wolves, racoons, bats, squirrels, rabbits, and chipmunks. The most common domestic animals reported to have rabies are dogs, cats, cattle, horses. mules, sheep, goats, and swine. It is possible for rabies to be transmitted if infective saliva enters a scratch or fresh break in the skin.

The development of the disease in a bitten person can be prevented by immediate and proper treatment, Once symptoms of rabies develop, death is virtually certain to result. Thus prevention of this disease is of the utmost importance.

Local port authorities should be informed of possible rabid animals, so that appropriate public health measures can be instituted.

Treatment

As soon as an individual aboard ship Is known to have been bitten by a dog or other possibly rabid animal, **RADIO MEDICAL ADVICE** should he obtained at once. Usually suspected cases are sent ashore to obtain the expert treatment and nursing care needed to prevent the disease.

Immediate local care should be given. Vigorous treatment to remove rabies virus from the bites or other exposures to the animal's saliva may be as important as specific anti-rabies treatment. Free bleeding from the wound should be encouraged. Other local care should consist of:

- thorough irrigation of the wounds with soap or detergent water solution;

- cleansing with antiseptic solution;

- if recommended by radio, giving an antibiotic to prevent infection:

- administering adsorbed tetanus toxoid, if indicated.

- Suturing of bite wounds should be avoided.

Prevention

When abroad, seamen should keep away from warm-blooded animals especially cats, dogs. and other carnivores. It is strongly advised that pets should not be carried on board ship as these may become infected unnoticed, through contact with rabid animals in ports.

Scarlet fever

French: *Scarlatine*   German: *Scharlach*   Italian: *Scarlattina*   Spanish: *Escarlatina*

Incubation Period: 1 to 3 days
Period of communicability: 3 days
Isolation Period: 14 days in untreated cases, 1 to 2 days if given antibiotics.
Quarantine Period: None

Scarlet fever is not often contracted by adults. It has features similar to those of measles and German measles; see the table of differences of symptoms.

The onset is generally sudden and the temperature may rapidly rise to 39.5 to 40°C on the first day. With the fever the other main early symptom is a sore throat, which in most cases is very severe. The skin is hot and burning to the touch. The rash appears on the second day and consists of tiny bright red spots so close together that the skin assumes a scarlet or boiled lobster-like colour. It usually appears first on the neck, very rapidly spreads to the upper part of the chest and then to the rest of the body. There may be an area around the mouth which is clear of the rash. The tongue at first is covered with white fur and, when this goes, it becomes a very bright red (strawberry). The high fever usually lasts about a week. As the rash fades the skin peels in circular patches.

The danger of scarlet fever arises from the complications associated with it, e.g. inflammation of the kidneys (test the urine for protein once a day), inflammation of the ear due to the spread of infection from the throat, rheumatism and heart disease. These complications can be avoided by careful treatment.

General treatment

The patient must stay in bed and be kept as quiet as possible. The patient can be given paracetamol to relieve the pain in the throat which may also be helped if he takes plenty of cold drinks. He can take such food as he wishes.

Specific treatment

As scarlet fever usually follows from a sore throat or tonsillitis you may already be giving him the relevant treatment. Otherwise give the specific treatment for tonsillitis.

Tetanus – lockjaw

French: *Tetanos*   German: *Wundstarrkrampf*   Italian: *Tetano*   Spanish: *Tetanos*

Incubation Period: 4 to 21 days
Period of communicability: No person to person transmission
Isolation Period: None
Quarantine Period: None

Tetanus is caused by the infection of a wound by the tetanus bacterium which secretes a powerful poison (toxin). This bacterium is very widespread in nature and the source of the wound infection may not always be easy to trace. Puncture wounds are particularly liable to be dangerous and overlooked as a point of entry. In the UK immunisation against the disease usually begins in childhood but it is necessary to have further periodic inoculations to maintain effective immunity. Fortunately the disease is a very rare condition on board ship.

The first signs of the disease may be spasms or stiffening of the jaw muscles and, sometimes, other muscles of the face leading to difficulty in opening the mouth and swallowing. The spasms tend to become more frequent and spread to the neck and back causing the patient's body to become arched. The patient remains fully conscious during the spasms which are extremely painful and brought on by external stimulus such as touch, noise or bright light. The patient is progressively exhausted until heart and lung failure prove fatal. Alternatively, the contractions may become less frequent and the patient recovers, but there is a high mortality.

Treatment

The patient should be isolated in a darkened room as far as possible from all disturbances. Get RADIO MEDICAL ADVICE. Give antibiotic treatment and give diazepam or chlorpromazine as sedation and to control spasms. The patient must be got to hospital as soon as possible.

Tuberculosis – TB, consumptlon

French: Tuberculose   German: Tuberkulose   Italian: Tuberculosis   Spanish: Tuberculosis

Incubation Period: 4 to 12 weeks
Period of communicability: indefinite, 2 weeks after antibiotics
Isolation Period: depends on the degree of infection, rarely necessary
Quarantine Period: None

This infectious disease is caused by the tubercle bacillus. Although the lung (pulmonary) disease is the most common, TB bacteria may attack other tissues in the body: bones. joints. glands, or kidneys. Unlike most contagious diseases, tuberculosis usually takes a considerable time to develop, often appearing only after repeated, close, and prolonged exposures to a patient with the active disease. A healthy body is usually able to control the tubercle bacilli unless the invasion is overwhelming or resistance is low because of chronic alcoholism, poor nutrition, or some other weakening condition.

The pulmonary form of the disease is spread most often by coughing and sneezing.

A person may have tuberculosis for a long time before it is detected. Symptoms may consist of nothing more than a persistent cough, slight loss of weight, night sweats, and a continual 'all-in' or 'tired-out' feeling that persists when there is no good reason for it. More definitive signs pointing to tuberculosis are a cough that persists for more than a month, raising sputum with each cough. persistent or recurring pains in the chest, and afternoon rises in temperature.

When he reaches a convenient port, a seaman with one or more of these warning signs should see a physician.

Treatment

Every effort should be made to prevent anyone who has active tuberculosis from going to sea. since this would present a risk to the crew's health as well as the individual's.

The treatment of tuberculosis by medication will not usually be started at sea, since the disease does not constitute an emergency.

To prevent the spread of tuberculosis, every patient with a cough, irrespective of its cause, should hold disposable tissues over his mouth and nose when coughing or sneezing and place the used tissues in a paper bag, which should be disposed of by burning.

The medical attendant should follow good nursing isolation techniques (see Isolation Chapter 3). No special precautions are necessary for handling the patient's bedclothes, eating utensils, and personal clothing.

Tuberculosis control

A tuberculosis control programme has three objectives: (I) to keep individuals with the disease from signing on as crew-members; (2) to locate those who may have developed the disease while aboard ship and initiate treatment: and (3) to give preventive treatment to persons at high risk of developing the active disease. The first objective can be achieved by periodic, thorough physical examinations including chest X-rays and bacteriological examination of sputum.

To identify those who might have developed active tuberculosis, a chest X-ray should be taken and a medical evaluation including bacteriological examination of sputum requested when in port, if a crew-member develops symptoms of a chest cold that persist for more than two weeks.

Also, when any active disease is discovered, survey should be made of close associates of the patient and others in prolonged contact with him. Such persons are regarded as contacts and are considered at risk from the disease; they should be given a tuberculin test and chest X-ray when next in port. If they develop symptoms, full medical examination, including bacteriological examination of sputum, should be requested.

Typhus fever

French: *Typhus exanth\Aematique*   German: *Flecktyphus*
Italian: *Tifo petecchiale*   Spanish: *Tifus petequial*

Incubation Period: 6 to 15 days, usually 12
Period of communicability: Not directly transmissible from person to person
Isolation Period: not required after de-lousing
Quarantine Period: 14 days

This disease should not be confused with typhoid fever. Typhus is caused by a small bacterium. The disease is conveyed by lice, fleas, ticks and mites. Treatment for the various types of typhus is the same and the symptoms are very similar. The main typhi are epidemic (from lice) and murine, or ship typhus, (from rat fleas).

Symptoms and signs

Onset is sudden with headache, vomiting, shivering and nausea. The temperature rapidly rises and may reach 40.0°C to 40.6°C. The patient suffers great prostration, and may be delirious or confused.

About the fifth day a rash appears on the front of the body, spreading to the back and limbs in the form of dusky red spots which give the skin a blotchy appearance. The disease if untreated lasts about two weeks. With tick or mite borne typhus there is usually a punched out black ulcer (eschar) which corresponds to the site of attachment.

Treatment

In the case of louse-borne typhus isolate the patient at once. Bedding and clothing of the patient and close contacts should be treated with a residual insecticide.

The patient should receive Doxycycline until his temperature settles plus one day. The response is normally prompt.

Whooping cough – pertussis

French: *Coqueluche*   German: *Keuchhusten*   Italian: *Pertosse*   Spanish: Tos *Ferina*

Incubation Period: 7 to 10 days, rarely exceeding 14 days
Period of communicability: 21 days, normally no more than 5 days after antibiotics
Isolation Period: 5 days after antibiotics
Quarantine Period: None

This disease occurs among unvaccinated children; unvaccinated adults may contract it. The disease in adults has no typical features.

Symptoms and signs

The onset occurs as a severe cough which after about 7 to 10 days is marked by a typical 'whoop', with or without vomiting. The whoop is caused by a convulsive series of coughs reaching a point where the patient must take a breath. It is this noisy indrawing of breath which produces the 'whoop'. The coughing bouts may be very distressing.

Treatment

Give erythromycin for 5 days. This is unlikely to affect the course of the disease unless given very early, but it will reduce the infectiousness of the patient.

In children, during the bouts of coughing, feeding may induce vomiting. It is best, therefore, to give light food in between the coughing bout and to keep the child quiet in bed.

Yellow fever

French: *Fièvre jaune*   German: *Gelbfieber*   Italian *Febbra gialla*   Spanish: *Fiebra amarilla*

Incubation Period: 3 to 6 days
Period of communicability: 6 days
Isolation Period: 12 days only if stegomyia mosquitoes are present in the port or on board
Quarantine Period: 6 days

This is a serious and often fatal disease which is caused by a virus transmitted to humans by a mosquito. The disease is endemic in Africa from coast to coast between the south of the Sahara and Kenya, and in parts of the Central and Southern Americas.

Prevention

Travellers to these areas should be inoculated against the disease. Many countries require a valid International Certificate of yellow fever inoculation for those who are going to, or have been in or passed through, such areas. See also the note on prevention of mosquito bites in the section dealing with malaria.

Features of the disease

The severity of the disease differs between patients. In general, from 3 to 6 days after being bitten the patient fluctuates between being shivery and being over hot. He may have a fever as high as 41°C, headache, backache and severe nausea and tenderness in the pit of the stomach. He may seem to get slightly better but then, usually about the fourth day, he becomes very weak and produces vomit tinged with bile and blood (the so-called 'black vomit'). The stomach pains increase and the bowels are constipated. The faeces, if any, are coloured black by digested blood. The eyes become yellow (jaundice) and the mind may wander. After the fifth or sixth day the symptoms may subside and the temperature may fall. The pulse can drop from about 120 per minute to 40 or 50. This period is critical leading to recovery or death. Increasing jaundice and very scanty, or lack of, urine are unfavourable signs. Protein in the urine occurs soon after the start of the illness and the urine should be tested for it.

General treatment

The patient must go to bed and stay in a room free from mosquitoes.
The patient must be encouraged to drink as much as possible, fruit juices are recommended.

The following diseases are transmitted by sexual contact: gonorrhoea, chlamydia infections, chancroid, genital herpes, trichomoniasis, syphilis, chlamydia lymphogranuloma, granuloma inguinale, genital warts, pubic lice, scabies, viral hepatitis B and human immunodeficiency virus,.

Sexually transmitted diseases in sailors are generally acquired through unprotected casual and promiscuous sexual contacts, often with prostitutes.

The most common symptoms of sexually transmitted diseases include discharge, redness and swelling of the genitalia, genital ulcers, lymph node enlargement, warts, and the presence of lice or mites on or in the skin. In some sexually transmitted diseases a single organ is affected. while in others the infection spreads. throughout the body.

Clinical and laboratory facilities are necessary for accurate diagnosis of sexually transmitted diseases. Since such facilities are not likely to be available on board ship, the medical attendant can make only a presumptive diagnosis, based on rough clinical criteria. If the ship is more than one day from port, the medical attendant should start antibiotic treatment immediately when a sailor is thought to be suffering from a sexually transmitted disease. The subjective and objective symptoms, treatment, and response to treatment should be carefully recorded.

On arrival in port, the patient should be referred as soon as possible to a specialist who can perform the appropriate diagnostic tests and, if necessary, give additional treatment.

If possible, all sexual contacts of the patient should be traced and told to seek medical advice.

In case of any doubt concerning diagnosis or treatment, RADIO MEDICAL ADVICE should be obtained.

Urethritis and urethral discharge

Urethritis is characterised by a discharge from the orifice of the urethra, a burning sensation and pain on urination, or an itch at the end of the urethra. Urethritis may be caused by the gonococcus (gonorrhoea) or chlamydia.

Gonococcal urethritis tends to produce more severe symptoms than non-gonococcal urethritis. The incubation time of gonococcal urethritis can range from I to 14 days, but is usually 2–5 days. The discharge is generally abundant, yellow, creamy and purulent.

Non-gonococcal urethritis is generally caused by chlamydia, but in some cases, no causative organism can be found. The discharge in non-gonococcal urethritis is usually scanty, watery, mucoid or serous.

In men, a careful distinction must be made between urethritis and balanitis or posthitis, in which there are secretions from the glans penis and the prepuce (foreskin). Wearing disposable gloves, carefully retract the prepuce to determine the origin of the discharge or secretions.

In women, the same organisms that cause urethritis can cause infection of the cervix of the uterus and the urethra. In more than 60% of women with such infections, there are no visible symptoms. In the remaining cases, the principal sign is an increase in the vaginal discharge (see also Vaginal discharge).

Sexually transmitted diseases

Associated infections

Rectal infection
The organisms that cause urethritis can also infect the rectum. The main symptoms are a discharge of pus, sometimes mixed with blood, and itching around the anus.
Conjunctivitis
Male and female patients with urethritis may also develop an infection of the conjunctivae of the eye.

Treatment

It is not generally possible to make a definitive diagnosis of the cause of urethritis without laboratory facilities. Treatment must therefore be effective for both gonococcal and non-gonococcal infections, and must take account of the facts that the patient may be infected with more than one type of organism, and that some strains of gonococcus are resistant to penicillin. Patients should be given Ciprofloxacin 250 mg as a single and Doxycycline, one 100 mg capsule or tablet twice daily for 7 days.

This treatment should be effective for all urethral and rectal infections. If the patient also has conjunctivitis, 1% tetracycline ointment should be applied to the eye 3 times daily for one week. About one week after completion of treatment, the patient should attend a specialist clinic to verify that he is no longer infected.

Swollen scrotum

A swollen scrotum can be defined as an increase in volume of the scrotal sac, accompanied by oedema and redness. It is sometimes associated with pain (or a history of pain), urethral discharge, and a burning sensation on urination (see Urethritis and urethral discharge). The swelling of the scrotum is usually confined to one side.

Among ships' crews most cases of swollen scrotum are caused by inflammation of the epididymis, produced by sexually transmitted organisms. Such a cause should be strongly suspected in patients with urethral discharge or a recent history of it. The onset of epididymitis is often acute, but in some cases, it may develop over 24–48 hours. There may initially be an 'unusual sensation' in the scrotum, which is rapidly followed by pain and swelling. The pain is of a dragging, aching nature.

This condition must be distinguished from testicular twisting (see testicular pain, Chapter 7). In the latter case, the testis can become non-viable within 4–6 hours of onset of vascular obstruction. This condition occurs most frequently in children and is very rarely observed in adults over the age of 25. The presence of a history of urethritis would exclude the diagnosis. In cases of testicular twisting the testicle is often slightly retracted and elevation of the scrotum does not decrease the pain. This condition needs urgent referral. Other conditions that may lead to scrotal swelling include trauma (injury), inguinal hernia, mumps, and tumours.

Balanitis and posthitis

Balanitis is an inflammation of the glans of the penis, and posthitis is an inflammation of the prepuce. The two conditions may occur simultaneously (balanoposthitis). Lack of good hygiene, in particular in uncircumcised males, is a predisposing factor, as is diabetes mellitus.

In balanitis and balanoposthitis, a mild to profuse superficial secretion may be present. This must be carefully distinguished from urethral discharge. Wearing disposable gloves, retract the prepuce in order to determine the origin of the secretion.

Other signs include itching and irritation, causing considerable discomfort. Sometimes, the penis is swollen and retraction of the prepuce may be painful. Redness, erosion (superficial defects), desquamation of the skin of the prepuce, and secretions of varying aspects and consistency can be observed.

Treatment

The glans of the penis and the prepuce should be washed thoroughly with warm water antiseptic three times daily. Fluconazole 150 mg as a single dose should be given. If there is no improvement within one week, the patient should be referred to a specialist ashore.

Genital ulcers

Genital ulcers are a common reason for consultation, particularly in tropical countries. If not treated appropriately serious complications may arise from some of these conditions. Ulcers may be present in a variety of sexually transmitted diseases, including chancroid, genital herpes, syphilis, chlamydial lymphogranuloma, and granuloma inguinale.

The prevalence of these diseases varies according to geographical area. In Africa and South-East Asia, for instance, chancroid is the most common cause of genital ulcers, whereas in Europe and the USA, herpes genitalis is most common. Chlamydial lymphogranuloma and granuloma inguinale are much less common, and occur mainly in specific areas of the tropics. Chlamydial lymphogranuloma is endemic in West Africa and South-East Asia, while granuloma inguinale is prevalent in east Africa, India, certain parts of Indonesia, Papua New Guinea, and Surinam. Each of these diseases is described in more detail in the following pages.

Patients with one of these diseases usually complain of one or more sores on the genitals or the adjacent area. If the ulcer is located on the glans penis or on the inside of the prepuce, uncircumcised males may complain of penile discharge or of inability to retract the prepuce. In females, ulcers may be situated on the vulva, in which case the patient may complain of a burning sensation on urination.

Disposable gloves should be worn when examining the ulcers. The medical attendant should note the number and the characteristics of the lesions and the presence of lymph node swellings in the groin. Painless, indurated lesions can generally be attributed to syphilis; painful sores that bleed easily are attributable to chancroid; vesicular lesions that develop into superficial erosions or small ulcerations probably indicate herpes infection. Double infections are not uncommon, however, the clinical symptoms are often not sufficiently discriminatory to enable a definite diagnosis to be made without the help of laboratory tests. Knowledge of the relative importance of each disease in the area is crucial for a specific therapeutic approach. The recommended regimen is therefore aimed at curing the most frequently encountered diseases, chancroid and syphilis.

Treatment

Give simultaneously: 2.5 million units of benzylpenicillin, in one dose, intramuscularly and ciprofloxacin 250 mg orally. If the patient is allergic to penicillin, give Doxycycline 100 mg, by mouth, 2 times a day for at least 2 weeks.

When patients with syphilis are treated with penicillin, the so-called Jarisch-Herxheimer reaction may occur (see Syphilis). Bed rest should be advised for patients suffering from very painful genital ulcerations and lymph node swelling, and for those feeling severely ill.

As soon as treatment has started, patients should no longer be regarded as infectious and no special hygienic measures need to be applied. On arrival at the next port patients should be referred to a specialist together with all relevant information concerning their medical history.

Chancroid

Chancroid, almost always acquired during sexual intercourse, is caused by a bacterium. The incubation period (the time following the infecting contact to the initial appearance of symptoms) is short, usually averaging 3–5 days. The lesions are usually only seen in men; in women, clinical lesions are rare, but ulcers may be located in the vagina. The first lesion usually appears as a small inflamed bump, soon forming a blister or pustule, which breaks down within 2–3 days to become a very painful ulcer.

The classic chancroid ulcer (primary lesion) is superficial and shallow, ranging from a few millimetres to 2 cm in diameter. The edge usually appears ragged and is surrounded by a red zone. The base of the ulcer is covered by a necrotic exudate and bleeds easily. In contrast to the syphilitic chancre, the lesion is soft, and extremely painful and tender.

In males the most frequent sites of infection are the inner and outer side of the prepuce and the groove separating the head from the shaft of the penis.

About 1~2 weeks after the appearance of the primary lesion, the glands in the groin become enlarged, painful, and tender (buboes) (see Lymph node swelling, and Lymphatic inflammation, Chapter 7). At first, the swellings appear hard and matted together, but they soon become painful and red. Some time later, the lymph nodes may enlarge, become fluctuant, and discharge pus.

Treatment

Give the patient Doxycycline 100 mg 2 times daily for 7 days. If the buboes persist or become fluctuant, RADIO MEDICAL ADVICE should be sought.

Genital herpes

Genital herpes is caused by a virus; the disease can follow an asymptomatic course, the virus being harboured within the nerves to the skin without producing symptoms. Usually, however, genital herpes in men appears as a number of small vesicles on the penis, scrotum, thighs, or buttocks. The fluid-filled blisters are usually painful, but sometimes produce only a tingling sensation. Within a day or two the blisters break, leaving tiny open sores which take 1–3 weeks to heal. Lymph glands near the site of infection may react by becoming swollen and tender.

In most cases, a clinical diagnosis can be made on the basis of the appearance of the lesions, in particular at the blister stage. At specialised clinics, laboratory tests may be used to confirm the diagnosis.

After the sores are healed, the virus remains dormant in the body. Weeks or months later, there may be recurrence of the active infection. These recurrent attacks tend to become less frequent with time and to be less severe than the initial attack, and the lesions tend to heal more quickly.

Treatment

A definite cure for genital herpes is not yet available. Lesions should be kept clean by washing the affected sites with soap and water, followed by careful drying. Analgesics may be given to reduce discomfort.

If you are in any doubt about whether the diagnosis of genital herpes is correct, the patient should be managed as described under Genital ulcers.

Syphilis

Syphilis is caused by a spirochaete which enters the body through the mucous membranes of the genitals, rectum, or mouth, or through small cuts or abrasions in ordinary skin.

The clinical course of syphilis is usually divided into three stages. The lesions of the primary and secondary stages are usually painless and cause little disability. They may heal without treatment, and the disease can lie dormant in the body for several years. In the late stages syphilis can cause serious damage to the brain, spinal cord, heart, and other organs.

The first stage, primary syphilis, is characterised by the presence of a sore (or chancre) at the point where the spirochaetes enter the body. There is a delay of 10–90 days (average 3 weeks) after contact before the onset of any visible sign of infection. Following the appearance of the initial chancre, there can be an additional delay of a few weeks before the blood test for syphilis will become positive. The typical chancre occurs in the groove separating the head from the shaft of the penis. However, a chancre may occur anywhere on the body where there has been contact with an infected lesion. Such lesions are usually single, but there may be more than one. The primary chancres are often smooth and clean-looking on the surface. Sometimes the lesion ulcerates and leaves a reddish sore with the base of the ulcer covered by a yellow or greyish exudate. Unless there is also infection with other bacteria or with herpes virus, the ulcer will be painless. The lesion has a characteristic firmness (like cartilage) when felt between the thumb and forefinger (gloves must be worn)

Often there will be one or more rubbery, hard, painless, enlarged lymph nodes in one or both groins, or in other regions if the sore is not on the genitals. In the presence of a secondary infection, the nodes may be tender. Usually these lesions will heal spontaneously within 6 weeks. At the chancre stage, the patient is highly contagious

The secondary stage of syphilis usually develops about 6–8 weeks after the appearance of the primary chancre. In fact, the primary syphilitic chancre may still be present at the time of onset of the secondary stage. However, the secondary stage may be the first manifestation, occurring some 10–14 weeks after the infected contact. The most consistent feature of secondary syphilis is a non-itching skin rash, which may be generalised in the form of small, flat or slightly elevated pink spots, which gradually darken to become dark red in colour. They may be particularly localised on the palms, soles, or genital areas. A less frequently encountered sign is patchy loss of scalp hair. Patients with secondary syphilis may complain of malaise (not feeling well), headache, sore throat, and a low-grade fever (38.5 C). The presence of these symptoms plus a generalised rash and/or a rash involving the palms and the soles, which does not itch, and is associated with enlarged small lymph nodes in the neck, armpits and groins, should arouse suspicion of secondary syphilis. Other signs of the secondary stage may be the occurrence of moist sores, particularly in the genital area, or of flat, moist warts in the anogenital region. It should be noted that moist lesions of secondary syphilis are teeming with spirochaetes and are thus highly infectious. In the untreated patient the diagnosis is confirmed by microscopic examination of the lesions and by a blood test for syphilis.

The symptoms of the secondary stage will eventually disappear without treatment. The disease then enters the latent (hiding) phase, before reappearing as tertiary syphilis many years later.

Treatment

Patients with suspected syphilis should be given 2.5 million units of benzylpenicillin in a single dose, administered intramuscularly. If the patient is allergic to penicillin, give either 100 mg of Doxycycline by mouth, 2 times a day for 14 days or 500 mg of erythromycin by mouth, 4 times a day for 14 days. The patient should be referred to a specialist clinic at the next port of call.

Caution. When treated with antibiotics, about 50% of patients with primary or secondary syphilis will develop the so-called Jarisch-Herxheimer reaction, which usually appears 6–12 hours after the injection. This reaction is characterised by fever, chills, joint pain, increased swelling of the primary lesions, or increased prominence of the secondary rash. It is caused by the sudden destruction of a great number of spirochaetes and should not give rise to alarm. Analgesics may help to reduce the symptoms.

Chlamydial lymphogranuloma

Chlamydial lymphogranuloma is a systemic disease of venereal origin. The incubation time ranges from 4 to 21 days. The primary lesion is usually an ulcer, a vesicle, a papule or a pustule, not more than 5–6 mm in size and often located on the groove on the head of the penis in the male patient. Commonly single, the lesion is painless, transient, and heals in a few days without scar formation. in most cases, the patient does not even notice this primary ulcerative lesion. After the lesion has healed, the commonest symptom in heterosexual men is acute swelling of the lymph nodes in the groin, often on one side only. The swelling starts as a firm hard mass, which is not very painful, and usually involves several groups of lymph nodes. Within 1–2 weeks, the glandular mass (bubo) becomes attached to the skin and subcutaneous tissue and painful fluctuation occurs, followed by formation of pus. Not all buboes become fluctuant, some evolve into firm masses. Perforation of a bubo may occur, whereupon pus of varying aspect and consistency will be discharged. If not treated, chlamydial lymphogranuloma can produce severe scarring in the urogenital and rectal regions.

Treatment

Rest in bed is recommended for patients with chlamydial lymphogranuloma. An ice-bag may be applied to the inguinal region for the first two or three days of treatment to help relieve local discomfort and tenderness.

The patient should be given 100 mg of Doxycycline by mouth, twice daily for at least 2 weeks or 500 mg of erythromycin by mouth, 4 times daily, for at least 2 weeks. Fluctuating buboes require aspiration. If the bubo persists, RADIO MEDICAL ADVICE should be sought.

Granuloma inguinale

Granuloma inguinale is an infectious bacterial disease, with insidious onset. The sites usually affected are the genitals, the groin, the upper legs next to the groin, and the perianal and oral regions. The incubation period ranges from 17 to 50 days.

The earliest cutaneous lesion may be a papule or a nodule, which ulcerates, producing a single, enlarging, beef-like, velvety ulcer, or a coalescence of several ulcers. The typical ulcer in this disease is a raised mass, looking more like a growth than an ulcer. It has a smooth, elevated edge, sharply demarcated from the surrounding skin. There is no lymph node swelling and the general health of the patient is good. If not treated, the lesions may extend to adjacent areas of the body.

The diagnosis can usually be made on the basis of the typical clinical picture. At specialised clinics microscopic examination of crushed tissue smears is used to confirm the diagnosis in the untreated patient.

Treatment

The patient should be given Doxycycline 100 mg 2 times a day for at least 2 weeks. The patient should be referred to a specialist clinic at the next port of call.

Lymph node swelling

Lymph node swelling is the enlargement of already existing lymph nodes. It is unusual for lymph node swelling to be the sole manifestation of a sexually transmitted disease. In most cases, inguinal lymph gland swelling is accompanied by genital ulcers, infection of the lower limbs, or, in a minority of cases, severe urethritis. The swelling may be accompanied by pain and may be on one or both sides. Pain and/or fluctuation can sometimes be evoked by palpation.

The lymph node swelling may be regional (for instance in the groin in the presence of genital ulcers, etc.) or may involve more than one region (for instance in the case of secondary syphilis or human immunodeficiency virus infection).

The prepuce of patients suffering from lymph node swelling should always be retracted during examination in order to detect genital ulcers or scars of genital ulcers.

Treatment

The patient should be treated as described under Genital ulcers. If no improvement is noted within one week, RADIO MEDICAL ADVICE should be obtained.

Vaginal discharge

Sexually transmitted diseases in women often produce an increase in the amount, or a change in the colour or odour, of vaginal secretions. Vaginal discharge is probably the most common gynaecological complaint. It may be accompanied by itching, genital swelling, a burning sensation on urination, and lower abdominal or back pain.

Various infections can produce such symptoms.

Trichomoniasis is a common disease, particularly in tropical areas. It is characterised by a sometimes foul-smelling, yellow, or green foamy discharge.

Vaginal candidiasis is also a very common disease throughout the world. It is characterised by a white, curd-like discharge, vulvar itching, and sometimes a red and swollen vulva and vagina.

Bacterial vaginosis is very common. In general, there is no itch. The typical discharge is a grey sometimes foamy, fishy-smelling paste.

Other infections, e.g., gonorrhoea, may produce a white or yellow, watery or purulent discharge.

Infection with herpes virus usually produces painful lesions (redness, blisters, ulcers) on the vulva.

It should be remembered that more than one infection may be present at a time.

Treatment

In a situation without gynaecological examination facilities and in the absence of laboratory equipment the following practical approach should be followed. First the patient should be treated for trichomoniasis and/or bacterial vaginosis (treatment A). If the condition does not improve, this treatment should be followed by an anti-gonococcal and anti-chlamydial treatment regimen (treatment B). If the symptoms still persist, an anti-candidiasis treatment (treatment C) should follow, or the patient should be referred to a specialist at the next port of call.

Treatment A

Give metronidazole 2.0 g, by mouth, in a single dose.

Treatment B

Give Doxycycline 100 mg , by mouth, 2 times a day for 7 days.

Treatment C

Fluconazole 150 mg, by mouth as a single dose.

Pelvic Inflammatory disease – Salpingitis

Pelvic inflammatory disease is a general expression covering various pelvic infections in women, caused by micro-organisms, which generally ascend from the lower genital tract (vagina, cervix) and invade the mucosal surface of the uterus, the fallopian tubes, and the peritoneum.

Pelvic inflammatory disease, caused by sexually transmitted pathogens, is a major cause of infertility and chronic abdominal pain, and may result in ectopic pregnancy. A vigorous approach to treatment is therefore justified.

The symptoms include mild to severe lower abdominal pain on one or both sides associated with fever and vaginal discharge (see Vaginal discharge).

The use of an intra-uterine (coil) device may be associated with the development of pelvic inflammatory disease. It should be noted that it is difficult to diagnose pelvic inflammatory disease without appropriate gynaecological and laboratory investigations; moreover, it is difficult to differentiate this disease from other causes of acute abdominal pain, e.g., appendicitis.

Treatment

In a case of suspected pelvic inflammatory disease, RADIO MEDICAL ADVICE should be obtained.

The treatment is Doxycycline, 100 mg twice daily for 14 days in combination with metronidazole, 1.0 g, by mouth, twice daily, for 14 days.

Caution. Patients should abstain from alcohol during treatment.

Genital warts

Genital warts are caused by a virus, and occur most frequently in young adults. In male patients, warts may be present on the penis, around the anus, and in the rectum. In females, the usual sites of infection are the vulva, the area surrounding the anus, and the vagina. Warts are soft, flesh-coloured, broad-based or pedunculated lesions of variable size. They may occur singly, or several may coalesce to form a large mass, often with a cauliflower-like appearance. Small warts cause little discomfort, but large genital or anal warts are embarrassing and uncomfortable to the patient and are liable to ulcerate; secondary infection and bleeding may then occur. Diagnosis is usually made on clinical grounds.

Treatment

There is no appropriate treatment that can be given on board ship. The patient should be referred to a specialised clinic at the next port of call.

Pubic lice

Pubic lice are nearly always sexually transmitted. The infection has become endemic in many countries, usually affecting young adults. The main symptom is moderate to severe itching. leading to scratching, redness, irritation and inflammation. The lice may be observed as small brown spots in the groin and around the genitals and anus. The nits attached to the hairs may be seen with the aid of a magnifying glass.

Treatment

Lindane cream, 1%, should be applied to the affected areas (pubic area, groin, and perianal region) at 8–hour intervals over a period of 24 hours. The patient should take a shower immediately before each application. At the end of the 24–hour period, the patient should again shower, and put on clean clothes.

Scabies

Scabies, caused by a mite, is now recognised as a sexually transmitted disease in industrialised countries. The most common symptom is itching, particularly at night. The lesions are roughly symmetrical.

The usual sites of infection are the finger webs, sides of the fingers, wrists, elbows, axillary folds, around the female breasts, around the umbilicus, the penis, the scrotum, buttocks and the upper part of the back of the thighs.

With the naked eye, only papules, excoriations and crusts may be seen. Using a magnifying glass, it is possible to detect the burrows of the mites.

Diagnosis is usually made on the basis of the clinical picture. At specialised clinics microscopic examination of skin samples can be performed, to detect the female scabies mite and her eggs.

Treatment

A thin layer of lindane cream, 1%, should be applied to the entire trunk and extremities and left for 8–12 hours. At the end of this period. the patient should take a shower or a bath, and change his clothes and bed linen.

Human Immunodeficiency Virus (HIV)

HIV infection is an increasing cause of premature death in both the developed and developing world. In the majority of cases spread is by sexual contact. HIV infects the white cells responsible for immunity to disease and as the infection develops so the patient's immunity to infection decreases and they become increasingly vulnerable to life-threatening infections. There are effective drugs which can slow down the progression of the disease very considerably. These drugs are expensive and only available to a small minority of patients. The majority of HIV infected patients in the developing world will not survive more than 5 years. HIV infection was originally called AIDS (acquired immune deficiency syndrome) because of the characteristic pattern of infections which developed in the first patients observed. This term is now of limited use as the original description of the disease bares little resemblance to the disease as it now exists outside the developed world.

HIV is present in the majority of the body fluids of an infected person. Nearly all infections result from contact with semen, vaginal secretions, blood or blood products. HIV is not transmitted through normal social contact, including kissing. All those with HIV infection should be regarded as infectious, whether or not they have symptoms of the disease.

Within a few weeks of infection the patient may experience a glandular fever like illness. Often this goes unnoticed, but occasionally the patient may be seriously unwell. At this point the HIV antibody test becomes positive. Following this the patient may be perfectly well for several years before developing serious infections. The first signs of HIV disease depend upon the exposure of the patient to infectious diseases. In poorer countries, where standards of housing and hygiene are low, patients will present, within 2 to 3 years, with diarrhoea, chest infections including tuberculosis and septicaemia. The patients have often lost a lot of weight and complain of fevers and tiredness. In developed countries patient may go many years before presenting with pneumonia, unusual skin cancers, meningitis and malignant tumours.

Treatment

Nearly all the infections that cause illness in patients with HIV can be treated with antibiotics. It is only the diseases that occur late on in HIV infection that require more complicated and expensive treatments. These diseases all require laboratory tests to make the diagnosis. Several drugs are effective at limiting the development of HIV and these have dramatically altered the natural course of the disease which usual ended in death within 10 years. The use of these drugs requires frequent monitoring of the HIV infection.

Prevention

There is no vaccine available. Appropriate anti-viral therapy can prevent the spread of disease from mother to baby. It can also reduce the chance of infection following a needlestick injury. The most common way in which infection is spread is by sexual contact. Many prostitutes in the developing countries of Asia and Africa are HIV positive. Unprotected sexual intercourse with one of these prostitutes carries a very considerable risk of HIV transmission. The risk of transmission is greatly increased if either partner has another sexually transmitted disease, particularly genital ulcers. One way of reducing HIV transmission is to detect and treat sexually transmitted diseases. Barrier contraceptives and spermicides provide very considerable protection to HIV infection, but are not foolproof.

Proctitis

Proctitis is an infection of the rectum, often caused by sexually transmitted pathogens. In symptomatic infections, a discharge of pus from the anus, sometimes mixed with blood, can be observed. Itching around the anus may be present.

In females, proctitis is usually due to a secondary infection with vaginal discharge containing gonococci (see Vaginal discharge and Rectal infection). In male homosexuals, proctitis is caused by anal sexual contact with an infected person.

Treatment

Patients should be treated according to the regimens outlined for urethritis and urethral discharge. If there is no response to treatment within one week, RADIO MEDICAL ADVICE should be obtained.

Treatment centres at ports

Many ports have one or more specialist centres, where seafarers can obtain treatment for sexually transmitted diseases. Where they exist, these centres should be used in preference to the services of a general practitioner, since they have ready access to the necessary laboratory facilities, and experience of dealing with a large number of cases of sexually transmitted disease.

The clinic staff will advise on any further treatment and tests that may be necessary. A personal booklet is given to the seaman, in which is recorded the diagnosis (in code) and the treatment given, and which he should take with him if he visits a clinic in another port.

Instructions for medical attendants

The medical attendant should wear disposable gloves when examining any infected site in patients suspected of suffering from sexually transmitted disease. If the attendant accidentally touches any genital ulcer or discharge, or any material contaminated with pus from ulcers or discharge, he should immediately wash his hands thoroughly with soap and water.

If there is a sore on the penis or discharge from the urethra, a clean gauze dressing should be kept on the penis. This dressing should be changed frequently. In female patients suffering from genital ulcers or vaginal discharge, gauze or sanitary pads should be used.

Contaminated materials should be discarded in plastic bags, so that they will not be touched or handled by others.

Instructions for patients

The patient should avoid all sexual contact until a medical specialist confirms that he is free from infection. He should also make a special effort to practice good personal hygiene; for instance, he should use only his own toilet articles (toothbrush, razor, towels, washcloth etc.) and his own clothes and linen.

During the examination and treatment, the opportunity should be taken to inform the patient about his condition, sexually transmitted diseases in general, and the precautions to be taken to minimise the risk of acquiring them (see below).

Prevention of sexually transmitted disease

Being outside their normal environment and often in circumstances that allow for promiscuity, sailors are at special risk of contracting sexually transmitted diseases.

Avoidance of casual and promiscuous sexual contacts is the best way of minimising the risk of infection. Failing this, a mechanical barrier, such as a condom, can give both heterosexual and homosexual men and women a certain degree of protection against a number of sexually transmitted diseases. A supply of condoms should be available on board ship. The condom or rubber, is a thin elastic covering that forms a protective sheath over the penis. If properly used, it should prevent infection during intercourse, unless the point of contact with an infected lesion is beyond the area covered by the condom The condom comes rolled before use. It must be placed over the penis before sexual contact. The tip of the condom should be held to form a pocket to receive the ejaculate and the rest of the condom unrolled to cover the entire penis. As soon as the male has had an orgasm, the penis should be withdrawn from the vagina before it softens, because loosening of the condom may expose the penis to infection. The condom is removed by grasping the open end with the fingers and pulling it down quickly so that it comes off inside out. The condom should be discarded without further handling in case it contains infectious material.

In women, the use of a diaphragm in combination with a spermicide cream offers some protection against the acquisition of some sexually transmitted diseases; however, condoms offer better protection. In risk situations, both partners should urinate at once after possible exposure. Each partner should subsequently wash his or her genitals and other possible infected areas.

CARDIOVASCULAR SYSTEM – HEART AND BLOOD VESSELS

Chest (heart) pain

High blood pressure – hypertension

Varicose veins

RESPIRATORY SYSTEM – CHEST AND BREATHING

Asthma

Bronchitis

Chest pain

Pleurisy

Pleurodynia

Pneumonia – lobar pneumonia

Pneumothorax

ABDOMINAL SYSTEM – GASTRO-INTESTINAL TRACT

Abdominal pain

Anal fissure

Anal itching (anal pruritus)

Appendicitis

Biliary colic (gallstone colic)

Cholecystitis (inflammation of the gall bladder)

Diarrhoea

Haemorrhoids (piles)

Hernia (rupture)

Intestinal colic

Jaundice

Peritonitis

Ulcers (peptic ulceration)

Worms

GENITO-URINARY SYSTEM

Paraphimosis

Testicular pain

Urinary problems

BRAIN AND NERVOUS SYSTEM

Mental illness

Neuralgia

Paralysis

Strokes

HEAD AND NECK

Ears

Eyes

Headache

Sinusitis

Teeth and gums

Throat

LOCOMOTOR SYSTEM – MUSCLES AND BONES

Backache

Gout – gouty arthritis

Rheumatism

SKIN AND SUPERFICIAL TISSUES

Bites and stings

Boils, abscesses and carbuncles

Cellulitis

Hand infections

Skin disease

GENERALISED ILLNESSES

Alcohol abuse

Allergy

Anaemia

Colds

Diabetes

Drug abuse

Hayfever

High temperature

Lymphatic inflammation

Oedema

Sea sickness

Other diseases and medical problems

CARDIOVASCULAR SYSTEM – HEART AND BLOOD VESSELS

Chest (Heart) pain

With any suspected heart pain get RADIO MEDICAL ADVICE.

When the calibre of the coronary arteries becomes narrowed by degenerative change, insufficient blood is supplied to the heart and, consequently, it works less efficiently. The heart may then be unable to meet demands for extra work beyond a certain level and whenever that level is exceeded, attacks of heart pain (angina) occur. This can be compared to a 'stitch' of the heart muscle. Between episodes of angina the patient may feel well.

Any diseased coronary artery is liable to get blocked by a blood clot. If that blockage occurs the blood supply to a localised part of the heart muscle is shut off and a heart attack (coronary thrombosis) occurs.

Angina (Angina Pectoris)

Angina usually affects those of middle age and upward. The pain varies from patient to patient in frequency of occurrence, type and severity. It is most often brought on by physical exertion (angina of effort) although strong emotion, a large meal or cold conditions may be additional factors. The pain appears suddenly and it reaches maximum intensity rapidly before ending after two or three minutes. During an attack the sufferer has an anxious expression, pale or grey face and may break out in a cold sweat. He is immobile and will never walk about. Bending forward with a hand pressed to the chest is a frequent posture. Breathing is constrained by pain but there is no true shortness of breath.

During the attack the patient will describe a crushing or constricting pain or sensation felt behind the breast bone. The sensation may feel as if the chest were compressed in a vice and it may spread to the throat, to the lower jaw, down the inside of one or both arms – usually the left – and maybe downwards to the upper part of the abdomen.

Once the disease is established attacks usually occur with gradually increasing frequency and severity.

General treatment

During an attack the patient should remain in whatever position he finds most comfortable. Afterwards he should rest. He should take light meals and avoid alcohol, tobacco and exposure to cold. He should limit physical exertion and attempt to maintain a calm state of mind.

Specific treatment

Pain can be relieved by sucking (not swallowing) a tablet of glyceryl trinitrate 0.5 mg or using the metered dose spray. The tablet should be allowed to dissolve slowly or the spray directed under the tongue. These tablets can be used as often as necessary and are best taken when the patient gets any symptoms indicating a possible attack of angina. Tell the patient to remove any piece of the tablet which may be left when the pain has subsided since glyceryl trinitrate can cause a throbbing headache. The glyceryl trinitrate 0.5 mg may also be taken before any activity which is known to induce an angina attack.

If the patient is emotional or tense and anxious, give him diazepam 5 mg three times daily during waking hours, and if sleepless 10 mg at bed time. The patient should continue to rest and take the above drugs as needed until he sees a doctor at the next port.

WARNING: Sometimes angina appears abruptly and without exertion or emotion even when the person is resting. This form of angina is often due to a threatened or very small coronary thrombosis (see below), and should be treated as such, as should any attack of anginal pain lasting for longer than 10 minutes.

Coronary thrombosis (myocardial infarction)

A heart attack happens suddenly and while the patient is at rest more frequently than during activity. *The four main features are pain of similar distribution to that in angina, shortness of breath, vomiting and degree of collapse which may be severe.* The pain varies in degree from mild to agonising but it is usually severe. The patient is often very restless and tries unsuccessfully to find a position which might ease the pain. Shortness of breath may be severe and the skin is often grey with a blue tinge, cold and covered in sweat. Vomiting is common in the early stage and may increase the state of collapse.

In mild attacks the only symptom may be a continuing anginal type of pain with perhaps slight nausea. It is not unusual for the patient to believe mistakenly that he is suffering from a sudden attack of severe indigestion.

General treatment

The patient must rest at once, preferably in bed, in whatever position is most comfortable until he can be taken to hospital. Exertion of any kind must be forbidden and the nursing attention for complete bed rest carried out. Restlessness is often a prominent feature which is usually manageable if adequate pain relief is given. Most patients prefer to lie back propped up by pillows but some prefer to lean forward in a sitting position to assist breathing. A temperature, pulse and respiration chart should be kept at ½ hourly intervals. Smoking and alcohol should be forbidden.

Specific treatment

If available, give one Aspirin tablet (150–300mg) by mouth. Oxygen should be given, in as high a flow rate as possible. Whatever the severity of the attack it is best to give all cases an initial dose of morphine 10 – 15 mg and an anti-emetic at once. In a mild attack it may then be possible to control pain by giving codeine 60 mg every 4 to 6 hours. If the patient is anxious or tense, in addition give diazepam 5 mg three times a day until he can be placed under medical supervision. In serious or moderate attacks, give morphine 15 mg with an anti-emetic three to four hours after the initial injection. The injection may be repeated every four to six hours as required to obtain pain relief. Get RADIO MEDICAL ADVICE.

Specific problems in heart attacks

If the pulse rate is less than 60 per minute get RADIO MEDICAL ADVICE.
If the heart stops beating get the patient onto a hard flat surface and give chest compression and artificial respiration at once.
If there is obvious breathlessness the patient should sit up. If this problem is associated with noisy, wet breathing and coughing give frusemide 40 mg intramuscularly, restrict the fluids, start a fluid balance chart and get RADIO MEDICAL ADVICE.

Paroxysmal tachycardia

This is a condition which comes in bouts (paroxysms) during which the heart beats very rapidly. The patient will complain of a palpitating, or fluttering or pounding feeling in the chest or throat. He may look pale and anxious and he may feel sick, light-headed or faint. The attack starts suddenly and passes off after several minutes or several hours just as suddenly. If the attack lasts for a few hours the patient may pass large amounts of urine. The pulse will be difficult to feel because of the palpitations, so listen over the left side of the chest between the nipple and the breast bone and count the heart rate in this way. The rate may reach 160 – 180 beats or more per minute.

General treatment

The patient should rest in the position he finds most comfortable. Reassure him that the attack will pass off. Sometimes an attack will pass off if he takes and holds a few very deep breaths or if he makes a few deep grunting exhalations. If this fails, give him a glass of ice cold water to drink.

Specific treatment

If these measures do not stop an attack, give diazepam 5 mg. Check the heart rate every quarter of an hour. If the attack is continuing get RADIO MEDICAL ADVICE.

Chest pain – associated signs

Diagram number	Position and type of pain	Age group	Onset	Breathless	General condition	Blue lips and ears	Pale colour
1	Behind breast bone – down left arm, up into jaw or down into abdomen. Constricting.	Middle age and upward	Sudden, usually after effort	No	Looks ill and anxious	No	Yes
2	Behind breast bone, up into jaw, down into abdomen. Down either arm, usually left. Crushing.	Middle age and upward. Can occur in younger people	Sudden often at rest	Yes (severe)	Looks very ill. Collapsed. Restless. Vomiting	Often	Yes
3	Burning sensation up behind the whole of breast bone.	Any	May follow mild indigestion	No	Good. May vomit	No	Not usually
4	Along line of ribs on one side. Aching.	Any but more likely in older people	Slow	No	Good	No	No
5	Any part of rib cage. Sharp stabbing. Worse on breathing and coughing.	Any	Sudden	Slight	Good	No	No
5	Any part of rib cage. Sharp stabbing. Worse on breathing and coughing.	Any	Gradual or sudden. Often follows a cold	Yes	Looks very ill. Flushed	Yes	No
6	Pain passes from right abdomen through to shoulder blade and to tip of right shoulder.	Usually middle aged	Slow	No	Ill, sometimes flushed. Vomiting	No	Not normally
6	Same distribution as for cholecystitis. Agonising colicky pain.	Any, often middle aged	Sudden	Yes when spasms are present	Ill, restless. Nausea and vomiting	No	Yes
7	Any part of rib cage. Sharp pain.	Any	Sudden	Yes	Good at first	Later	Yes
7	At site of injury. Sharp stabbing made worse by breathing.	Any	Sudden	No	Normally good, but may be shocked	No	Yes (when shocked)
8	Any part, often in back. Dull aching.	Any	Slow	No	Good	No	No
8	Any part of rib cage. Continuous ache made worse by breathing.	Any	Sudden	No	Good	No	No

Sweating	Temperature	Pulse rate/min	Respiration rate/min	Tenderness	Additional information	PROBABLE CAUSE OF PAIN
Yes	Normal	Normal	18	Nil	Can be brought on by effort, eating a large meal, and by cold or strong emotion. Passes off in two to three minutes on resting. Patient does not speak during an attack.	**Angina page 128)**
Yes	Normal	Raised 60–120	Increased 24+	Nil	Pulse may be irregular – heart may stop.	**Coronary Thrombosis (page 128)**
No	Normal	Normal	18	Nil	Patient may notice acid in mouth.	**Heartburn (see Peptic ulcer) (page 150)**
No	Usually normal	Normal	Normal	Often between ribs in affected segment	Small spots similar to those of chickenpox appear along affected segment. Breathing will be painful. May affect other parts of the body.	**Shingles (page 178)**
No	Elevated 37.8°C – 39.4°C (100–103°F)	Raised 100–120	Increased 24	Nil	May be the first sign of pneumonia.	**Pleurisy (page 135)**
Yes	Elevated 39.4°C – 40.6°C (103–105°F)	Raised 110–130	Greatly increased 30–50	Nil	Dry persistent cough at first, then sputum becomes 'rusty'.	**Pneumonia (page 136)**
No	Elevated up to 30°C (101°F)	Raised to 110	Slightly increased 18	Over gall bladder area	Note that pain in the right shoulder tip may result from other abdominal conditions causing irritation of the diaphragm.	**Cholecystitis (page 145)**
Yes	Usually normal	Raised 72–110	Increased up to 24 or more during spasms	Over gall bladder area		**Biliary colic (page 145)**
No	Normal	Raised 72–100	Increased 18–30	Nil	May be caused by penetrating wound of chest or occur spontaneously. Symptoms and signs depend on the amount of air in the pleural cavity. The affected side moves less than the normal side.	**Pneumothorax (page 137)**
Only if shocked	Normal	Raised if shocked	Increased	At affected area	Fractured ribs may penetrate lung. Look for bright red frothy sputum and pneumothorax.	**Fracture of the rib (page 38)**
No	Normal	Normal	Normal	At affected areas	'Nodules' may be felt. Common site around the upper part of the back.	**Muscular rheumatism (page 169)**
No	Normal	Normal	Normal	At affected areas	Do not confuse with pleurisy.	**Pleurodynia (page 136)**

High blood pressure – hypertension

As blood is pumped by the heart, it exerts a pressure on the walls of the arteries. This pressure, blood pressure, varies within normal limits. During activity it tends to be higher; during sleep, lower. It also shows a tendency to be slightly higher in older people.

The blood pressure is temporarily raised when a person is exposed to anxiety, fear or excitement, but it reverts rapidly to normal when the causal factor is removed. It is more permanently raised when the artery walls are hardened or otherwise unhealthy, in kidney disease, and in long standing overweight. In respect of the latter, an improvement in blood pressure can often be achieved by a reduction in weight.

The onset of high blood pressure is usually slow. The early symptoms may include headaches, tiredness, vague ill-health and lassitude. However, high blood pressure is more often found in people who have no symptoms, and a sure diagnosis is only possible with a sphygmomanometer. A patient with suspected high blood pressure should be referred for a medical opinion at the next port.

If the degree of hypertension is more severe, then the symptoms of headache, tiredness and irritability become more common and there may be nose bleeding, visual disturbances and anginal pain. Occasionally, however, the first sign of hypertension is the onset of the complications such as stroke, breathlessness (through fluid retention in the lungs), heart failure or kidney failure. You should check for the latter by looking for oedema , (water retention in the legs) and testing the urine for protein.

Treatment

Temporary hypertension, due to anxiety, should be treated by reducing any emotional or stress problems which exist, as outlined under mental illness. Anyone thought to be suffering from severe hypertension, or who gives a history of previous similar trouble, should be kept at rest, put on a diet without added salt, and given diazepam 5 mg three times daily until he can be referred for a medical opinion ashore.

Persons suffering from a degree of hypertension which requires continuous medication are not suitable for service at sea.

Varicose veins

Veins have thin walls which are easily distended by increased pressure within the venous system. When pressure is sustained, a localised group of veins may become enlarged and have a knotted appearance in a winding rather than straight course. Such changes, which usually take place slowly over a period of years, commonly affect the veins of the lower leg and foot and those in the back passage (piles). The surrounding tissues often become waterlogged by seepage of fluid from the blood in the engorged veins (oedema). Gravity encourages the fluid to gather in the tissues closest to the ground.

When the leg veins are affected, there are no symptoms at first but, later, aching and tiredness of the leg invariably appear with some swelling (oedema) of the foot and lower leg towards evening.

General treatment

In most cases the patient is able to continue to work, provided the veins are supported by a crepe bandage during the daytime. This should be applied firmly from the foot to below the knee on getting up in the morning.

After work the swelling may be reduced by sitting with the leg straightened, resting on a cushion or pillow and raised to at least hip level. Swelling is usually considerably reduced after the night's rest. If swelling is persistent and troublesome, bed rest may be indicated. The patient should be seen by a doctor when convenient.

A bleeding varicose vein

Varicose veins are particularly prone to bleed either internally or externally if knocked or scraped accidentally. The leg should be raised then a sterile dressing should be applied to the affected place and secured in position by a bandage. Varicose veins are prone to inflammation (phlebitis see below), so it is best for the patient to remain in bed with the leg elevated for several days.

Phlebitis

Inflammation of a vein (phlebitis) with accompanying clotting of the blood within the affected vein is a common complication of varicosity. The superficial veins or the veins deep within the leg may be affected and more often those of the calf than the thigh.

In superficial inflammation the skin covering a length of vein becomes red, hot and painful and it is hard to the touch. Some localised swelling is usually present and sometimes the leg may be generally swollen below the inflammation. A fever may be present and the patient may feel unwell. Inflammation of a deep vein is much less frequent but it has more serious consequences. In such cases there are no superficial signs but the whole leg may be swollen and a diffuse aching will be present.

General treatment

In all cases of deep vein phlebitis, the patient should be confined to bed and the affected leg should be kept completely at rest. A bed-cradle should be used. Bed rest should continue until the patient is seen by a doctor at the next port.

Mild cases of superficial phlebitis need not be put to bed. The affected leg should be supported by a crepe bandage applied from the foot to below the knee. Swelling of the leg should be treated by sitting with the leg elevated and supported on a pillow after working hours. Anti-inflammatories such as Diclofenac may be useful.

Cases of more extensive superficial phlebitis may require bed rest if the symptoms are troublesome or if feverish.

Varicose ulcer

When varicose veins have been present for a number of years the skin of the lower leg often becomes affected by the poor circulation. It has the appearance of being thin and dry with itchy red patches near the varicosity. Slight knocks or scratching may then lead to the development of ulceration, which invariably becomes septic.

General treatment

The patient should be nursed in bed with the leg elevated on pillows to reduce any swelling. The ulcer should be bathed daily using gauze soaked in antiseptic solution. A paraffin gauze dressing, covered by a dry dressing thick enough to absorb the purulent discharge, should be applied under a bandage after the bathing. Varicose ulcers are often slow to heal and the patient should see a doctor at the next port.

RESPIRATORY SYSTEM – CHEST AND BREATHING

Asthma

Asthma is a complaint in which the patient suffers from periodic attacks of difficulty in breathing out and a feeling of tightness in the chest, during which time he wheezes and feels as if he is suffocating. The causes of asthma are unknown but there is abnormal airway sensitivity to irritants. These may be:

- inhaled, e.g., dust, acrid fumes, solvents or simply cold air, *or*

- ingested, e.g., shellfish or eggs;

- acute anxiety;

- certain chest diseases, e.g. chronic bronchitis, acute viral or bacterial chest infection.

Asthma may begin at any age. There is usually a previous history of attacks which have occurred from time to time in the patient's life.

The onset of an attack may be slow and preceded by a feeling of tightness in the chest, or it may occur suddenly. Sometimes the attack occurs at night after the patient has been lying flat particularly at 0400 when the body's natural steroids are at their lowest.

In the event of a severe attack, the patient is in a state of alarm and distress, unable to breathe properly, and with a sense of weight and tightness around the chest. He can fill up his chest with air but finds great difficulty in breathing out, and his efforts are accompanied by coughing and wheezing noises due to narrowing of the air tubes within his lungs. His distress increases rapidly in severe cases and he sits or stands, as near as possible to a source of fresh air, with his head thrown back and his whole body heaving with desperate efforts to breathe. His lips and face, at first pale, may become tinged blue and covered with sweat, while his hands and feet become cold. His pulse is rapid and weak, and may be irregular. Fortunately, less severe attacks, without such great distress, are more common. He may only manage short sentences or odd words in a staccato fashion.

An attack may last only a short while, but it may be prolonged for many hours. After an attack, the patient may be exhausted, but very often he appears to be, and feels, comparatively well. Unfortunately this relief may only be temporary and attacks may recur at varying intervals.

Asthma must not be confused with suffocation due to a patient having inhaled something e.g., food into his windpipe.

General treatment

The patient should be put in a position he finds most comfortable which is usually half sitting up. If he is emotionally distressed try to calm him.

Specific treatment

A person who knows that he is liable to attacks has usually had medical advice and been supplied with a remedy. In such cases the patient probably knows what suits him best and it is then wise merely to help him as he desires and to interfere as little as possible. He should be allowed to select the position easiest for himself.

Otherwise advise the patient to inhale 2 puffs (1 puff for children) from a salbutamol inhaler, ('puffer' often blue), every six hours. To use the inhaler:

- Shake the container thoroughly;

- Hold the container upright;

- Tilt the head back and breathe out fully;

- Close the lips over the inhaler, start to breathe in, then activate the inhaler; some are now breath activated.

- Inhale slowly and deeply, hold the breath for ten seconds and then breathe out through the nose;

- Wait for 30 seconds before repeating the procedure.

If the patient does not respond to this treatment seek RADIO MEDICAL ADVICE as additional treatment will be required. In any event the patient should see a doctor at the next port. Unstable asthmatics should not be at sea.

Bronchitis

Bronchitis is an inflammation of the bronchi, which are the branches of the windpipe inside the lungs. There are two forms, acute (i.e. of recent origin) and chronic (i.e. of long standing).

Acute bronchitis

This may occasionally occur as a complication of some infectious fever (e.g. measles), or other acute disease. More usually, however, it is an illness in itself, being commonly known as a 'cold on the chest'. It usually commences as a severe cold or sore throat for a day or two, and then the patient develops a hard dry cough, with a feeling of soreness and tightness in the chest which is made worse by coughing. Headache and a general feeling of ill-health are usually present. In mild cases there is little fever, but in severe cases the temperature is raised to about 37.8°C – 38.9°C, the pulse rate to about 100 and the respiration rate is usually not more than 24.

In a day or two the cough becomes looser, phlegm is coughed up, at first sticky, white and difficult to bring up, later greenish yellow, thicker and more copious, and the temperature falls to normal. The patient is usually well in about a week to ten days, but this period may often be shortened if antibiotic treatment is given.

NOTE:

- the rise in temperature is only moderate;
- the increase in the pulse and respiration rates is not very large; and
- there is no sharp pain in the chest.

These symptoms distinguish bronchitis from pneumonia which gives rise to much greater increases in temperature and pulse with obviously rapid breathing and blue tinge of the lips and sometimes the face. The absence of pain distinguishes bronchitis from pleurisy , for in pleurisy there is severe sharp pain in the chest, which is increased on breathing deeply or on coughing.

General treatment

The patient should be put to bed and propped up with pillows because the cough will be frequent and painful during the first few days. A container should be provided for the sputum which should be inspected. Frequent hot drinks and steam inhalations several times a day will be comforting. Smoking should be discouraged.

Specific treatment

Give 2 tablets of paracetamol every 4 hours. That is sufficient treatment for milder cases with a temperature of up to 37.8°C which can be expected to return to normal within 2 to 3 days. If the temperature is higher than 37.8°C give antibiotics, e.g. Ciprofloxacin, Trimethoprim or erythromycin.

Should there be no satisfactory response to treatment after three days, seek RADIO MEDICAL ADVICE.

Subsequent management

The patient should remain in bed until the temperature has been normal for 48 hours.
Examination by a doctor should be arranged at the next port.

Chronic bronchitis

This is usually found in men past middle age who are aware of the diagnosis. Exposure to dust, fumes and tobacco smoking predisposes to the development of chronic bronchitis. Sufferers usually have a cough of long standing. If the cough is troublesome give codeine.

Superimposed on his chronic condition, a patient may also have an attack of acute bronchitis, for which the treatment above should be given. If this occurs the temperature is usually raised and there is a sudden change from a clear, sticky or watery sputum, to a thick yellow sputum. Every patient with chronic bronchitis should seek medical advice on reaching his home port.

Chest pain

When you have examined the patient and recorded temperature, pulse and respiration rates, use the chart to help you diagnose the condition.

More information about each condition and the treatments are given separately under the various illnesses.

Pleurisy

Pleurisy is an inflammation affecting part of the membrane (the pleura) which covers the lungs and the inner surface of the chest wall. The condition is usually a complication of serious lung diseases such as pneumonia and tuberculosis. In a typical case arising during the course of pneumonia, the breathing movements rub the inflamed pleural surfaces together, causing severe chest pain which is usually felt in the armpit or breast area. It is described as a stabbing or tearing pain which is made worse by breathing or coughing and relieved by preventing movement of the affected side. Occasionally the rubbing can be felt by the hand placed over the site of pain.

If a pleurisy occurs without the other signs of pneumonia get RADIO MEDICAL ADVICE. All cases of pleurisy, even if recovered, should be seen by a doctor at the first opportunity.

Shingles, severe bruising or the fracture of a rib or muscular rheumatism in the chest wall may cause similar pain but the other features of pleurisy will not be present and the patient will not be generally ill.

Pleural effusion – fluid round the lung

In a few cases of pleurisy the inflammation causes fluid to accumulate between the pleural membranes at the base of a lung. This complication should be suspected if the patient remains ill but the chest pain becomes less and chest movement on the affected side is diminished in comparison with the unaffected side.

General treatment

If pneumonia is present follow the instructions below. Otherwise, confine the patient to bed. If there is difficulty in breathing, put the patient in the half sitting-up position or in the leaning forward position, with elbows on a table, used for people who have difficulty in breathing, give oxygen. Get RADIO MEDICAL ADVICE

Pleurodynia and Chostochondritis

This is a form of rheumatism affecting the muscles between the ribs or the joints between the ribs and breast bone, respectively. In this condition, there is no history of injury and no signs of illness; pain along the affected segment of the chest is the only feature. The pain is continuous in character and may be increased by deep breathing, by other muscular movement and by local pressure.

It should not be confused with pleurisy or herpes zoster (shingles). Treatment should consist of two tablets of paracetamol every four hours. Local heat may be helpful. Read the section of MSN 1726 on analgesics if the above treatment is ineffective.

Pneumonia – lobar pneumonia

Lobar pneumonia is an inflammation/ infection of one or more lobes of a lung. The onset may be rapid over a period of a few hours in a previously fit person or it may occur as a complication during the course of a severe head cold or an attack of bronchitis.

The patient is seriously ill from the onset with fever, shivering attacks, cough and a stabbing pain in the chest made worse by breathing movements or the effort of coughing. The breathing soon becomes rapid and shallow and there is often a grunt on breathing out. The rapidity of the shallow breathing leads to deficient oxygenation of the blood with consequent blueness of the lips. The cough is at first dry, persistent and unproductive but within a day or two thick, sticky sputum is coughed up which is often tinged by blood to give a 'rusty' appearance. The temperature is usually as high as $39.4° – 40.6°C$, the pulse rate $110 – 130$ and the respiration rate is always increased to at least 30 and sometimes even higher.

General treatment

Put the patient to bed at once and follow the instructions for bed patients. The patient is usually most comfortable and breathes most easily if propped up on pillows at 45 degrees. Provide a beaker for sputum, and measure and examine the appearance of the sputum. Oxygen may be required.

Encourage the patient to drink because he will be losing a lot of fluid both from breathing quickly and from sweating. Encourage him to eat whatever he fancies.

Specific treatment

Give antibiotics e.g. Ciprofloxacin 500 mg every 12 hours for 5 days. Paracetamol can be given to relieve pain. Get RADIO MEDICAL ADVICE.

Subsequent management

The patient should be encouraged to breathe deeply as soon as he is able to do so and be told not to smoke. Patients who have had pneumonia should be kept in bed until they are feeling better and their temperature, pulse and respiration are normal. Increasing activity and deep breathing exercises are beneficial to get the lungs functioning normally after the illness. Patients who have had pneumonia should not be allowed back on duty until they have been to see a doctor.

Pneumothorax (Collapsed lung)

A pneumothorax results when air gets between the pleura (two membranes covering the outside of the lungs and the inside of the chest). Air gets into the pleural cavity usually as a result of a penetrating chest wound or a localised weakness in the lung (often in skinny asthmatics or chronic bronchitis / emphysema. When pneumothorax arises without association with an injury, it is called spontaneous pneumothorax. Sometimes, but not always, as the air escapes into the cavity a short sharp pain may be felt, followed by some discomfort in the chest. The effect of the air is to deflate the lung and thus cause breathlessness. The extent of the deflation, and the consequent breathlessness, will depend upon the amount of air in the cavity. The patient's temperature should be normal but his pulse and respiration will reflect the extent to which he is breathless.

When any associated wound or lung weakness starts to heal, the air in the cavity will gradually be absorbed and the lung will eventually re-inflate.

General management

Following the emergency treatment for pneumothorax associated with an injury and with cases of spontaneous pneumothorax, put the patient to bed in the sitting-up position used for breathlessness , give oxygen. He should see a doctor at the next port. If the patient suffers from more than slight breathlessness when he is resting in bed get RADIO MEDICAL ADVICE.

ABDOMINAL SYSTEM – GASTRO-INTESTINAL TRACT

Abdominal pain

Minor abdominal conditions

This group includes indigestion, 'wind', mild abdominal colic (i.e. spasmodic abdominal pain without diarrhoea and fever), and the effects of over-indulgence in food or alcohol. The patient can often tell quite a lot about the possible causes of his minor abdominal condition or upsets, so always encourage him to tell you all he can. Ask about intolerance to certain foods, such as fried foods, onions, sauces, and other spicy foods and any tendency to looseness, diarrhoea or constipation or any regularly felt type of indigestion and any known reasons for it. Mild abdominal pain will usually cure itself if the cause(s) can be understood and removed.

Guard against total acceptance of the patient's explanation of the causes of his pain until you have satisfied yourself after examination of his abdomen that he is not suffering from a serious condition. Note that a peptic ulcer may sometimes start with symptoms of slight pain .

General management

The patient should be put on a simple diet for 1 to 2 days and given magnesium trisilicate compound 500 mg three times a day. Repeat at night if in pain. Paracetamol may be safely given, not exceeding 8 x 500 mg in 24 hours. If the condition does not resolve within two days of starting this regime. get RADIO MEDICAL ADVICE. Anyone who has persistent or unexplained mild abdominal symptoms should be seen by a doctor at the next port.

Severe abdominal pain

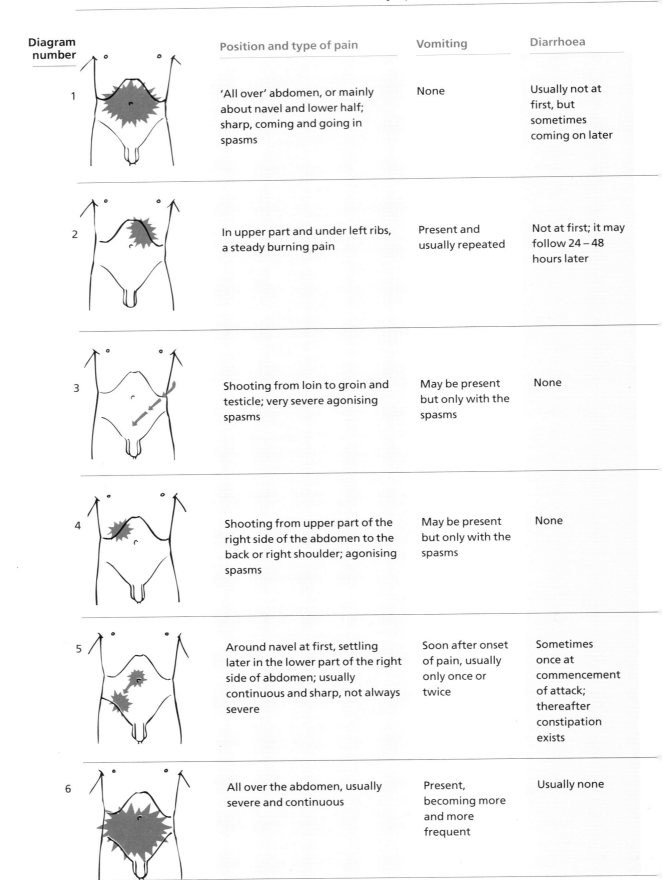

Diagram number		Associated symptoms		
		Position and type of pain	Vomiting	Diarrhoea
1	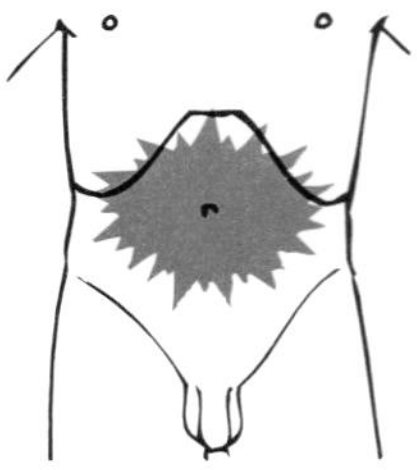	'All over' abdomen, or mainly about navel and lower half; sharp, coming and going in spasms	None	Usually not at first, but sometimes coming on later
2	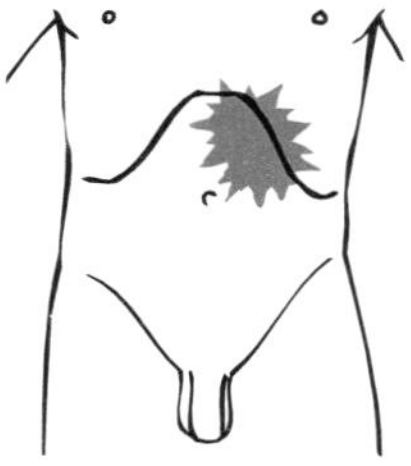	In upper part and under left ribs, a steady burning pain	Present and usually repeated	Not at first; it may follow 24 – 48 hours later
3	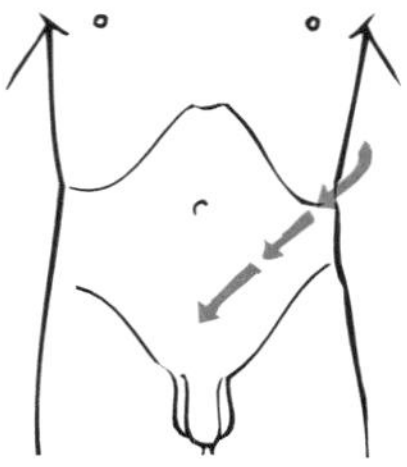	Shooting from loin to groin and testicle; very severe agonising spasms	May be present but only with the spasms	None
4	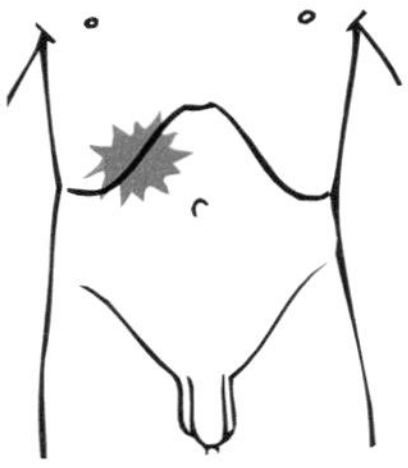	Shooting from upper part of the right side of the abdomen to the back or right shoulder; agonising spasms	May be present but only with the spasms	None
5	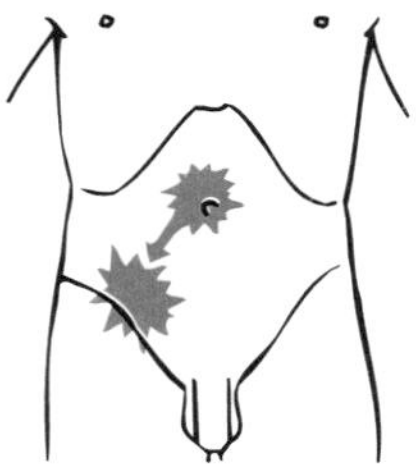	Around navel at first, settling later in the lower part of the right side of abdomen; usually continuous and sharp, not always severe	Soon after onset of pain, usually only once or twice	Sometimes once at commencement of attack; thereafter constipation exists
6	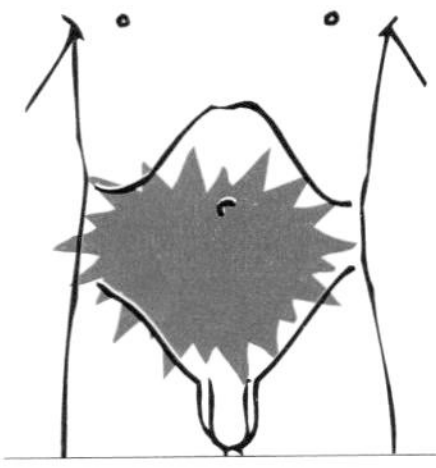	All over the abdomen, usually severe and continuous	Present, becoming more and more frequent	Usually none

Associated signs

General condition of Patient	Temperature	Pulse rate	Abdominal tenderness	PROBABLE CAUSE OF THE PAIN
Not ill; usually walks about, even if doubled up	Normal	Normal	None: on the contrary pressure eases the pain	**Intestinal colic (page 149)**
Wretched, because of nausea, vomiting and weakness, but soon improving	Usually normal; may be raised up to 37.8°C (100°F) in severe cases	Slightly raised, up to 80 – 90	Sometimes but not severe & confined to upper part of abdomen	**Acute indigestion (page 137)**
Severely distressed	Normal or below normal	Rapid as with shock	Over the loin	**Renal colic (kidney stones) (page 155)**
Severely distressed	Normal or below normal	Rapid as with shock	Just below the right ribs	**Gallstone (biliary colic) (page 145)**
An ill patient tends to lie still	Normal at first but always rising later up to 37.8°C (100°F); it may be raised more	Raised all the time (over 85) and tending to increase in rate hour by hour	Definitely present in the right side of the lower part of the abdomen	**Appendicitis (page 143)**
An extremely ill patient with wasted appearance, afraid to move because of pain	Present up to 39.4°C (103°F) or more except in final stage near death	Rapid (over 110) and feeble	Very tender, usually all over; wall of abdomen tense	**Peritonitis (page 150)**

Severe abdominal pain *(continued)*

Associated symptoms

Diagram number		Position and type of pain	Vomiting	Diarrhoea
7		Spasmodic at first, but later continuous	Increasing in frequency with brown fluid later	None; complete constipation exists
8		In the groin, a continuous and severe pain	Not at first but later as with obstruction	None, as with obstruction
9		Severe and continuous pain, worst in the upper part of the abdomen	Rare	None
10A		Lower abdominal pain – one or both sides just above midline of groin	Sometimes with onset of pain	Usually none
10B		Sudden onset of lower abdominal pain which may be severe	Sometimes with onset of pain	None
11		Lower abdominal pain. Spasms like labour pains	None	None
12		A continuous discomfort in pit of the abdomen and the crutch. Scalding pain on frequent urination	None	None

Associated signs

General condition of Patient	Temperature	Pulse rate	Abdominal tenderness	PROBABLE CAUSE OF THE PAIN
Very ill	Normal	Rising steadily; feeble	Slightly all over wall of abdomen, not hard but distended	**Intestinal obstruction (page 149)**
Very ill	Normal	Rising steadily; feeble	Over the painful lump in the groin	**Strangulated hernia (rupture) (page 148)**
Severely distressed at first, then very ill; afraid to move because of the pain	Normal or below normal at first; rising about 24 hours later	Normal at first, rising steadily a few hours later	All over; worst over site of pain. Wall of abdomen rigid	**Perforated ulcer of stomach (page 151)**
An ill patient – there may be vaginal discharge or bleeding	Tends to be high	Raised all the time	Lower abdomen, one or both sides	**Salpingitis (page 123)**
An ill patient may collapse if internal bleeding and pain are severe. There may be vaginal bleeding	Normal at first. May show slight rise later	Moderately raised but may be rapid and weak if internal bleeding continues	Tenderness in the lower abdomen	**Ectopic pregnancy (page 194)**
Anxious and distressed. May show some collapse if vaginal bleeding is severe	Normal	Normal or moderately raised. Rapid if vaginal bleeding	Tenderness in the lower abdomen	**Abortion Miscarriage (page 194)**
Made miserable by frequent painful urination	Normal but can be raised in severe infection	Normal or slightly increased	Moderate tenderness in central lower abdomen	**Cystitis (page 155)**

Abdominal emergencies

Introduction

Abdominal emergencies such as appendicitis and a perforated gastric or duodenal ulcer are high on the list of conditions, which, ashore, would be sent to hospital for surgical treatment. While there is no doubt that early surgical treatment is usually best, this does not mean that other forms of treatment are unsuitable or ineffective. In most abdominal emergencies on board a ship at sea, surgical treatment is usually neither advisable nor possible. Note that in the very early stages of abdominal conditions such as appendicitis or perforated ulcers, diarrhoea, vomiting, headaches or fevers are seldom present other than in a mild form. If these symptoms are present, the illness is much more likely to be a diarrhoea and vomiting type of illness.

Examination of the abdomen

The abdomen should be thoroughly examined. The first thing to do is to lay the patient down comfortably in a warm, well-lit place. He should be uncovered from his nipples to the thigh and the groin should be inspected (see Hernia). Look at the abdomen and watch if it moves with the patient's breathing. Get the patient to take a deep breath and to cough; ask him if either action causes him pain and if so, where he felt it and what it was like. Probably, if the pain is sharp he will point with his finger to the spot, but if it is dull he will indicate the area with the flat of his hand. A definite 'spot' or area of pain is of greater concern than a generalised one.

Look for any movement of the abdominal contents and note if these movements are accompanied by pain and/or by loud gurgling noises. Note if the patient lies very still and appears to be afraid to move or cough on account of pain or if he writhes about and cries out when the pain is at its height. Spasmodic pain accompanied by loud gurgling noises usually indicates abdominal colic or bowel obstruction. When the patient lies still with the abdomen rigid, think in terms of perforated appendix or perforation of a peptic ulcer.

Bowel sounds

When you have completed your inspection, listen to the bowel sounds for at least two minutes by placing your ear on the abdomen just to the right of the navel.

- Normal bowel sounds occur as the process of normal digestion proceeds. Gurgling sounds will be heard at intervals, often accompanied by watery noises. There will be short intervals of silence and then more sounds will be heard – at least one gurgle should be heard every minute.

- Frequent loud sounds with little or no interval occur when bowels are 'working overtime', as in food poisoning and diarrhoea, to try to get rid of the 'poison'; and in total or partial intestinal obstruction, to try to move the bowel contents. The sounds will be loud and frequent and there may be no quiet intervals. A general impression of churning and activity may be gained. At the height of the noise and churning, the patient will usually experience colicky pain which if severe may cause him to move and groan.

- No bowel sounds means that the bowel is paralysed. The condition is found with peritonitis following a perforated ulcer or a perforated appendix or serious abdominal injuries. The outlook is serious. RADIO MEDICAL ADVICE is required. The patient should go to a hospital ashore as soon as possible.

When you have learned all that you can by looking and listening – and this takes time – you should then feel the abdomen with a warm hand. Before you start, ask the patient not to speak, but to relax, to rest quietly and to breathe gently through his open mouth in order that his abdominal muscles are as relaxed as possible. Then begin your examination by laying your hand flat on the abdomen away from the areas where the patient feels pain or complains of discomfort. If you examine the pain-free areas first you will get a better idea of what the patient's abdomen feels like in a part which is normal. Then, with your palm flat and your fingers straightened and kept together, press lightly downwards by bending at the knuckle joints. Never prod with finger-tips. Feel systematically all over the abdomen, leaving until last those areas which may be 'bad' ones. Watch the patient's face as you feel. His expression is likely to tell you at once if you are touching a tender area. In addition you may feel the abdominal muscles tensing as he tries to protect the tender part. When you have finished your examination ask him about the pain and tenderness which he may have felt. Then make a written note of all that you have discovered.

Examination of urine

The urine of any patient suffering from abdominal pain or discomfort should always be examined and tested .

When you have completed the examination of the abdomen and recorded temperature and pulse rate, use the table and diagrams to diagnose the condition or to confirm your diagnosis.

More information about each condition and the treatments are given separately under the various illnesses.

Anal fissure

An anal fissure is an ulcer which extends into the back passage from the skin at the anal margin. The fissure is usually narrow, elongated and purple-coloured. When passing faeces intense pain is experienced, which can continue for half an hour or more. A little slime and blood may be noticed.

Place the patient in the position advised under haemorrhoids (piles). Put on polythene gloves before examining the anus. With one finger gently open out a small segment of the anal edge. Continue until the whole circumference has been inspected. This may give rise to intense pain and make a complete examination impossible.

Thrombosed external piles or an abscess in this region are the only other likely reasons for such pain.

Treatment

Relieve pain with paracetamol. An anti-haemorrhoidal preparation, (e.g: Anusol) should be used if available. Laxatives and plenty of liquids should also be taken to soften the stool.

If the pain is severe, lignocaine gel may be smeared around the fissure prior to passing faeces. The area should be washed with soap and water, then carefully dried after each bowel action.

This treatment should be continued until the patient is seen by a doctor at the next port.

Anal itching (anal pruritus)

Localised itching around the anus is commonly caused by excessive sweating, faecal soiling or a discharge from haemorrhoids.

The skin has a white, sodden appearance bordered by a red inflamed zone. The skin surface is typically abraded by frequent scratching which prolongs and worsens the condition. Dry toilet tissue can also exacerbate the irritation, the use of wet wipes is preferable.

Threadworm infestation should be excluded as a cause.

Treatment

Any haemorrhoids should be treated.

After the bowels have moved, the area around the anus should be washed gently with soap and warm water, then patted dry with a towel before applying zinc ointment. Loose fitting cotton boxer trunks should be worn. Scratching must be strongly discouraged. If the impulse to scratch becomes irresistible the knuckles or back of hand, never the fingers, should be used. Consult a doctor at the next port.

Appendicitis

Appendicitis is the commonest abdominal emergency and mostly occurs in people under 30 years old but it can appear in people of all ages. When considering appendicitis as a diagnosis, always enquire whether the patient believes that he has already had his appendix removed. It can be difficult to diagnose in children and the elderly, where a high index of suspicion is needed.

The illness usually begins with a combination of colicky abdominal pain, nausea and perhaps mild vomiting. The pain is usually felt first in the mid line just above the navel or around the navel. Later, as the illness progresses, *the pain moves* from the centre of the abdomen to the right lower quarter of the abdomen. *The character of the pain changes* from being colicky, diffuse and not well localised when it is around the navel to a pain which is sharp, distinctly felt and localised at the junction of the outer and middle thirds of a line between the navel and the front of the right hip bone (Figure 7.1).

The person usually loses his appetite and feels ill. The bowels are sluggish and the breath is rather bad or even foul. Often the pain is exacerbated by movement, so the person prefers to lie still.

Examine the patient. If the patient complains of sharp stabbing pain when you press gently over the right lower quarter of his abdomen, and especially if you feel his abdominal muscles tightening involuntarily when you try to press gently, you can be fairly sure that the appendix is inflamed. The temperature and the pulse rate will rise as the inflammation increases.

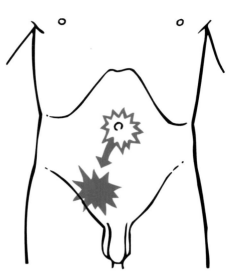

Figure 7.1 Appendicitis – movement of pain.

Treatment

Once you suspect a patient has appendicitis GET RADIO MEDICAL ADVICE AND GET THE PATIENT TO HOSPITAL AS SOON AS POSSIBLE. DO NOT GIVE A PURGATIVE.

If the patient can reach hospital within 4 to 6 hours, give him no food or liquid and *no drugs* as he will probably require a general anaesthetic. Keep him in bed until he is taken off the ship. Keep a record of the temperature, pulse and respiration rates and send these and your case note to the hospital with the patient.

If the patient cannot get to hospital within 4 to 6 hours, put him to bed and take his temperature, pulse and respiration rates hourly. The patient should have no food, but can have non-alcoholic drinks. You should start a fluid input/output chart and follow the instruction about fluid balance and treat and manage the patient as below.

■ *Specific treatment after four hours* Give benzyl penicillin 600 mg intramuscularly and metronidazole 400 mg at once, *and* then repeat both every 8 hours for 5 days. For patients allergic to penicillin, give erythromycin 500 mg and metronidazole 400 mg at once and then repeat both every 8 hours for 5 days. Treat severe pain.

■ *Subsequent management* If the patient is still on board after 48 hours, he should be given some fluids such as milk, sweet tea and soup until he can be put ashore.

Anyone who was thought to have appendicitis but seems to have improved should be seen by a doctor at the next port. Improvement is shown by diminution of pain and fall in temperature.

Diagnoses which may be confused with appendicitis in men and women include

■ *Urinary infection*. Always test the urine for protein in any case of suspected appendicitis and look for the presence or absence of urinary infection.

■ *A perforated duodenal ulcer*. This may cause sharp abdominal pain felt on the right, but the pain is usually all over the abdomen which is held rigid. The onset of the pain is usually more sudden and there is normally a past history of indigestion after eating.

■ *Other causes of colicky abdominal pain*. Renal colic, biliary colic and cholecystitis. These can cause severe colicky pain, but usually show other features which are unlike appendicitis. Severe constipation, especially in children may mimic appendicitis.

■ *Ectopic pregnancy (tubal pregnancy).* Always ask the date of the last menstrual period and whether the periods are regular or irregular. If there may be a possibility of pregnancy on the sexual history, always consider that ectopic pregnancy may be possible. Approximately 1 pregnancy in 100 is ectopic. Severe one sided abdominal pain usually precedes vaginal blood loss.

■ *Salpingitis (Tubal infection).* This is infection of the fallopian tubes. Always enquire about evidence of infection such as history of sex contacts, pain on urinating and vaginal discharge and bleeding. The fever is usually higher than in the case of appendicitis. They may have an offensive vaginal discharge.

Biliary colic – gallstone colic

Biliary colic is usually caused by a gall stone stuck in the neck of the gall bladder or in a bile duct. There is usually a history of vague indigestion and intolerance to fat. An attack starts very suddenly without warning symptoms and it may cease just as abruptly.

The bouts of colic, often very severe, are felt in the right upper abdomen just below the lowest rib but occasionally at the same level only more towards the mid line. Sometimes pain is also felt passing inwards through the body to the angle of the shoulder blade. The patient feels cold, sweats profusely and is extremely restless. Nausea is always present and vomiting may occur. The abdomen feels bloated and the bowel is constipated. The pulse is rapid and the temperature is normal or slightly raised. A moderately raised temperature may indicate that the gall bladder is also inflamed.

Examine the abdomen, look for jaundice, take the temperature, pulse and respiration rate, note the colour of the urine and test for protein and examine the faeces. Rigid abdominal muscles prevent examination during an acute spasm of pain. Between spasms feel for tenderness at the gall bladder area. When the outflow of bile is blocked the faeces become pale or putty coloured because bile pigment is deficient. However, the urine, containing excess bile pigment, becomes much darker in colour. Look for jaundice each day. If protein is present in the urine, consider renal colic.

General treatment

Put the patient to bed. Record the temperature, pulse and respiration rates every four hours. If feverish, give only fluids for the first 48 hours. A fat-free diet should be provided thereafter.

Specific treatment

As soon as possible give morphine 15 mg with an anti-emetic. The morphine will relieve the pain and the anti-emetic reduce vomiting. Reassure the patient that the injection will act in about 15 minutes. If the pain returns the injection should be repeated after four hours and RADIO MEDICAL ADVICE should be sought.

If gall bladder inflammation (cholecystitis) is also present, give antibiotics. GET RADIO MEDICAL ADVICE.

Subsequent management

Isolate any jaundiced patient and get RADIO MEDICAL ADVICE. All cases should see a doctor at the next port.

Cholecystitis – inflammation of the gall bladder

Cholecystitis may occur in either acute or chronic form and nearly always the inflammation is associated with the presence of stones in the gall bladder. The patient is usually middle aged or upwards, overweight and often in a chronic case has a history of long-standing indigestion with flatulence made worse by fried or fatty foods. In a typical acute attack there is a sudden onset of pain in the right, upper quarter of the abdomen in the gall bladder area. The pain is usually moderately severe, constant rather than colicky, and may spread through the body towards the right shoulder blade and sometimes to the right shoulder tip. Fever, nausea and vomiting are present and the patient tends to lie still in bed rather than roll about. This stillness is an important diagnostic sign in distinguishing cholecystitis from biliary colic where the patient is extremely restless during the spasms of colic.

On feeling the abdomen, local tenderness over the gall bladder is often found with an associated hardness of contracted, right, upper abdominal muscles.

If the hand is slid gently under the rib margin at the gall bladder area while the abdominal muscles are drawn in during a deep breath, it is usually possible to find a localised and very tender place, the person will groan as they breath in, with an examining hand on the right upper quadrant.

In diagnosis, cholecystitis must not be confused with biliary colic, right-sided pneumonia, hepatitis, perforation of a peptic ulcer or right-sided pyelitis (see diagnostic charts for abdominal and chest pain).

General treatment

The patient should be confined to bed, solid food should be withheld until the nausea subsides but adequate fluids (except milk) should be given. Thereafter, a bland diet without fried or fatty foods should be offered. A hot water bottle applied to the gall bladder area will alleviate pain. The temperature, pulse and respiration should be recorded. The white of the eye should be inspected for jaundice each day and the urine and faeces examined for changes associated with jaundice.

Further management

All cases, even if recovered, should be seen by a doctor when convenient.

Specific treatment

Give Ciprofloxacin 500 mg twice daily for five days. In an uncomplicated case the condition should be improved after two days. If the pain and fever increase or gall stone colic starts or jaundice appears, get RADIO MEDICAL ADVICE.

Diarrhoea

Diarrhoea is a symptom, not a disease. Seafarers are particularly prone to it because of the climatic changes to which they are subject.

In acute cases of diarrhoea you should consider the possibility of enteric fever , cholera or malaria.

All cases of diarrhoea should be treated as an infectious condition. If the condition does not settle within 48 hours, get RADIO MEDICAL ADVICE.

Acute gastro-enteritis

The commonest cause is 'food-poisoning' and the diarrhoea will often be associated with vomiting, abdominal colic (griping) and a raised temperature. This type of diarrhoea can be mild to very severe but will nearly always settle with simple treatment.

A lot of outbreaks of gastro-enteritis can be prevented by good hygiene in galleys and sensible eating and drinking ashore.

Treatment

- Rest in bed for at least 24 hours *without solid foods* in severe cases, plenty of clear fluids, small amounts, frequently. Mild cases need only a restricted, light diet.

- Fluids should be given in as large a quantity as the patient will tolerate. Oral rehydration salts are recommended.

- Antacids such as Magnesium trisilicate will often help to relieve symptoms.

When the diarrhoea appears to have settled, then a slow return to normal diet can be made.

In a very small number of cases there is an associated high temperature and general malaise. In these cases the antibiotic regime, and the sodium chloride and dextrose recommended below for dysentery may be undertaken.

Bacillary dysentery

This condition is difficult to differentiate from acute gastro-enteritis without laboratory investigations. It is an infection of the bowel caused by eating or drinking food contaminated by infected excreta. Flies are often the means of conveying the infection.

The symptoms are usually more severe than in the case of gastro-enteritis and tend to last for several days. It is more often associated with moderate to severe malaise and high temperature and the passage of slimy blood-stained faeces than is gastro-enteritis.

Treatment

- Moderate to severe cases should be treated in the same manner as for gastro-enteritis.

- In severe cases of diarrhoea and dysentery give sodium chloride and dextrose compound oral powder (oral rehydration salts) dissolved in water, to which fruit juices can be added. Give about 4 litres a day in addition to other fluids.

- Severe cases with high temperatures should also be given Ciprofloxacin 500 mg twice daily, for five days. This should not be continued beyond this period as the drug itself may cause diarrhoea.

Amoebic dysentery

A chronic condition which is seen in tropical countries. The general symptoms are much the same but may recur over a period. The diarrhoea is not as frequent as with bacillary dysentery and may often be mixed with blood and mucous.

Treatment

Give metronidazole 800 mg every 8 hours for 5 days.

Haemorrhoids – piles

Haemorrhoids are varicose veins found around the anus. They may be external or internal. External haemorrhoids are found below the anal sphincter (the muscle that closes off the anus). They are covered by skin and are brown or dusky purple colour. Internal haemorrhoids may protrude through the anal sphincter. These are covered by a mucous membrane, and are bright red or cherry coloured.

Haemorrhoids are usually noticed because of bleeding, pain or both after the bowels have moved. Hard faeces can scrape the haemorrhoids and will increase discomfort and bleeding. Faecal soiling of underclothes may occur if the anal sphincter is lax. Occasionally, the blood in an external haemorrhoid may clot and give rise to a bluish painful swelling about the size of a pea, or grape, at the edge of the anus – a thrombosed external haemorrhoid.

To inspect the anus, the patient should be instructed to lie on his left side with both knees drawn up to his chin. When in this position, separate the buttocks. The anus should be carefully inspected for swellings caused by external haemorrhoids or by internal haemorrhoids which have come down through the anus.

Treatment

The patient should be advised to eat wholemeal bread, breakfast cereals containing bran, vegetables and fruit in order to keep the faeces as soft as possible. Fluid intake should be increased. After a bowel action the patient should wash the anus with soap and water, using cotton wool. He should then thoroughly wash his hands using a soft nail brush to ensure cleanliness of the nails.

In the case of extremely painful *external haemorrhoids*, bed rest may be advisable. Taking a hot bath after passing a motion can be comforting. Lignocaine gel may give some relief. The condition usually subsides in about seven to ten days.

The patient should be told if he has *internal haemorrhoids*, so that he can push them back after washing his back passage. If they are painful and bleeding, standard piles medications, such as Anusol or Germaliods, should be used according to the instructions.

If the haemorrhoids cannot be pushed back (prolapsed internal haemorrhoids) the patient should be put to bed face downwards with an ice pack over the prolapsed haemorrhoids. After some time, 30 minutes to one hour or upwards, the prolapsed haemorrhoids should have shrunk and can usually be pushed back.

Bleeding from haemorrhoids is usually small in amount. Local discomfort around the anus may be relieved by calamine lotion or zinc ointment. Any patient with haemorrhoids should always be seen by a doctor at the next port for treatment and to exclude any more serious disease of the bowel.

Hernia – rupture

The abdominal cavity is a large enclosed space lined by a sheet of tissue. The abdominal wall muscles resist the varying changes of pressure within the cavity. Increased pressure may force a protrusion of a portion of the lining tissue through a weak spot in the muscles of the abdominal wall. This forms a pouch and usually, sooner or later, some part of the abdominal contents will be pushed into the pouch. It may appear at the navel or through an operation scar but the commonest position is in the groin. The weakness may have been present from birth but it may be brought on by a chronic cough or strain. At first, a rupture is noticed under the skin as a soft rounded swelling which is often no larger than a walnut but it may become very much bigger after some months. The swelling tends to disappear when the patient is lying down but it reappears when he stands up or coughs. Normally there is no severe pain but, usually, a sense of discomfort and dragging is present.

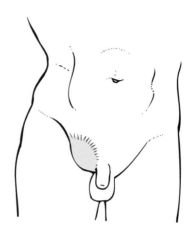

Figure 7.2 Inguinal hernia

When a hernia is suspected, the patient must always be examined while standing. In the groin, the swelling of a rupture must not be confused with swollen lymph glands, the latter tend to feel irregular and rubbery. Usually there are several swollen tender glands and they never disappear when the patient lies down.

It is sometimes possible to see and to feel an impulse transmitted to the hernia swelling if the patient is asked to cough forcibly several times.

Treatment

A person who knows he is ruptured has often learned to push the swelling back for himself. He should be removed from heavy work. An operation to cure the weakness is necessary. If the hernia is painful, the patient should be put to bed. Often the swelling can be replaced into the abdomen by gentle pressure when the patient is lying on his back with his knees drawn up. Keep him in bed until he can be seen by a doctor at the next port. Relaxation in a warm bath or even oral Diazepam 5 mg may be necessary.

Strangulation or Rupture

Most hernias, whatever their size, manage to pass backwards or forwards through the abdominal wall weakness without becoming trapped in the opening. However, the contents of the hernia pouch may occasionally become trapped and compressed by the opening and it may be impossible to push them back into the abdomen. The circulation of blood to the contents may be cut off and if a portion of intestine has been trapped, intestinal obstruction may occur. This is known as a strangulated hernia and unless attempts to return the abdominal contents through the hernia weakness are successful, surgical operation will become urgently necessary.

Get **RADIO MEDICAL ADVICE.**

An injection of morphine 10 – 15 mg intramuscularly should be given at once. The patient should then lie in bed with his legs raised at an angle of 45° and his buttocks on a pillow. In about 20 minutes, when the morphine has completely relieved the pain, try again by *gentle manipulation* to coax the hernia back into the abdomen. If you are not successful within 5 minutes, stop.

Intestinal colic

Intestinal colic causes a griping pain which comes and goes over the whole abdomen. The pain is due to strong contractions of the muscle around the bowel.

Intestinal colic is not a diagnosis; it is a symptom of many abdominal conditions but commonly it is associated with food poisoning, the early stages of appendicitis and with any illness which causes diarrhoea. However, the most serious association of severe intestinal colic is with intestinal obstruction.

Intestinal obstruction

Get RADIO MEDICAL ADVICE.

Intestinal obstruction may come on either slowly or suddenly; a common cause is a strangulated hernia. The bowel will always try to push intestinal contents past any obstruction, and in doing so the bowel muscle will contract strongly causing colicky pain. These strong contractions may be seen and also heard as loud gurgling noises.

In the early stages, the patient may often complain of an attack of wind and constipation. Later on he cannot even pass wind (absolute constipation). The patient's abdomen may distend and harden due to gas production which he cannot get rid of by passing wind and the bowel sounds become louder. The patient may vomit, at first the stomach contents and later faecal matter. The bowel sounds may eventually become absent, but should be listened for, for a full 5 minutes.

General treatment

As one of the causes of obstruction is a strangulated hernia, look carefully for this and do everything possible to alleviate this condition. Whatever the cause, it is essential that the patient is removed as quickly as possible to a place where surgical treatment can be carried out to relieve the obstruction. Delay can be fatal. Get RADIO MEDICAL ADVICE.

In the meantime, put the patient to bed. Give him nothing by mouth except water to wash out his mouth if he vomits. Rectal fluids will be required to maintain fluid balance. This should be started immediately.

Specific treatment

The patient may be given morphine 10 – 15 mg intramuscularly.

Jaundice

Jaundice is a yellow discoloration of the skin and of the whites of the eyes due to an abnormally high accumulation of bile pigment in the blood.

If the patient is fair-skinned jaundice will give it a yellow tinge which will not be obvious in those of tanned or darker colour. In all people the yellow colour can be seen in the white of the eye. It is best to look for jaundice in the corners of the eye in natural daylight, as some forms of artificial lighting can impart a yellow tinge.

A patient with jaundice will often complain of an itching skin, and state that he has had nausea and vomiting for 2 to 4 days before the colouring was noticed. His urine will be the colour of strong tea and his faeces will be putty-coloured. The colour and quantity of both should be recorded. On a ship the most likely causes of jaundice are ineffective hepatitis and gallstones or alcoholic liver cirrhosis. If the patient has jaundice get RADIO MEDICAL ADVICE.

General treatment

The patient should be put to bed and given a fat-free diet. Unless the Radio Medical Doctor advises otherwise it should be assumed that the patient has infective hepatitis and this means that he should be in strict isolation. There is no specific treatment for jaundice which can be given on board ship. Any patient with jaundice should see a doctor at the next port.

Peritonitis

Get RADIO MEDICAL ADVICE

This is inflammation of the thin layer of tissue (the peritoneum) which covers the intestines and lines the inside of the abdomen. It may occur as a complication of appendicitis after about 24 – 48 hours or certain other serious diseases of the contents of the abdomen.

The onset of peritonitis may be assumed when there is a general worsening of the condition of a patient already seriously ill with some abdominal disease. It commences with severe pain all over the abdomen – pain which is made worse by the slightest movement. The abdomen becomes hard and extremely tender, and the patient draws up his knees to relax the abdominal muscle. Vomiting occurs and becomes progressively more frequent, large quantities of brown fluid being brought up without any effort. The temperature is raised (up to 39.4°C) and the pulse is feeble and rapid (110 – 120), gradually increasing in rate. The pallid anxious face, the sunken eyes and extreme general weakness all confirm the gravely ill state of the patient. If hiccoughs begin, this must be regarded as a very serious sign.

Treatment

Peritonitis is a very serious complication of abdominal disease so get RADIO MEDICAL ADVICE and deliver the patient into hospital as soon as possible. Until this can be done manage the illness as follows:

- *Treat the infection.* Give benzyl penicillin 600 mg intramuscularly and metronidazole 400 mg at once and repeat both every 8 hours for 5 days. For patients allergic to penicillin give erythromycin 500 mg and metronidazole 400 mg at once, and repeat both every 8 hours for 5 days. (If vomiting is a problem, see elsewhere).

- *Correct the dehydration.* Give water per rectum and keep a fluid input /output chart. If thirst continues, cautiously allow sips of water.

- *Keep regular records.* Make notes of the patient's temperature, pulse and respiration every 1/2 hour, and any change, for better or worse, in his condition.

Ulcers

Peptic ulceration – duodenal and stomach ulcers

This is a special type of ulcer which develops in the wall of the stomach or duodenum. A shallow ulcer may heal within a short time but more often it becomes deep seated and causes recurring bouts of indigestion with pain.

At first, discomfort is noticed about three hours after meals at a point half way between the navel and the breastbone in the mid-line or slightly towards the right side. Within days or weeks the discomfort develops into a gnawing pain associated with a feeling of hunger occurring 1 – 3 hours after meals. Sleep is often disturbed by similar pain in the early part of the night. The pain is relieved temporarily by taking food or indigestion medicine. Vomiting is uncommon but acid stomach fluid is sometimes regurgitated into the mouth – the so-called heartburn. The appetite is only slightly diminished and weight loss is not marked. Bouts of indigestion lasting weeks or months alternate with symptom-free periods of varied length. Gastric ulcer pain tends to come on sooner after a meal and vomiting is more common than with duodenal ulceration.

On examination of the abdomen, tenderness localised to the area mentioned above will be found by gentle hand pressure.

Treatment

The patient should rest in bed but may be allowed up for washing and meals. Frequent small meals of bland food should be provided with milk drinks in between. Tobacco and alcohol should not be allowed. Antacids such as Magnesium trisilicate should be given half way between meals also Cimetidine 400 mg 12 hourly. Pain relief tablets are not necessary and aspirin, which often irritates the gut, should never be given. The patient should be sent for full investigation to a doctor at the next port.

Complications

The ulcer may extend through the thickness of the gut wall causing a hole (perforation) or it may erode the wall of a blood vessel causing serious internal bleeding.

Bleeding peptic ulcers

GET IMMEDIATE RADIO MEDICAL ADVICE.

Most peptic ulcers, gastric or duodenal, have a tendency to bleed, especially if they are long standing. The bleeding may vary from a slight oozing to a profuse blood loss which may endanger life. The blood always appears in the faeces. Small amounts may not be detected but larger amounts of digested blood turns the faeces, which may be solid or fluid, black and tarry. In some cases fresh, bright red blood may be vomited; but, if it is partially digested, the vomit looks like coffee grounds.

The patient usually has had a history of indigestion and sometimes the symptoms may have increased shortly before haemorrhage takes place.

General treatment

The patient must be put to bed at once and should be kept at rest to assist clot formation, see internal bleeding. Get RADIO MEDICAL ADVICE and get the patient to hospital as soon as possible.

A pulse chart should be started to watch for a rising pulse rate which would be an indication for urgent hospital treatment. The patient should be given nothing by mouth during the first 24 hours except sips of iced or cold water. After the first 24 hours small amounts of milk or milky fluids can be given with 15 to 30 ml of milk each hour for the first 12 hours. This amount can then be doubled if the patient's condition is no worse.

Specific treatment

Give morphine 15 mg intramuscularly at once, then give 10 to 15 mg every 4 to 6 hours, depending on the response to treatment which aims at keeping the patient quiet, at rest and free from worry.

If bleeding continues at a worrying rate, which will be indicated by a rising pulse rate and a deterioration in the patient's condition, all that can be done is to increase, if possible, the efforts to get the patient to hospital and attempt to meet fluid requirements by giving rectal fluids . A fluid input/output chart should be started.

Perforated ulcer

GET URGENT RADIO MEDICAL ADVICE.

When perforation occurs there is a sudden onset of agonising abdominal pain felt at once in the upper central part before spreading rapidly all over and being accompanied by some degree of general collapse and sometimes vomiting. The patient is very pale and apprehensive and breaks out in a profuse cold sweat. The temperature usually falls but the pulse rate is at first normal or slow, although weak. The patient lies completely still either on his back or side, with his knees drawn up, and he is afraid to make any movement which might increase his agony – even talking or breathing movement are feared and questioning is often resented.

Large perforations produce such dramatic symptoms that the condition is unlikely to be mistaken for other causes of abdominal pain where the patient is likely to move about in bed and cry out or complain when pain increases. The pain is most severe just after perforation has occurred when the digestive juices have escaped from the gut into the abdominal cavity. However, after several hours the pain may become less severe and the state of collapse be less marked but this apparent recovery is often short-lived.

On feeling the abdomen with a flat hand the abdominal muscles will be found to be completely rigid – like feeling a board. Even light hand pressure will increase the pain and be resented by the patient, especially when the upper abdomen is felt. It will be seen that the abdomen does not take part in breathing movements. The patient *cannot* relax the abdominal muscles which have been involuntarily contracted by pain.

As the size of a perforation can vary from a pinhole to one of much larger diameter, a small perforation may be confused with appendicitis because the pain begins centrally. But:

■ with a perforated ulcer, the pain is usually in the upper middle abdomen at first and not around the navel as in appendicitis;

■ with a perforated ulcer, the central upper pain remains as the main source when the pain starts to be experienced elsewhere, whereas in appendicitis the pain moves – the central colicky pain becoming a sharp pain in the right lower quarter of the abdomen; *and*

■ a patient with a perforation usually has a history of previous indigestion but this does not apply to patients with appendicitis.

General treatment

It is essential that the patient should be transferred to hospital as quickly as possible. Get RADIO MEDICAL ADVICE. The patient should be confined to bed on strict bed rest. A temperature, pulse, respiration chart should be started with hourly readings for the first 24 hours and then four hourly.

The perforation may close naturally if nothing is given by mouth for the first 24 hours. Fluid requirement during this period can be met by giving fluid per rectum if the patient is thirsty and pain relief has been adequate. A fluid input/output chart should be started.

Specific treatment

It is essential to achieve adequate pain relief so give morphine 15 mg intramuscularly with an anti-emetic at once. In a case of severe pain not satisfactorily controlled by that injection, a further injection may be given within the first hour. Thereafter, the injection should not be repeated more frequently than every four hours. Aspirin or drugs containing aspirin must never be given.

All patients, unless sensitive to penicillin, should be given benzyl penicillin 600 mg intramuscularly at once, followed by 300 mg every six hours until the patient is seen by a doctor. If the patient is sensitive to penicillin, seek advice urgently regarding use of alternative antibiotics.

Subsequent management

After the first 24 hours, if progress is satisfactory, a small amount of milk or half milk/half water can be given. Start with 15 to 30 ml of such fluid each hour for the first 12 hours. The amount can then be doubled provided the pain does not become worse. If milk is well tolerated, increasing amounts can be given frequently. Apart from milk and water, the patient should consume nothing until he is in hospital ashore.

Worms

Infestations can be caused by threadworms, roundworms or tapeworms. Identification of worms in the faeces is dealt with elsewhere.

Threadworms – pinworms

This is the most common infestation. The gut is infested with many small worms measuring up to 1.2 cm (½ in) in length which resemble short lengths of white cotton. There is marked irritation around the anus caused by the migration of the female worms which pass through the anus to lay eggs on the surrounding skin. This irritation occurs particularly at night when warm in bed and the impulse to scratch becomes almost irresistible. Worm eggs then contaminate the anal skin and are deposited on clothing and bedclothes. Failure to wash the hands each time after contact can then result in personal reinfection or the contamination of foodstuff or conveying the eggs to another person.

General treatment

Prevention of reinfection is essential. The nails should be kept short and the hands should be washed scrupulously after defecation or scratching. Underclothes, pyjamas and bedclothes should be boiled.

Specific treatment

The patient should be given, with the evening meal, a single dose sachet of mebendazole 100 mg once and repeat 2 weeks later.

If there should be evidence of reinfection, the treatment may be repeated after a fortnight.

Roundworms

Roundworms are similar in appearance to the earthworm. Infection usually results from eating contaminated salads or vegetables which have been insufficiently cooked. The worm eggs may also contaminate drinking water. The first sign of infestation may be the presence of a worm in the faeces but vague abdominal pain and either diarrhoea or constipation may occur.

Specific treatment

The patient should be treated with Mebendazole in the same dosage as that advised for threadworms.

Tapeworms

Infestation is conveyed by eating infected pork or beef which has been cooked insufficiently to kill the worm eggs. The worm usually grows to a length of many feet made up of white flat segments. There may be no symptoms but, in some cases, there is an increased appetite with vague abdominal pains and occasional diarrhoea.

Treatment on board is not advised and should only be carried out under medical supervision.

GENITO-URINARY SYSTEM

Paraphimosis (Penile swelling)

A condition where a naturally tight foreskin is retracted over the head of the penis and cannot be pulled forward. It can occur in some individuals following sexual intercourse. The head of the penis becomes constricted by the tight band of foreskin, and then swollen, congested, and painful.

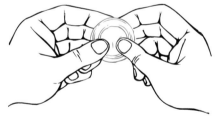

Treatment

Put the patient to bed. The congestion should be relieved by application of ice packs until the foreskin can

Figure 7.3 Replacement of foreskin.

be manipulated over the head of the penis again. This is done by pressing the head of the penis backwards with the thumbs and, at the same time, drawing the foreskin over and forward with the fingers (Figure 7.3). If this fails seek RADIO MEDICAL ADVICE.

Testicular pain

In all cases of disease or injury to the testicles, the man should be referred to a doctor for examination at the next port, even if the condition appears to be better.

Twisted or inflamed testicle (Torsion)

- Twisting of the testicle can follow a sudden effort causing the testicle to twist on its cord and cut off the blood supply. This is an uncommon condition and, when it occurs, frequently affects a testicle that is suspended in an abnormal (horizontal) line. Seek RADIO MEDICAL ADVICE.

- Inflammation of the testicle may be caused by an infection. Always remember this can be a complication of gonorrhoea, see urethritis or mumps .

Both conditions show many similar features. The testicle becomes painful, swollen, and very tender. The scrotum also becomes inflamed and fluid will collect inside it adding to the swelling and pain. It may be difficult to tell the difference between the two conditions but the following facts will be of help.

With twisting (Figure 7.4) the patient is usually young and, although in great discomfort, does not feel ill. There may be a history of physical effort. The onset of pain is very sudden. Check the position and lie of the other testicle. With inflammation, there may be a history of infection. The patient feels ill, he is feverish and the pulse rate is increased. He may pass urine frequently causing a burning sensation.

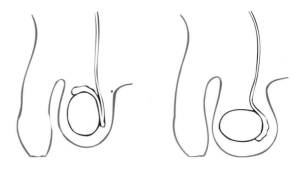

Figure 7.4 Twisted testicle.

A useful test is to support the testicles in a crutch bandage for one hour. Do not give any pain-killers. If within the hour the pain is partially relieved, you are probably dealing with an inflammation; if not, or the pain is worse, the condition is a twisting of the testicle.

Treatment

Get **RADIO MEDICAL ADVICE** at once.

Put the patient to bed and support the testicles by placing a pillow between the legs and letting the scrotum rest on this. Relieve pain by giving codeine 30 mg every 6 hours. If an infection is suspected give Doxycycline 100 mg every 12 hours for 10 days in addition to the painkillers.

Injury to the testicles

This not uncommon condition is usually the result of falling astride a rope under tension or a hard surface.

The testicles become very swollen and tender and there is a great deal of pain. Depending on the severity of the injury bruising will appear on the scrotum and can extend up the shank of the penis, up the abdominal wall and down into the thighs.

General treatment

The patient should be put to bed with the testicles supported on a pillow. Depending on the severity of the pain he should be given either two paracetamol tablets or one codeine 30 mg tablet every 6 hours. The urethra may be bruised or more severely injured. Always check that the patient can pass urine. If difficulty is found get **RADIO MEDICAL ADVICE**.

Other swellings of the scrotum

Two conditions should be borne in mind:

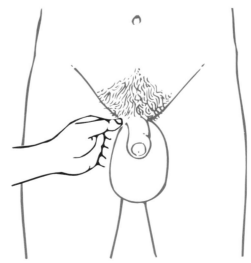

- A large hernia which has passed down from the groin into the scrotum;

- A hydrocoele.

Both these swellings can become very large, but there is no great tenderness, no inflammation, no rise in temperature or pulse rate, and the patient does not feel ill.

A hydrocoele is a collection of fluid in the scrotum, often caused by a minor injury which the patient may not remember. In contrast to those caused by twisting or infection, these swellings are not inflamed or tender, and the

Figure 7.5 Hydrocoele

patient does not feel ill or feverish. However, there is one exception to this general rule (strangulated hernia).

There are two ways to distinguish a hydrocoele from a hernia in the scrotum:

■ In a darkened room, place a lighted torch behind the swelling. If there is fluid present, i.e. a hydrocoele, the swelling will become translucent (light up).

■ Grasp the top of the swelling with the thumb and forefinger and judge if it is confined to the scrotum or if it is continuous up into the groin. If it is entirely in the scrotum suspect a hydrocoele; if it is continuous with a swelling in the groin, then it is a hernia (Figure 7.5).

Treatment

The treatment for both these conditions is surgical and the man should be seen at the next port by a doctor. In the meantime some relief may be obtained by supporting the scrotum in a crutch bandage, particularly if the man has a hydrocoele.

Urinary problems

See also female disorders and sexually transmitted diseases.

Renal colic

A stone may remain in the kidney without causing any trouble but often it causes a dull pain in the loin accompanied on occasion by passing blood in the urine. Acute pain (renal colic) does not arise until a stone enters the tube (the ureter) leading from the kidney to the bladder.

The pain, which is agonising, comes on suddenly. It starts in the loin below the ribs then shoots down to the groin and testicles. Each bout may last up to ten minutes with a similar interval between bouts. The patient is unable to keep still and rolls about calling out with each paroxysm of pain. Vomiting and sweating are common. The pulse is rapid and weak but the temperature usually remains normal. An attack usually lasts for several hours before ending, often abruptly, when the stone moves downwards to the bladder.

General treatment

The patient should be put to bed but often wishes to get out and move about.

Always examine a specimen of urine, when it is available, for clots of blood. Test also for protein. Examine every specimen for grit or stones that have been passed.

Specific treatment

As soon as possible give morphine 15 mg intramuscularly with an anti-emetic. The acute pain once relieved may not recur, but renewed paroxysms of pain are an indication to repeat the injection at intervals not shorter than four hourly, encourage fluids.

Inflammation of the bladder and kidneys – cystitis and pyelitis

This relatively common inflammation which may affect the bladder alone (cystitis) or the bladder together with the kidneys (pyelitis) occurs more often in women than men. Predisposing factors are poor hygiene, co-existing disease of the urinary system or genitalia, kidney or bladder stones, urethritis, vaginal discharge, or partial obstruction of the outflow of urine (enlarged prostate gland).

The usual symptoms of cystitis are dull pain in the pit of the abdomen and in the crutch, with a frequent or constant need to pass small quantities of urine which causes a burning sensation when passed. The temperature is moderately raised and the patient feels generally unwell.

A specimen of the infected urine may contain matter or small amounts of blood. A cloudy appearance and an unusual odour may be noticed.

In contrast to this usual pattern of disease, cystitis can occur without temperature change or general symptoms so that, apart from frequent urination, the patient may not realise that infection is present.

When the kidneys are also inflamed, there will in addition be pain in one or both loins with a high temperature 38.9° – 40°C. The patient will feel very ill with widespread aching, shivering attacks and even vomiting.

General treatment

All save the mildest cases should be put to bed. The temperature, pulse and respiration should be recorded and the urine examined daily and tested for protein.

At least 3 litres of bland fluid should be drunk each 24 hours. Hot baths and heat applied to the lower abdomen will ease the bladder discomfort.

Specific treatment

Give Trimethoprim 200 mg every 12 hours for five days. If the response to treatment is unsatisfactory, get RADIO MEDICAL ADVICE.

Acute stoppage or retention of urine

A stoppage is present when a person is unable to urinate even though the bladder is full. Much pain and suffering are caused as the bladder becomes increasingly distended. It can be felt in the lower abdomen as a rounded, tender swelling above the pubic bone and, in severe cases, can extend upward as far as the navel.

There is always some degree of blockage somewhere in the tube (urethra) between the bladder and the external opening. Common causes include localised injury, a scar within the tube (stricture), urinary stone stuck in the tube, holding the water too long particularly during or after heavy drinking and, most common in men past middle age, an enlargement of the prostate gland. This enlargement may have caused previous difficulty with urination such as a poor stream, trouble starting and stopping, dribbling and a frequent, urgent need to urinate during both day and night.

Acute retention of urine is rare in women.

Treatment

The patient should lie in a hot bath where he should try to relax and to pass urine. If he has severe discomfort give morphine 15 mg intramuscularly before he gets into the bath. Any constipation should be relieved. Give nothing to drink. Keep the bath water really hot. If urination has not occurred within half-an-hour the penis and genital area should be washed thoroughly in preparation for catheterisation.

Catheterisation – male

In extreme cases of urine retention, catheterisation will be necessary. Passing a catheter must be done with local anaesthesia and also with great attention to cleanliness so that urinary infection is not produced. If morphine has not been given, give diazepam 10 mg by mouth while he is still in the bath (see paragraph above). This will take effect while preparations are being made.

Collect together all the necessary equipment:

- clean towels;
- a catheter (Foley, size 16 Charriere gauge);
- a large receiver for the urine;
- antiseptic solution or soap and water;
- anaesthetic (lignocaine gel 2%);
- 20 ml syringe (to inject water into the retaining bag of the catheter);
- nozzle, drainage bag and holder;
- sticking plaster or tape to retain catheter and drainage bag.

Prepare to pass the catheter:

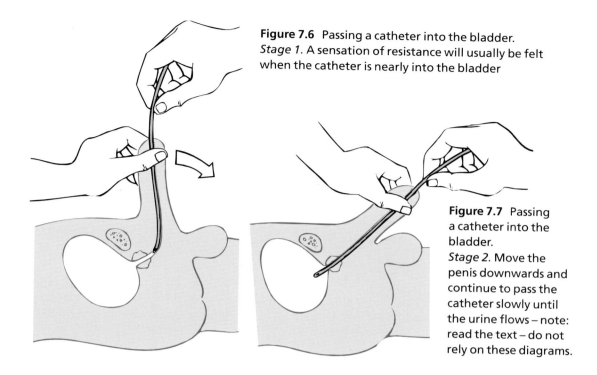

Figure 7.6 Passing a catheter into the bladder. *Stage 1.* A sensation of resistance will usually be felt when the catheter is nearly into the bladder

Figure 7.7 Passing a catheter into the bladder. *Stage 2.* Move the penis downwards and continue to pass the catheter slowly until the urine flows – note: read the text – do not rely on these diagrams.

- tell the patient what you are going to do when he leaves the bath;
- help him to leave the bath and to lie down;
- wash your hands;
- place clean (sterile if possible) towels around the patient's thighs and lower abdomen so that only his penis is showing;
- retract the foreskin fully and swab the head of the penis with antiseptic solution
- wash your hands thoroughly;
- holding the penis vertically, insert lignocaine gel 2% into the urethra and massage it down inside the penis to between the legs;
- use plenty of lignocaine because it acts both as an anaesthetic and as a lubricant. *The commonest cause of failure to catheterise successfully is insufficient anaesthesia* leading to spasm of muscle at the base of the bladder;
- *wait for 5 minutes* for the anaesthetic to act;
- place a receiver between the patient's legs ready to receive the urine;
- wash your hands again;
- open the catheter package onto a new clean towel spread over the patient's abdomen just above the penis;
- hold the catheter about 20 cm from its tip, and have someone else squirt some lignocaine gel onto a sterile swab *without touching the swab* and use this to spread lignocaine along the catheter. Make sure that the catheter does not touch anything else while you spread the lignocaine;
- stand on the right side of the patient, hold the penis vertically by the sides using your left hand, and pass the catheter slowly into the penis;
- when the catheter tip has passed into the urethra and is lying between the legs, about 15 cm of catheter passed, a sensation of resistance will usually be felt;
- move the penis downwards towards the feet and continue to pass the catheter slowly until urine flows into the receiver;
- make sure that the catheter does not slip out and insert the recommended volume of water into the catheter balloon to retain the catheter;

- pull the foreskin completely forwards, connect the catheter to the drainage bag and fix the catheter and the drainage tube to the patient's thigh. Make sure that the catheter cannot be tugged by making and fixing to the patient a loop in the drainage tube near the catheter end;

- test the urine for protein and record the result;

- keep the catheter in place;

- give Trimethoprim 200 mg every 12 hours until the patient is handed over to the care of a doctor;

- empty the urine collecting bag as required. Be especially careful about cleanliness so that infection cannot travel up from the bag to the patient.

BRAIN AND NERVOUS SYSTEM

Mental illness

Many people feel low in mood or irritable when physically ill but this gets better as the illness improves. What we may term true mental illness occurs on its own, but also often as a result of distressing news. There is a difference in behaviour which may be slightly unusual, or bizarre and completely abnormal. It is important to realise that the person who is mentally ill may or may not know he is acting in an abnormal way.

To diagnose mental illness is a highly skilled job, but all that can be done at sea is to recognise that something is wrong and seek expert help as soon as possible. Meanwhile handle the situation firmly and tactfully. This may require time and effort, as the patient may be irrational, violent and/or suicidal.

How to cope with a person who appears mentally ill

Try to keep calm and friendly, remember that what the person is experiencing is very real to him. Try to establish a trusting relationship and allow him to talk and express his feelings. Try not to contradict or argue as this might provoke withdrawal or even aggression. Offer comfort and help if necessary. If possible, ask the patient if he has suffered previous episodes of a similar nature.

Three types of mental illness may be seen at sea; anxiety, depression and obvious madness. It should also be recognised that excessive alcohol intake or use of illicit drugs can produce bizarre symptoms, as can withdrawal from these substances.

Depression

Two kinds of depression are usually described. The first has *obvious cause* such as the death of a close friend or relative. The second kind occurs *without apparent cause*.

In both kinds of depression the symptoms are similar, from feeling miserable to being suicidal. Every intermediate stage can occur. The patient may be emotionally up one day and down the next. *Early wakening* (e.g. 0200) and staying awake is the usual sleep disturbance. In appearance, morose and even sullen, he retires within himself and speaks only when spoken to. It may be difficult to get a clear story from him because he is sunk in misery and simply wants to be left alone. When he is alone, he may sit and cry, so enquire sympathetically about this because it helps to indicate the level of depression.

Very depressed people may commit suicide. It is essential to recognise those at risk so that correct precautionary measures can be taken. By a natural progression of questioning about the patient's general feelings, it should be possible to establish whether suicide has been contemplated.

Obvious madness

Any person who is obviously mad will require a good deal of looking after. In such cases it is always wise to assume that the person's behaviour is so unpredictable that he may at any time become violent or suicidal, often without provocation or warning. Anyone who shows signs of severe mental illness should at once be sedated with Chlorpromazine and kept under close observation. He should in the early stages be approached by *two* people. *Failure to observe these precautions can result in tragedies.*

How to deal with potential suicide

Anyone who appears to be deeply depressed or who talks of suicide or threatens suicide should never be left alone. This is not an easy thing to accomplish in practice. The person should be confined to a cabin and kept there under supervision. The deck is a dangerous place and the ship's side may be a temptation to suicide. The person must be escorted, even to the toilet and the door left ajar. All drugs and medicines must be removed and all string, rope and sharp, or potentially sharp objects should be taken away. He should eat with a spoon.

Specific treatments

Anxiety

For anxiety without depression, the drug of choice is diazepam. Begin with 5 mg three times a day. If after 24 hours of treatment the anxiety is not controlled increase the dose to 10 mg three times a day. The dose can be adjusted up or down according to the effect observed over 24 hours.

For a person who is mildly anxious and not very restless a dose of 5 mg of Diazepam can be given at night only to help them sleep.

Depression

Seek RADIO MEDICAL ADVICE. Diazepam in the doses described for anxiety can be given for a person who is very agitated as well as depressed.

Obvious madness

If there are signs of severe mental illness, Chlorpromazine 25 mg should be given at once by intramuscular injection. Seek RADIO MEDICAL ADVICE.

Neuralgia (Nerve pain)

Nerves

- *sensory* (incoming) nerves to the brain and spinal cord, relay sensations of pain, touch, sight, hearing, smell, etc.

- *motor* (outgoing) nerves activate muscles to initiate movement.

As some nerves contain both sensory and motor fibres, disease or damage will cause loss of sensation to an area of skin with paralysis of the muscles.

Neuralgia causes pain in part or whole of an area supplied by sensory nerves. The pain may vary from slight to disabling. For relief of pain, see analgesics .

All severe or recurrent cases of neuralgia should be referred to a doctor as soon as practicable. Radio medical advice may be required.

Brachial neuralgia

This causes pain in the shoulder and down the arm. It often also affects the neck and spreads from the neck over the head from back to front. It is usually due to acute or chronic intervertebral disc damage and/or arthritis in the neck. If pain is severe and disabling, bed rest and analgesics will be necessary . In milder cases, appropriate analgesics will be all that is required. A neck collar may be applied .

Dental neuralgia – see toothache

Facial neuralgia *Trigeminal neuralgia – ('Tic Douloureux')*

The patient is usually *past middle age* and develops intermittent intense pain in one side of the face. The pain can be devastating. In severe cases it can be triggered by chewing, washing the face or even by draughts of cold air. Always examine the mouth to exclude a dental cause.

The patient may need to rest in a darkened, draught-free, room. Medical advice by radio may be necessary in severe cases if the usual analgesics are ineffective .

Post-herpetic neuralgia

Following an attack of shingles (herpes zoster) some patients experience a persistent mild to severe and disabling neuralgic pain which will require alleviation with analgesics.

Sciatica

This is pain radiating into the buttock and/or down the back of the leg. Treat as for fibrositis.

Paralysis

Paralysis occurs when the muscles cannot work and the patient complains that the affected part feels heavy and dead, and he is unable to move it. It can be a complication of many diseases but the commonest aboard ship is stroke.

Strokes

A stroke occurs when the blood supply to a part of the brain is suddenly cut off. This is caused by a clot in, or breakage of a blood vessel inside the brain. It usually happens in middle-aged and old people and can be a complication of high blood pressure. The symptoms will vary according to the extent and severity of the clot or bleeding inside the brain and the site.

In a mild stroke the patient may feel suddenly confused, dizzy, sick, and unwell. He may notice a feeling of weakness and heaviness of the limbs on one side of the body (hemiplegia). The face on that side may also feel weak and appear to sag. Saliva may dribble from the corner of the mouth and the speech is usually slurred. Recovery may occur within 24 hours, if so this is known as a Transient Ischaemic Attack (TIA)

In a severe stroke there is loss of consciousness, the breathing is heavy and laboured, and the patient may lapse into a deepening coma and die.

Treatment

Regardless of his condition, put the patient to bed and get RADIO MEDICAL ADVICE as soon as possible. If unconscious or paralysed he should be nursed as described in Chapter 3.

Injury to spinal cord

Paralysis may also occur when the spinal cord is injured.

If the spinal injury is situated in the small of the back it will result in a paralysis from the waist down (*paraplegia*). If the spinal injury is situated in the neck all four limbs will be paralysed (*quadriplegia*).

It is important to remember that in spinal injuries there will be paralysis of the bladder and bowel and control will be lost over the excretion of urine and faeces.

There is no specific treatment for paralysed patients, other than nursing care described in Chapter 3. Figures 3.1 and 3.2 show how to rest the patient in bed and support the paralysed limbs. Gentle movement of the joints should be carried out several times a day to prevent them seizing up.

Facial paralysis – Bell's palsy

This is paralysis of one side of the face. It is usually of rapid onset and it can be complete in a few hours. The patient cannot close the eye or blink. Food may collect in the affected cheek and there may be dribbling from the corner of the mouth which tends to droop. Recovery over a period of time is the rule in the majority of cases.

The loss of blinking may lead to dryness of the eyeball and contamination by dust, an eye pad should be worn, for protection. Conjunctivitis may develop and it should be treated with antibiotic eye ointment. Otherwise the patient feels well and his general health is unaffected.

HEAD AND NECK

Ears

The parts of the ear (Figure 7.8)

There are three main parts:

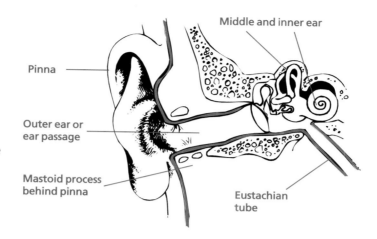

Figure 7.8   Diagram of the ear.

a. *The outer ear* is that part which can be seen on the outside of the head together with the passage which leads inward to the ear drum. The pinna is the correct term for the external ear.

b. *Middle ear* is a small cavity in the skull beyond the ear drum at the end of the ear passage.
A narrow tube (the eustachian tube) runs between the middle ear and the back of the nose and throat to keep the cavity at atmospheric pressure.

c. *Inner ear* is a complicated, deep seated arrangement of tissues concerned with the senses of balance and hearing. Inner ear disease is beyond the scope of this guide.

The mastoid process is the rounded, large bony prominence behind the pinna. It contains many tiny cavities resembling a honeycomb. It is sometimes inflamed by the spread of infection from the middle ear.

How to examine an ear

Compare the appearance of both ears. Look for swelling or redness of the pinna and the surrounding area, and for discharge from the ear passage. Feel for tender or enlarged lymph nodes around the affected ear and compare them with those of the other ear.

In a good light pull the pinna gently backwards and upwards to enable inspection further inside the ear passage.

Press firmly on both mastoid processes. Tenderness of one may indicate middle ear or mastoid infection.

Check the duration, intensity and nature of any earache. Establish if hearing has been diminished or if there are added noises in the ear and if the sense of balance has been impaired.

Wax in the ear

Accumulated wax may cause only slight discomfort in the ear passage but if it has hardened and is near the ear drum, pain may be felt when swallowing or blowing the nose. Hearing is often diminished and especially so if water gets into the passage. It is often possible to see the wax plug when the entrance to the ear passage is examined in good light.

Treatment

No attempt should be made to scrape out the wax. If treatment is felt to be necessary, the patient should lie down with the affected ear uppermost. Slightly warmed vegetable oil should be put into the ear passage and left for five minutes before wiping away any drops which run out when the head is tipped sideways.

Repeat this treatment twice a day for three days. Do not put a cotton wool plug in the ear. If relief of symptoms is not satisfactory, advice should be sought at the next port.

Infection of the outer ear (otitis externa)

This is a common infection in hot weather or after swimming, especially in the tropics and sub-tropics. The condition frequently affects both ears whilst boils and middle ear infection occur mainly in one ear. Pain is not a feature of the disease but the ear may be uncomfortable and itch, with a discharge from the ear passage. The skin of the ear passage is liable to bleed slightly and appears red, shiny and abraded.

Treatment

The ear passages should be gently mopped out with cotton wool swabs, not cotton buds, until dry. Sometimes it is better for the patient to do this for himself under supervision. When dry, three drops of antibiotic ear drops should be put in one ear passage while the patient is lying on one side. After five minutes in that position, the ear should be dried before the other ear is similarly treated. Repeat the treatment three times per day for 3 to 7 days.

The patient must not swim or get water into his ears when washing until he has been seen by a doctor or his ears have been normal for two weeks. Under no circumstances should cotton wool or other ear plugs be used.

Boil in the ear

A boil in the ear passage causes a throbbing pain which increases in severity over several days. When the boil is about to burst, there is a sudden stab of pain followed by a small discharge of blood-stained pus with much relief of pain. If the pinna is gently drawn upwards and backwards, it is often possible to see the boil in the ear passage. Pulling the pinna in this manner usually increases the pain and confirms the diagnosis. An inflamed middle ear causes similar pain but, pulling the pinna does not make the pain worse.

The ear passage of the affected side may be obviously narrowed and red in comparison with the other side. The lymph glands draining the infected area may be swollen and tender.

Treatment

Give paracetamol or codeine every 4 to 6 hours until the pain is controlled. Use antibiotic ear drops three times per day until the pain goes. If the boil bursts, clean the ear passage which should be kept clean and dry subsequently.

Infection of the middle ear (otitis media)

An infection of the nose or throat may spread to the middle ear cavity via the eustachian tube (Figure 7.6).

When normal drainage of the middle ear through the eustachian tube is impaired, pressure within the small cavity increases. Bulging of the ear drum can cause severe pain, which can be very distracting for the sufferer. Infected secretions will then burst through the ear drum causing a perforation.

At first there is deep seated earache, throbbing and nagging like toothache, with some deafness and maybe noises in the ear. The patient feels ill and the temperature is raised. As pressure rises the pain becomes worse until the ear drum perforates. Discharge through the perforation brings relief of pain and fever. The lymph glands around the ear are not enlarged .The mastoid bone may be tender to pressure firmly applied. The sequence of events may be modified if the infection responds readily to the antibiotic treatment.

General treatment

The patient should be put to bed and the temperature, pulse and respiration rates recorded four-hourly. Codeine tablets should be given six-hourly until the pain is controlled.

Specific treatment

Even if you only suspect that the patient may have otitis media you should give, *as soon as possible*, in order to prevent perforation of the drum either:

- if the patient is not allergic to penicillin – benzyl penicillin 600 mg intramuscularly followed by the antibiotics by mouth e.g. Ciprofloxacin; *or*

- to patients allergic to penicillin – erythromycin 500 mg followed by 250 mg every six hours for five days.

  If the patient is not better at the end of the 5 days, seek RADIO MEDICAL ADVICE.

Subsequent management

When antibiotic treatment is completely successful, the inflammation will settle, pain and fever will subside and there will be no perforation or discharge.

If perforation does occur the ear passage should be dried every two hours. Perforation does not imply that the antibiotic has not worked. The full five day course of treatment must be given.

When the patient feels better and has no fever he can be allowed out of bed but the ear must be kept as clean and dry as possible. Warning: swimming or air travel are not advised until approved by a doctor, to whom all cases should be sent when next in port.

Infection of the mastoid cells

A middle ear infection sometimes spreads to the mastoid cells. This can happen at any time during the course of a long-standing middle ear infection when a perforated ear drum together with a septic discharge have been present for months or years.

In new middle ear infections mastoids should be suspected whenever a patient continues to feel unwell, complains of earache and continuing discharge and is feverish 10 to 14 days after the onset. There will be extreme mastoid tenderness even though a full course of antibiotics has been given. There may be a tender, red swelling behind the ear and the pinna may be pushed forwards. This is a serious complication which may require specialised treatment ashore. Get RADIO MEDICAL ADVICE.

Eyes

Introduction

Figure 4.15 shows a diagram of the eye and how to examine an eye is described in Chapter 4.

Styes

A stye is an inflammation around the root of an eyelash. It begins as a general swelling and redness of the eyelid near the affected eyelash accompanied by pain. It later takes on the appearance of a small boil. Very often when one stye disappears, another appears. The condition requires little treatment as the stye usually bursts of its own accord. Any discharge should be wiped away with sterile water of saline, and the surrounding skin should be kept as clean and dry as possible. If the eyelid swells only slightly, there is no cause for concern. When the yellow 'head' appears, bathe the stye with cotton wool swabs soaked in hot water. This will encourage the stye to discharge.

To prevent conjunctivitis in the affected eye, put antibiotic eye ointment onto the inner surface of the lower lid every 6 hours. The patient should blink to spread the ointment after it is applied. The vision may be blurred on doing this and it may sting. This treatment should be continued until the stye has stopped discharging. If the stye is still present on reaching port the patient should see a doctor.

Chalazion

A chalazion is a cyst of the eyelid. An infected cyst is almost as common as a stye and can develop in a matter of a few days. Put antibiotic eye ointment on to the inner surface of the lower lid every 6 hours. The patient should blink to spread the ointment after it is applied. This treatment should be continued until the condition clears. As there is a tendency to recurrence, the patient should see a doctor at the next port.

Acute red eye – Conjunctivitis (inflammation of the eye)

The thin membrane (conjunctiva) which covers the eyeball (except the cornea) and the inside of the eyelids is particularly liable to infection by germs. The condition is contagious and nearly always affects both eyes. One red and painful eye is more likely to be caused by a foreign body or by some other condition. Therefore examine the eyes, look for corneal damage and check for a history of an obvious alternative cause such as dust, smoke or a foreign body. At first conjunctivitis causes the eyes to water, feel gritty, and look bloodshot. There is usually considerable discomfort from pain and a sensation of heat. The watering soon thickens to a yellow discharge, which tends both to stick the eyelids together during sleep, and to form crusts at the lid margins when it dries.

Treatment

Advise the patient to use disposable paper towels or tissues for his face and eyes and to wash his hands thoroughly after any contact with his eyes. Dark glasses should be worn and the eyes must not be covered by a dressing. Bathe away the debris with sterile water or saline.

Specific treatment

Put antibiotic eye ointment on the inner surfaces of the lower lids and instruct the patient to spread the ointment by blinking several times. This treatment should be continued once every six hours until the eye has been white and clean for 24 hours.

Deep inflammation of the eye

This is suggested by severe pain in or around the eye, marked redness of the eyeball, blurring of vision and profuse watering (as distinct from a sticky, yellow, discharge).

Treatment

RADIO MEDICAL ADVICE should be sought at the earliest opportunity. Meanwhile dark glasses should be worn. Codeine 30 mg should be given six hourly, depending on the degree of pain. A course of antibiotic treatment should be given.

Headache

A headache is a symptom of an illness and is not a disease in itself. Some of the more common causes of headache are listed below and reference should be made to the relevant pages in the guide.

Common causes:

- The onset of an acute illness and is then almost always associated with fever and feeling ill. Examples are influenza and infectious diseases such as measles, typhoid, etc.
- Common cold with associated sinusitis.
- Over indulgence in alcohol.
- Tension headache caused by worry, work or family difficulties. They are not associated with fever or feeling ill. This type of headache is sometimes associated with eye strain.

Less common causes:

- Migraine which usually occurs only on one side of the head and is associated with vomiting and visual disturbances such as flashing lights.
- Disease of the brain; acute, as with meningitis, and less acute as seen with raised blood pressure (by no means a common symptom), and a stroke.

Treatment

Always take the patient's temperature and, if raised, put to bed and watch for the possible development of further signs and symptoms. Otherwise, give two paracetamol tablets, which may be repeated four hourly. In cases of more severe pain read the section on analgesics.

All cases of persistent headache should be referred to a doctor at the first convenient opportunity.

Sinusitis

Sinusitis is the inflammation of the accessory sinuses of the skull. These communicate with the nose through small openings. The larger sinuses in both cheek bones (maxillary) and in the forehead (frontal) are most commonly affected. Sinusitis usually begins suddenly, often during or just after a head cold. The small opening of one or more sinuses becomes blocked and pus will be trapped in the cavity causing local tenderness, pain and fever. The condition is often worse on waking and gradually diminishes throughout the day.

Maxillary sinusitis – The pain is felt in the cheek bone and is increased by pressing firmly on the bone or by tapping with a finger on the bone. The pain is usually made worse when the patient bends forward. A foul tasting and smelling discharge into the back of the mouth and nose is often present. Sometimes the eye of the affected side is bloodshot.

Frontal sinusitis – The pain is felt around the bony ridge which lies under the eyebrow and firm pressure there and, sometimes, inward pressure on the corner of the eye socket next to the nose will cause tenderness. There may be an intermittent nasal discharge of pus from the infected sinus. The patient is usually feverish and feels unwell. Sometimes the eye of the affected side is bloodshot.

General treatment

The patient should be put to bed and kept there until his temperature has been normal for 24 hours.

The patient may find steam inhalations helpful. Boiling water can be poured into a jug and the steam inhaled, preferably with the head covered by a towel. Proprietary solutions are available to add to the water, but are not essential. The patient should be told not to blow his nose but to wipe it. Apart from being painful, blowing the nose may force the infection further back and make the disease worse.

The patient should be told not to travel by air or to skin-dive until allowed to do so by a doctor.

Specific treatment

If the patient appears to have mild pain, his temperature is less than 38°C, and he does not feel ill, give him the antibiotic treatment, e.g. Doxycycline.

If the patient has a lot of pain, is ill and has a temperature of 38°C or above, give him benzlypenicillin 600 mg intramuscularly followed by 300 mg every 6 hours for 5 days; if the patient is allergic to penicillin give him erythromycin 500 mg followed by 250 mg every 6 hours for 5 days. If by the end of 5 days his temperature has not been normal for at least 24 hours seek RADIO MEDICAL ADVICE.

For pain relief see Analgesics.

Teeth and gums

Dental pain

Dental pain may be caused by disease of the tooth (usually dental decay, i.e. caries) or by disease of the gums (gingivitis).

Toothache

Toothache can arise from two basic causes, although the intensity of the pain may appear to be similar. To provide relief it is important to distinguish between the two causes:

Toothache associated with a 'live' tooth

Pain may occur from a tooth as a result of the live nerve inside the tooth being irritated by dental decay, sweet foods, or sudden temperature changes by food or hot drinks. Its constancy will vary from minutes to hours. There is usually a cavity resulting from decay or from loss of a filling. Touching the cavity will often cause a sudden sharp pain. The pain in a live tooth can often be relieved by inserting into the cavity a wisp of cotton wool soaked in clove oil and giving analgesics. If this fails a temporary filling may be attempted but how much of the following you can do will depend upon the amount of pain caused to the patient and the position of the cavity.

Remove from the cavity any soft decayed tooth substance or loose filling, or food. Then make a temporary filling to protect the sensitive part of the tooth. To do this, put on a glass slab enough zinc oxide powder, if available, to cover a 5p piece. Add 6 drops of oil of cloves, and mix the two ingredients thoroughly; the mixture should have a consistency similar to putty. A wisp of cotton wool can be added if the cavity is large. Before putting this filling into the cavity dry the cavity with a small plug of cotton wool held in tweezers.

Toothache associated with a dental abscess

This will occur when the nerve in the tooth is dead and an abscess forms round the root of the tooth in the jaw. The pain is not started or affected by sweet foods or changes of temperature. Pressure applied to the tooth by a finger, or by clenching the teeth, or by tapping the tooth, will usually give rise to greatly increased pain which will be of a throbbing or boring nature. The face may become swollen and the abscess may 'point' on the gum. If this looks like bursting the pus can be helped to escape and the pain relieved by making a small stab with a scalpel into the centre of the abscess. Give the standard antibiotic treatment. The patient should see a dentist at the next port of call.

Pain can be relieved by simple pain relievers, such as paracetamol (2 tablets of either every four hours). Hot salt water mouthwashes are also helpful.

Gingivitis

Gingivitis is inflammation of the gums, and most adults suffer this complaint without feeling any pain. If the patient feels some degree of pain, and there is a little bleeding, he should clean his teeth carefully with a brush and use floss to clean in between them; he should massage his gums with his fingertips, and wash his mouth regularly with slightly salty warm water or antiseptic mouthwash.

If the gums become really painful, bleed easily and produce an offensive odour combined with ulceration and a discharge of pus at the gum margin, an acute infection is probably present.

Antibiotic treatment may be given, such as metronidazole 400 mg 3 times per day for 3 days. The patient should also be told to use a mouth wash and clean his teeth as above. He should consult a dental surgeon at the next port. Note that alcohol taken during the course of treatment with metronidazole may be followed by severe nausea.

All patients with this type of painful or bleeding gums should use disposable crockery and eating utensils if possible; otherwise, they should be allocated crockery and eating utensils which should be boiled for 10 minutes, or placed in disinfectant solution and rinsed well after each use.

Peridontal disease – pyorrhoea

This is an advanced type of gingivitis which can cause pus to discharge around the tooth and the tooth to become loose.

The patient should see a dental surgeon at the next port; but, in the meantime he should wash his mouth regularly with slightly salty warm water, or antiseptic mouth wash, and be given antibiotic treatment.

Ulcers of the mouth and gums

These ulcers may be caused either by an infection or by an injury (e.g. from a fish bone, or from ill-fitting dentures). Inadequate cleaning of dentures may lead to mouth infections. Most mouth ulcers will heal within a short time and medication will not accelerate this healing. A mouth wash of slightly salty warm water or an antiseptic mouth wash may make the condition more comfortable.

If the ulcer is due to a rough denture, the denture should not be worn until the ulcer heals – in the meantime you may be able to make the rough part smooth.

Dental advice should always be sought if a mouth ulcer does not get better within a week.

Throat

Sore throat

Most sore throats are associated with the winter ailments of coughs and colds. Some are caused by the inhalation of irritants or the consumption of too much tobacco. Most are relatively mild but in others the tonsils or larynx may be inflamed.

Tonsillitis – This is the inflammation of the tonsils, the fleshy lumps on either side of the back of the throat. The symptoms are soreness of the throat, difficulty and pain in swallowing, and a general feeling of being ill with headache, chilliness, aches all over, all of which come on fairly suddenly. The patient may find it difficult to open his mouth. He also looks ill and has a flushed face. The tonsils will be swollen, red and sometimes covered with many yellow spots or streaks of pus. The tonsillar lymph glands become enlarged and can be felt as tender swellings behind the angles of the jaw on one or both sides. The temperature and pulse rates are normally raised. If treatment does not appear to be helping after 2 to 3 days, glandular fever should be considered as an alternative diagnosis. Feel for enlarged glands in the armpits and groin which indicate glandular fever.

Laryngitis – This is inflammation of the voice box (larynx). In addition to the causes mentioned for a sore throat the inflammation may be caused by over-use of the voice. There is generally a sense of soreness of the throat, pain on swallowing, a constant dry irritating cough and the voice is usually hoarse and may be lost altogether. Usually the temperature is found to be normal and the patient does not feel ill. Occasionally however there is a slight fever and in other cases bronchitis may be present.

Treatment for sore throats

Look at the throat for signs of infection; take the patient's temperature, and feel for tender enlarged glands in the neck.

Patients with sore throats should not smoke.

Give patients with only a mild sore throat and no general symptoms of illness and fever paracetamol to relieve the pain. The patient may find it helpful to gargle with antiseptic mouth wash. *Mild sore throats should not be treated with antibiotics.*

Patients with tonsillitis, or a sore throat accompanied by a fever, and whose glands are swollen and who feel generally unwell should be put to bed and can be given paracetamol and a gargle as above. Give patients not allergic to penicillin, benzyl penicillin 600 mg intramuscular followed by oral antibiotic treatment.

Subsequent management

Keep a check on the general condition of the patient and keep a record of his temperature, pulse and respiration. Recovery will usually begin within 48 hours and the patient can be allowed up when his temperature is normal and he feels better.

Peritonsillar abscess (see below) can be a complication following tonsillitis

Peritonsillar abscess – quinsy

This is an abscess which can follow tonsillitis. It forms behind one tonsil, and the swelling pushes the tonsil downwards into the mouth. The patient may find it so difficult and painful to swallow that he may refuse to eat. He may have earache on the affected side. The swelling on the tonsil will be extremely tender, and a finger pressing gently inwards just below and behind the angle of the jaw will cause pain. There is usually fever, sometimes quite high. The throat will be red and a swelling will be seen above the tonsil on the affected side.

General treatment

The patient should be put to bed and his temperature, pulse and respiration taken and recorded every 4 hours. Give liquid diet or minced food in a sauce as solids are usually painful to swallow. Ice cold drinks are much appreciated as they dull the pain and thus allow some fluid and nourishment to be taken. Gargling with antiseptic mouth wash may be comforting.

Specific treatment

Give the patient benzyl penicillin 600 mg intramuscularly at once, and repeat every 6 hours until the patient is able to swallow; then continue with oral antibiotic treatment for 5 days.

If the patient is allergic to penicillin give erythromycin 500 mg every 6 hours for 5 to 7 days; if necessary, crush the tablets in a teaspoonful of honey or jam, which the patient can wash down with sips of water. Give 2 paracetamol tablets every 6 hours to relieve pain.

Subsequent management

A peritonsillar abscess may settle down with treatment or it may burst. If improvement is not rapid seek RADIO MEDICAL ADVICE. The patient should be told that the abscess will be very painful before it bursts, and that there will be severe pain, followed by a discharge of pus which should be spat out, when the abscess does break. The patient should be given a mouth wash to gargle with after the abscess breaks. Soon after the abscess has broken the patient will feel much better and he can be allowed up when his temperature has remained normal for 24 hours.

LOCOMOTOR SYSTEM – MUSCLES AND BONES

Backache

Pain in the small of the back is a symptom of many conditions which affect the spine, spinal ligaments, back muscles and nerves. Pain is usually the only symptom and the general health remains normal. However, backache can be an indication of more serious underlying disease, especially kidney disease, so in every case the urine should be tested for protein and the temperature and pulse rate taken.

Simple backache

This is usually of sudden onset and it may follow a period of heavy work or some quick movement of the back but it can appear for no known reason. The pain may vary from a dull ache to a severe disabling pain. Some degree of spasm of the back muscles, which is made worse by movement, is always present. With proper rest and appropriate treatment (muscular rheumatism) the pain will settle down within several days. The patient may then be allowed to be more active but heavy work is inadvisable.

Some patients have severe backache from the onset and, occasionally, the main leg nerve becomes affected (sciatica). A sensation of numbness and tingling or a burning pain travelling down the leg will then be present. If there is numbness or tingling around the genital area or there is loss of control of the bowel action or urination seek RADIO MEDICAL ADVICE.

Treatment

It is essential that the patient should keep the spine straight at all times. If a board to lie on can be fitted to the bed, he should remain in bed in the position which is most comfortable. Otherwise, he should lie on a hard, flat, surface with minimal padding until the pain eases. Whenever possible, he should eat meals while standing with a straight back. He should be washed in bed, but allowed to go to a lavatory rather than use a bed pan. Local application of heat to the back (hot water bottle) will help to relieve muscle spasm and pain. If pain is severe give Codeine Phosphate 60 mg at once. If pain continues it should be controlled with Morphine. Treatment should be continued and the patient kept at rest until a doctor can be consulted at the next port.

Gout – gouty arthritis

This is a disturbance of kidney function in which the excretion of a particular acid in the urine is impaired. Crystals formed from the acid are deposited in, and cause inflammation of, tissues such as cartilage and ligaments.

Gout often runs in families and affects men at or over middle age more frequently than women. The first attack usually affects the big toe but recurrent attacks occur which may involve any of the elbow or hand joints or those of the ankle or foot. It can even involve the ear cartilage. The attack often happens during the night when the affected joint suddenly swells up and becomes severely painful, especially on movement. The overlying skin becomes very red and shiny. The patient often feels irritable and short-tempered before and during the attack. Mild fever may be present but the general health is unimpaired. Attacks usually last for two or three days, then the joint returns to normal. There may be a white/ yellow hard centre to the swelling, a gouty tophus.

General treatment

The patient should rest in bed. The application of either heat or ice to the affected joint may be comforting.

An affected foot joint should be protected from pressure of bed clothes by the use of a bed cradle. **Alcoholic drinks should not be allowed.**

Specific treatment

Give codeine 60 mg every six hours to relieve pain. The patient should insert into the rectum one suppository of diclofenac 100 mg daily for two or three days.

Rheumatism

Acute rheumatism – rheumatic fever

This is an acute, feverish illness affecting young persons which is quite separate from rheumatism in the popular sense (see muscular rheumatism).

Rheumatic fever starts fairly suddenly, although it may be preceded by a sore throat and a general sense of illness together with pains flitting from joint to joint. The temperature rises rapidly to between 38.9-40°C and then one or more of the joints becomes hot, swollen, red and painful, especially on movement.

The joints most commonly affected are the knees, ankles, shoulders and wrists but not all the joints are affected at once. The disease tends to attack first one and then another over a period of two to six weeks. The patient sweats profusely and suffers the usual symptoms associated with a high temperature.

There is a milder form of rheumatic fever in which the general symptoms and fever are less severe although the characteristics of the disease remain unaltered. The most important aspect of rheumatic fever is that more often than not it affects the heart as well as the joints. In that event heart valve disease may develop later in life.

Treatment

The main objective is to avoid undue damage to the heart and to this end the patient must be kept at absolute rest in bed in whatever position he finds most comfortable. He must not be allowed out of bed for any purpose whatever. He should be fed and washed and he should use a bedpan and urine bottle. General nursing principles must be followed closely. He should be encouraged to drink plenty of water, fruit juice, milk or soup. The affected joints should be wrapped in cotton wool for comfort. Diclofenac has a specific anti-rheumatic property and should be give daily until the patient can be transferred to medical care as soon as possible.

Restlessness and sleeplessness should be treated with diazepam 5 mg at intervals of either four or six hours according to the response to treatment.

Muscular rheumatism – fibrositis

Muscular rheumatism is a general term used to describe many aches and pains of uncertain cause in the soft tissue of the trunk or limbs. There is usually muscular stiffness in the affected part associated with local tender points (nodules). The general health is unaffected.

An attack often follows a period of physical or mental stress and it can vary from a mild ache to a disabling pain. The shoulder region and neck or the lower back and buttocks are commonly affected.

Treatment

When discomfort is severe the affected part must at first be rested. Two paracetamol tablets should be given four times a day until the pain is eased.

The affected part should be wrapped warmly and the application of local heat is beneficial. Gentle massage will often bring relief especially after taking a hot bath. Normal activity should be encouraged as soon as the acute symptoms subside.

Chronic rheumatism – osteo-arthritis

This term is often used to describe the stiffness and pain felt in a joint and nearby muscles when degenerative change (wear and tear) has affected the joint. It is the commonest form of arthritis affecting those of middle age and upward.

The weight-bearing joints of the lower trunk and spine are most often affected. Gradually increasing pain and stiffness with some restriction of movement is noticed in one or more joints. The symptoms are often worse after a period of inactivity. Although of gradual onset, the condition may flare up during periods of over activity when symptoms resembling muscular rheumatism may become more troublesome. Then rest is necessary to remove strain from the joint. Local applications of heat together with diclofenac and/or paracetamol will relieve symptoms. Medical advice on long-term treatment should be sought when convenient.

SKIN AND SUPERFICIAL TISSUES

Bites and stings

Animal bites

All animal bites should be treated by thorough washing (not scrubbing) with soap and water and swabbing with antiseptic solution. All traces of soap should be removed before using the antiseptic solution. The wound is then covered with a dressing. You should check that the patient is protected against tetanus. If an hour or more later the wound is throbbing, the patient should be given antibiotic treatment. Also read the section on rabies.

Rat bites

If a seafarer is bitten by a rat antibiotic treatment should be given.

Snake bites

Many snakes are harmless but there are three poisonous types:
- cobras, mambas, African spitting cobras, etc.;

- vipers and adders; *and*

- the highly poisonous sea snakes of the Pacific and Indian Oceans.

Snake bites are likely to occur ashore or from cargo. Unprovoked bites of humans never occur. Even where a snake is disturbed and bites, shoes will usually give complete protection against fang penetration.

There is usually local pain and swelling around a snake bite, except sea snake bites which cause no local reaction but generalised muscle pains.

If large amounts of venom have been injected, shock occurs, with heart palpitations, difficulty in breathing, collapse and sometimes convulsions. Delayed blood clotting may occur. These symptoms can present within 15 minutes to an hour of the bite.

General management

The common symptom in snake bite is *fright and fear of sudden death*. Research has shown that serious poisoning is rare in humans and death is *highly exceptional. Reassurance is therefore most important*. Diazepam or alcohol in moderation are helpful for their calming effects.

If vomiting occurs, guard against inhalation, if necessary by putting the patient in the unconscious position.

If the snake has been killed, it should be lifted with a stick into a container and retained for identification. Do not attempt to find or kill a snake as this might result in further bites. *Do not handle a dead snake* as head reactions can persist for up to one hour.

Treatment

If bites occur ashore or in port, *transport to hospital immediately*. In other cases, seek RADIO MEDICAL ADVICE giving, where possible, a description of the snake and the nature of the bite.

If the bite is on the hand, arm, foot or leg the best immediate treatment is to wipe the site of the bite, cover with a dressing and apply a broad firm, but not tight, crepe bandage above the bite. Alternatively, immobilise the whole limb by the same means. The bitten limb should be moved as little as possible because movement spreads the venom.

Sucking the venom out of a bite is not generally recommended because of the danger of aggravating bleeding, introducing infection and poisoning the person giving the treatment. Vigorous sucking at frequent intervals may, however, be used for bites on the face and body where immobilisation is not possible. The person sucking should spit out extracted venom.

If venom from a spitting cobra enters the eye, bathe the eye thoroughly with water.

Jellyfish

It is sensible not to swim in waters where jellyfish abound. If someone has a part of a jellyfish stuck to him, this could contain sting cysts. Alcohol or methylated spirits should be applied to the affected part to kill the undischarged sting cysts. The tentacles and slime should then be scraped off. If no alcohol or methylated spirit is available, dry sand or any dry powder should be thrown onto the sting. *Do not rub the sting with wet hands or a wet cloth* as this will aggravate the sting.

In severe cases, with rapid collapse, resuscitation may have to be carried out .

Poisonous fish

These exist in most tropical waters especially around the islands of the Pacific and Indian Oceans. They have long spines covered by venom-secreting tissues. The stings cause an intense and often agonising local pain.

If possible, immerse the affected part in the hottest water the patient can bear. The pain is then relieved within seconds. Remove the limb quickly from the water to avoid blistering. Re-immerse as pain recurs (usually after about 30 minutes). If the affected part of the body cannot be immersed in hot water (face or trunk) the puncture wound should be injected with lignocaine 1% as follows.

Prepare a syringe containing lignocaine 1%. Swab the skin with antiseptic, and push the point of the needle just under the skin. Inject sufficient lignocaine to raise a small blob under the skin. Wait for a few minutes to allow the anaesthetic to act. Lower the barrel of the syringe so that the needle is kept just under the skin, push it forward and inject a further small amount of lignocaine (Figure 7.9). Pull the needle back, move the barrel round through about 60 degrees push the needle forward and inject again. By repeating this process an area of about 3 to 4 cm in diameter can be anaesthetised (Figure 7.10).

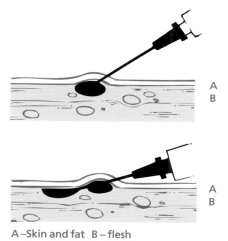

A –Skin and fat B – flesh

Figure 7.9 Injecting small quantities of lignocaine around the site of a sting or wound.

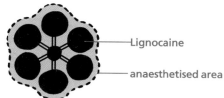

Lignocaine

anaesthetised area

Figure 7.10 Pattern of Lignocaine injections as in Figure 7.9.

Sea urchins

The spines of sea urchins can produce painful injuries when they pierce the skin. This is particularly true of the sea urchin found in the Mediterranean, off the coast of France, Spain and in the South of England. This sea urchin has a black body 30 mm in diameter which is covered with sharp purple spines about 25 mm long. Parts of the spines are left in or under the skin. Remove these, after injecting lignocaine 1% if necessary. Wait for at least five minutes before you start to cut the skin. If the patient complains of pain in any part, give a further injection. Try to use the smallest possible amount to gain the maximum effect.

After removal, swab the skin with antiseptic solution and apply a dry dressing. If you think that you have left part of the spine in the skin, refer the patient to a doctor at the next port, as small cysts may develop which, when burst, can cause a recurrence of the severe burning pain.

Scorpions, centipedes and spiders

Local pain and fright are the commonest, and often the only, results from bites by these insects. Stings and bites by a few varieties can, however, sometimes be painful, particularly in children. In such cases apply pressure above the bite and suck the wound vigorously for five minutes spitting out frequently anything sucked out of the bite. Wash the wound well with soapy water and apply a dressing to the wound. If the pain remains severe, inject lignocaine 1% in the manner suggested for poisonous fish spines.

Bee, wasp, hornet and ant stings

These are often painful and may be followed by considerable swelling. A sting in the throat may cause obstruction to breathing. If you are in port and the swelling looks likely to be severe or the sting is in the throat send the patient to hospital.

If the sting is still in the wound, try to remove it. If part of the sting is above the skin surface, try to expel any remaining poison by running your thumbnail along the length of the sting starting from its base. Wash with a cupful of water in which a teaspoonful of sodium bicarbonate (baking soda) has been dissolved. A person who has been stung in the mouth or throat should be given the sodium bicarbonate solution to drink and an ice cube to suck.

Some patients are very susceptible to stings. Allergic symptoms can start very quickly, including rapid collapse.

Boils, abscesses and carbuncles (see also cellulitis and whitlows).

Boils

A boil is an area of inflammation which begins at the root of a hair. It commences as a hard raised red tender spot which enlarges. It may subside in two or three days but more often it softens on the top and forms a yellow 'head'. The top breaks, the pus drains out, after which the boil heals. Normally the boil does not cause an increase in body temperature but lymphangitis may occur. Even a small boil can be very painful.

Carbuncles

A carbuncle is a collection of small boils very close together. The boils cause a large swelling which is very painful. There may be a temperature rise to 38°C and the patient will feel ill.

Abscesses

An abscess is a localised collection of pus which gives rise to a painful throbbing swelling. At first the swelling is red, hot, hard and very tender and after a day or two it becomes distended with pus and increasingly painful. At this stage, the skin over it becomes thinned and purplish in colour and it 'gives' slightly when it is lightly touched. There is usually a rise in temperature to 38 to 40°C.

The commonest sites for abscesses are on the arm, in the armpit, on the neck, in the groin and beside the anus.

General treatment

Where there is a small boil with localised inflammation and no rise in temperature, there is no need to give antibiotics. The area round the boil should be swabbed with antiseptic solution and dried and a light dry dressing applied.

Where there is a large boil, a carbuncle or an abscess, any hair around the area should be clipped short before swabbing. In these cases the specific treatment described below is required. No boil, carbuncle or abscess should be squeezed.

Always test the urine for glucose in any patient who has an abscess, carbuncle or bad boil. The test is best carried out on a specimen of urine which is passed about 2 – 2½ hours after a substantial meal. If glucose is found in the urine the patient should see a doctor at the next port because he may have diabetes mellitus.

Specific treatment

For patients not allergic to penicillin, give benzyl penicillin 600 mg intramuscularly. *At the same time*, start oral antibiotic treatment.

Subsequent management

The dressing should be changed daily. If a yellow 'head' appears it can be punctured with a sterile scalpel to drain the pus. If the patient feels ill and has a temperature, he should be put to bed and given two paracetamol tablets every 4 to 6 hours in addition to the specific treatment.

As the discharge is infected, you should dispose of the dressing carefully, sterilise any instruments or bowls you have used, and wash your hands thoroughly.

Cellulitis

This is a septic skin condition but, unlike an abscess, the inflammation spreads under the skin without becoming localised. The skin is red and swollen and, when the infection has taken hold, the skin will pit on pressure as in oedema. The patient will usually feel unwell and shivery, and often has a headache and fever. The nearby lymph nodes will become enlarged and painful.

General treatment

All patients with fever should be put to bed. If the swelling is other than very slight, the part should, if possible, be elevated.

Specific treatment

Give benzyl penicillin 600 mg intramuscularly if the patient is not allergic to it, and then oral antibiotic treatment.

Hand infections

Many infections of the hands could have been prevented by simple measures which are often neglected in practice. Small scratches, cuts, abrasions or pricks should never be ignored and they should be treated by thorough washing in soap and water before being covered by a protective dressing. Patients with hand infections must not handle/prepare food.

Inflammation and suppuration of a hand or finger wound may lead to internal scarring which could result in some loss of hand function. It is always advisable to start a course of standard antibiotic treatment as soon as the signs of inflammation affect a hand or finger.

For more than just a minor hand infection, get RADIO MEDICAL ADVICE.

Some common finger infections are described in this section.

Pulp infection

The top segment of a finger (with the nail on one side and the fleshy pulp on the other side) is completely shut off inside from the rest of the finger. An infection of the pulp will cause a rapid increase of internal pressure in the segment which can result in lasting damage unless treatment is promptly given. Infection may follow quite a trivial injury such as a needle prick , thorn scratch, or other minor puncture wounds. Slight soreness of the pulp within a few hours of injury may quickly progress to a severe throbbing pain accompanied by redness and tense swelling of the whole pulp.

Treatment

When symptoms start give benzyl penicillin 600 mg intramuscularly and begin oral antibiotic treatment. The patient should remain at rest with the hand elevated above shoulder height. Pain should be relieved by two paracetamol tablets every 4 to 6 hours but, if the pain is severe in the early stages, codeine 30 mg, six hourly may be necessary.

Inflammation around the base of a nail (Paronychia or Whitlow)

Infection has usually entered through a split at one corner of the nail skin fold, and spreads round the nail base. The semicircle of skin becomes shiny, red, swollen and painful.

General treatment

The arm should be kept at rest in a sling.

Specific treatment

A course of antibiotic treatment should be given. With treatment, the infection usually subsides without pus formation. If pus should form it can often be seen as a small 'bead' just under the skin. The pus should be released by making a tiny cut over the 'bead', with a scalpel blade or large injection needle. A paraffin gauze dressing under a dry dressing should be applied twice daily until the discharge has finished. Protective dry dressings should then be applied until healing is completed.

Skin diseases

The skin may be affected in many diseases. This is especially so in infectious diseases such as chickenpox and measles. Recognition and treatment of the underlying condition will be the appropriate cure for such skin eruptions. Any patient with a skin problem should therefore be questioned on his general state of health and, if necessary, an appropriate examination should be made.

Some skin diseases remain localised but, as their spread may be unrecognised by the patient, it is usually best to inspect the skin as a whole. The origin, and the later distribution, together with the duration and nature of the eruption, should be noted.

Barber's rash – sycosis barbae

This is an infection of the hair roots (follicles) of the beard area of the face and neck which is caused by shaving. The area affected is usually small at first but is spread more widely by an infected razor, shaving brush, hand towel or by rubbing the face with the hand. At the onset each affected hair root is surrounded by a small, red spot which soon develops into a septic blister. The blisters invariably break and form crusts.

General treatment

The patient should stop shaving at once and, if desired, facial hair should be kept short by clipping with scissors. The razor should be replaced or sterilised in boiling water for at least ten minutes before use after the condition has cleared. Rubbing or scratching the face should be discouraged. Disposable paper tissues or towels should be used.

Specific treatment

Give oral antibiotic treatment. If weeping is present, the affected area should be bathed several times a day with a solution of a small pinch of potassium permanganate in one litre of water. This may cause a temporary discoloration of the skin which will soon disappear when treatment ends.

Chaps

These are cracks on the backs of the hands, feet, lips, ears or other parts of the body caused by exposure to cold wind or salt water, or by washing in cold weather without drying the skin properly. There is often much irritation and pain. The affected parts should be freely smeared with vaseline and kept warm. Gloves should be worn.

Chilblains

The chilblain is a painful, red swelling of the skin caused by exposure to cold. The ears, fingers and toes are most often affected.

Susceptible persons should always be warmly clad in cold conditions because this is the one effective preventive measure. Most sufferers have learned by experience the type of treatment which suits them. However, as a general measure the chilblain should be kept clean by washing with soap and water, then smeared with zinc oxide ointment.

Dermatitis

Most of the dermatitis seen on board ship is due to irritation of the skin by substances which have been handled or misused. In a much smaller number of cases, the cause is allergy. The common irritants which cause dermatitis are detergents, cleaning powders, solvents, oil and paraffin.

There are various types of dermatitis but, in most cases, the condition starts as a diffuse reddening of the affected skin. Soon small blisters form on the reddened area and, later, these blisters break, releasing a thin, yellowish fluid which forms crusts. There is usually considerable irritation of the skin.

An attempt should be made to identify the irritant which has caused the dermatitis. The patient should then avoid contact as far as possible with any known cause. It should be borne in mind that a substance, e.g. detergent, with which the patient has been in contact for some time without any adverse effect may suddenly become an irritant.

Specific treatment

Apply a thin smear of hydrocortisone 1% ointment to the affected part three times daily. If the skin is weeping it should be bathed in a solution of a small pinch of potassium permanganate in 1 litre of water then patted dry with a paper tissue before the hydrocortisone is applied.

Athlete's foot

The web between the little and adjacent toe on both feet is first affected. The skin is thickened and split but later becomes white, sodden and looks dead. The condition may spread to other toe webs and also to the tops and soles of the feet. In severe infections the affected area may be red, inflamed and covered with small blisters which may weep or become septic. Itching is usually present. This condition can be passed from person to person through wearing others' seaboots and in bathrooms. Personal hygiene to avoid the spread of infection is therefore important.

Treatment

The feet should be washed morning and night with soap and water before each treatment. Loose shreds of white sodden skin should be removed gently using paper tissues before applying a thin smear of benzoic acid compound ointment or miconazole cream. In severe cases, before applying the ointment, the feet should be bathed in a solution of a small pinch of potassium permanganate in 1 litre of water. If benzoic acid compound ointment causes smarting and irritation, miconazole nitrate cream may be used instead. Cotton socks which can be boiled should be used.

Dhobie itch

This is a form of ringworm (caused by a fungus). The inner surfaces of the upper thighs are affected by intensely itchy, red, spreading patches which often extend to the crutch and involve the scrotum. The patches have a well-defined, slightly scaly, raised margin. The armpits may be similarly affected.

Always look for the presence of athlete's foot which may be the source of infection. If this is present, it must be treated at the same time to prevent reinfection.

Treatment

Cotton underpants, preferably boxer shorts, should be worn and changed daily. They should be boiled after use. Benzoic acid compound ointment or miconazole cream should be applied to the affected area twice daily and treatment should continue for two weeks after the condition has cleared. The ointment should not be applied to the scrotum but, if it is affected, miconazole cream should be used alone.

Ringworm – tinea

See also dhobie itch.
Ringworm is a fungus infection which produces rings on the skin. Each ring is red with a peeling and slightly swollen outer edge where the live fungus is advancing towards uninfected skin. The normal-coloured area in the centre of the ring is skin healed after the fungus has passed. The rings may join or overlap each other.

General treatment

The fungus cannot survive on cold dry skin, but thrives on hot sweaty skin. Anything which can be done to keep the temperature down and the skin dry is beneficial. Sunlight, provided the patient does not sweat, is of help. Air conditioning and cool breezes are always beneficial.

If the affected area is normally covered, cotton clothes should be worn and boiled for 10 minutes each day after use.

Specific treatment

Apply a small amount of benzoic acid compound ointment to the advancing edge of each ring twice a day until the condition clears.

Impetigo

This skin infection usually affects the exposed parts such as the face and hands. It starts as a thin-walled blister which soon breaks and becomes covered with an amber-coloured crust which gives the impression of being 'stuck on'. The surrounding skin is often not reddened. The eruption spreads rapidly, especially on the beard area of the face and neck. It sometimes affects the skin folds around the mouth, nose and ears, where it may cause red, sodden cracks. In severe cases the scalp may be affected. It is a highly contagious disease which is easily spread by the patient to other parts of his body, or to other persons, unless strict precautions are taken.

General management

The high risk of contagion should be explained to the patient who should not touch the eruptions. For a male patient, if the face is affected he should not shave and the beard should be clipped using scissors. Disposable paper tissues or towels should be used and any bedding, clothing or equipment likely to have been in contact with the eruption should be thoroughly boiled after use. The hands should be washed thoroughly after the affected area has been bathed, or unintentionally touched.

Infected food handlers in the catering department should be removed from duty until the condition has cleared.

Specific treatment

Give oral antibiotic treatment. If the condition has not responded satisfactorily after 5 days, give an alternative antibiotic treatment and seek RADIO MEDICAL ADVICE. The affected area should be bathed twice a day for about 10 minutes using a solution of a small pinch of potassium permanganate in 1 litre of water. The skin should be dried using disposable paper tissues. Facial eruptions should be left uncovered but those on the hands or any part covered by clothing should be protected with a dry dressing which should be changed daily.

Pediculosis – lice

Three varieties of lice live on human beings – head lice, body lice, and crab (pubic) lice. They bite the skin to obtain blood for nourishment, thereby causing itching with consequent scratching and sometimes infection in the bite marks. Female lice lay many eggs which hatch out within a fortnight. The eggs (nits) are pin-head sized objects which adhere either to hair shafts (head and crab lice) or to seams of underclothes (body lice).

Head lice

The hair at the back and sides of the head is usually more heavily infested. If scratching has caused infection this may be seen as septic places which resemble impetigo. The adjacent lymph glands in the neck may be enlarged and tender .

Treatment for head lice

Wet the patient's hair and rub in Permethrin cream rinse. Do not wash the head until 24 hours later. Anyone who has lain on the patient's bed should be told that he or she may catch the infestation and should be treated as above if there is any doubt. Change the bed linen.

Combing wet hair with plenty of conditioner applied, using a nit comb, will help to detect lice and eggs.

Other body lice – including crab lice

Crab lice (pubic lice) – see Sexually Transmitted Diseases – Chapter 6

Other body lice. These lice spend most of their time on bedding and underclothing where their eggs are laid. They crawl to the skin to feed and sometimes attach eggs to the body hair before returning. Itching may be persistent and scratch marks, especially at the back of the shoulder, the waist and the buttocks may be found. If infestation is suspected, it is essential that the seams of the underwear should be carefully inspected for the presence of eggs and lice.

Treatment for lice other than head lice

The skin of the affected areas should be washed thoroughly with soap and water and then dried. Lindane 1% lotion should be applied thinly to the skin of the whole body (this preparation is not included in the scale of medical stores but Permethrin in isopropylalcohol is not suitable for treating body/pubic lice). The patient should not have a bath or shower for 24 hours. A single application is usually sufficient.

After this treatment, bedding should be changed and clean clothes worn. Used bedding and clothing should be suitably disinfested.

Prickly heat

This complaint commonly affects persons on first entering tropical climates and particularly when heat is associated with high humidity. It usually affects those areas where clothing rubs or is tight, such as the waist line and neck, but skin folds and the limbs may also be involved. The rash appears at first as scattered, small red pimples which prick or sting rather than itch, to the extent that sleep may be disturbed. In the centre of the pimples very tiny blisters may develop which may be broken and infected by scratching.

Prickly heat may be associated with heat illness, when a complaint of tiredness, loss of appetite and a headache may be made.

Treatment

The patient should avoid vigorous exercise or any activity that leads to increased sweating. Clothing should be light, porous and loose fitting. Sufficient cold showers should be taken to relieve symptoms and remove sweat but soap should not be used on the affected part because frequent use may remove the natural skin oils.

Afterwards, the skin should be dried by gentle patting rather than rubbing. The eruption should be dabbed with calamine lotion, if available. The condition may be expected to disappear if the patient can move to a cooler climate or remain in air conditioned surroundings.

If sleep is disturbed, diazepam 5 mg may be given.

Scabies

See Sexually Transmitted Diseases – Chapter 6.

Shingles – herpes zoster

Shingles is a painful disease in which whitish blisters with red margins occur on the skin along the course of a nerve – usually a single nerve in the wall of the chest, but sometimes a nerve of the face or thigh normally one side of the body only. The first symptoms of shingles are much like those of any feverish attack. The person may feel unwell for a few days with a slight rise of temperature and vague pains all over. The pain then settles at a point on one side of the body, the skin is red and tender there, and on examination the blisters are discovered varying in size from a pin's head to a pea. These increase in number and spread for a day or two until, quite often, there is a half-ring round one side of the affected part of the body. The blisters burst within about a week or ten days, and dry up with scabbing, but, particularly in more elderly persons, the pain may continue long after the scabs have fallen off.
NOTE: This condition can affect the eye causing severe pain and potential blindness – SEEK RADIO MEDICAL ADVICE.

Treatment

The affected skin should not be washed. Dust the area frequently with talc or apply calamine lotion, if available, and allow to dry. Some further slight relief of discomfort may be given by covering the area with dry lint. Give pain relief.

Urticaria – nettle rash

This is a sensitivity reaction of the skin in which itchy, raised weals similar to nettle stings appear. The cause may be apparent when the reaction is localised and is a response to an insect bite or jellyfish sting but any part of the skin may be affected and no precipitating cause may be found. Sometimes nettle rash appears suddenly if a particular food (e.g. shellfish or fruit) has been eaten. The patient is usually aware of similar episodes in the past. In like manner, medicines or injections may cause skin reactions and nettle rash is a common manifestation. The penicillin family of antibiotics is the most common offender and when these are given by injection, a severe reaction may occur. Other commonly used medicines, which either cause nettle rash or make it worse, are aspirin and codeine.

Nettle rash is usually easy to recognise as a slightly raised, reddened area with a hard white centre. Weals usually appear quickly, then subside only to be replaced by other weals at another part of the skin. This pattern may be present over a few hours or days and then cease. The patient does not usually feel ill but is often alarmed and should be reassured that the condition is seldom dangerous.

General treatment

Always enquire from the patient if he knows of any possible cause for the rash and check on all drugs which the patient is now taking or has been taking in the last few weeks and on all substances which he has handled or touched. If the cause can be identified and removed, no further attacks will occur. Should the cause not be removed, treatment by medicines can only suppress or damp down the reaction without curing the condition.

Specific treatment

To alleviate the rash give anti-histamines e.g. Astemizole for 5 days depending upon the severity of the rash. If the patient has not seen a doctor continue treatment until the condition subsides. Always warn the patient that the drug may sooner or later make him sleepy and that alcohol will increase the side effects.

GENERALISED ILLNESSES

Alcohol abuse

Warning

Breath smelling of alcohol means that a drink has been taken; it does not tell how much has been consumed, nor does it mean that the condition of the patient is due to alcoholic intoxication. Head injuries, certain drugs such as sleeping tablets, and some illnesses can make a patient behave as if he were drunk (Note, low blood sugar is easily missed). Therefore, always assume that the person may have other injuries or may be ill until you have examined him carefully.

Deaths of seafarers are recorded every year either as a direct result of the excessive drinking of liquor, or from accidents, such as falling from wharves and gangways, whilst under the influence of drink. In addition there have been cases where seafarers, brought on board in a semi-comatose condition, have been simply put to bed and have been found dead some hours later either as a result of absorbing a fatal quantity of alcohol from their stomachs or being choked, i.e. asphyxiated, by their own vomit.

Being extremely drunk may therefore place a person in a critical condition. Accordingly, drunkenness, common though it may be, should never be ignored or regarded as merely funny. On the contrary, anyone returning on board in a severely drunken state should be treated as sick persons, requiring close watching and careful nursing if their lives are not to be further jeopardised.

Ordinary drunkenness

A description of this is scarcely necessary except for the sake of comparison with other forms of drunkenness. The person has poor control of his muscles, finding it difficult to walk or talk properly and being unable to perform commonplace actions such as lighting a cigarette. The face is flushed and the whites of the eyes may be 'bloodshot'. He may vomit. He may be in a happy, excited mood, or fighting drunk, or he may cry and be very depressed owing to the loss of his normal controlling powers of reason and judgement.

Dead drunk

Alcohol in any form is a poison; and when a large amount has been taking during a short time, especially on an empty stomach, serious poisoning or intoxication may develop. This may prove fatal as a result of respiratory or heart failure. The drinking of alcohol in ports abroad, where poisonous spirit of illicit origin is frequently offered to seafarers, is especially dangerous. Someone who is 'dead drunk' lies unconscious with slow noisy breathing, dilated pupils, a rapid pulse, and some blueness of the lips. The breath will smell of alcohol but beware that stupor or coma may not always be solely due to drink. The signs of a drunken stupor are much like those of other conditions causing unconsciousness. The person must be examined carefully to make as sure as possible that it really is a case of alcoholic poisoning.

Treatment

People who are drunk but conscious should be encouraged to drink a pint of water to prevent a hangover caused by alcoholic dehydration and to go to bed. If they are seriously drunk they should not eat anything until they have recovered. It is advisable that someone stays with a person who is seriously drunk because he may inhale his vomit whilst asleep.

If in port, a person unconscious from alcohol should be sent to hospital. If the patient has to be kept on board, he should be put to bed and managed as in the routine for unconscious patients. Remember that he should never be left alone in case he moves out of the unconscious position and then dies from inhaling vomit.

Hangover

A hangover is usually made up of a headache, a general feeling of being unwell and a stomach upset. The patient should not take further alcohol. He should take plenty of non-alcoholic fluids to combat the dehydration caused by the alcohol, paracetamol tablets and, if necessary, an antacid, e.g. magnesium trisilicate compound 250 mg.

The stomach upset and other complaints will usually settle within 24 to 36 hours if the patient takes no more alcohol, very little if any food and plenty of fluid.

The shakes

The shakes is a sign of withdrawal of alcohol in a person who has, over a long period of time, become dependent on, and habituated to, alcohol. Trembling of the hands, shaking of the body, and sweating will appear in the morning when a person has not had alcohol since the previous evening. The alcoholic, for that is what he is, usually prescribes his own cure by taking a further drink. On board ship during a voyage it is reasonable to allow a small dose of alcohol in such circumstances provided that the patient is not showing any sign of mental or emotional imbalance. The patient should be referred for treatment of his alcoholism at the earliest opportunity.

DT's (Delirium Tremens)

An attack of the DT's can be a serious medical emergency. It occurs only in people who have been regular heavy drinkers for many years. Attacks do not follow a single 'blind' by someone who normally takes only a small or moderate amount of alcohol. On the other hand, it is often a bout of drinking (such as a seafarer, who is a chronic alcoholic, may indulge in after a prolonged voyage) which leads to an attack, or it may be brought on when a heavy drinker has an injury or illness which results in the sudden cessation of his excessive 'normal' intake.

The patient with delirium tremens is at first irritable and restless, and will not eat. These early signs are followed by shaking all over, especially of the hands. He is confused and may not know where he is and may not recognise those around him. He perspires freely, the temperature may rise to 39.4°C, the face is flushed, and the tongue is furred. He may be extremely disturbed, or even raving; this is usually worse at night (night terrors) when he is unable to sleep, and sees imaginary creatures like snakes, rats and insects, which frighten him and which he may try to pursue. He may deteriorate to a state of delirium in which there is a danger of his committing suicide or even homicide. This condition usually lasts for three or four days, after which the patient either improves and begins to acquire natural sleep, or else passes into coma, complete exhaustion and death.

It is the mental and emotional imbalance which differentiates the DT's from the shakes.

General treatment

The patient should be confined and nursed as described for the mentally ill. There should be subdued lighting by day and by night to reduce as far as possible the imaginary visions he is likely to see. He should be encouraged to drink plenty of sweetened fluid and, if he will eat, should be given food. The attack may end with the patient sleeping for up to 24 hours.

Specific treatment

First try to calm the patient with a glass (50 ml) of whisky. If this proves unsuccessful, physical restraint will be necessary. In either event then give chlorpromazine 50 mg by intramuscular injection. This may be repeated after 6 hours if the patient is still uncontrolled. In addition give diazepam 10 mg by mouth or per rectum and repeat 4 hourly until the patient is calm. Once treatment is started, it is essential that no more alcohol is given.

If in any doubt about diagnosis or treatment get RADIO MEDICAL ADVICE. In any event refer the patient for treatment of his alcoholism at the earliest opportunity.

Subsequent management. When a person has got over an attack of DT's it is vital to make sure that no further access to alcohol is possible. Alcoholics are often very cunning and devious. They frequently have hidden bottles in their cabin and work areas and may try to get to these bottles or may 'con' other people into fetching their bottle of 'medicine' to them. They are also very over optimistic about their chances of changing and abstaining.

Allergy

Allergy is caused by hypersensitivity to one or more of a very wide range of substances. Common causes are dust, pollen, strawberries, nuts and shellfish which may provoke reactions which include asthma, dermatitis/eczema urticaria ('nettle rash') and penicillins.

Major allergic reaction

Major reactions occur within seconds or minutes of contact with the incompatible substance which may have been taken by mouth or inhalation or introduced by medical injection, bite or sting. In the very worst type of allergic attack, the patient may suddenly begin to wheeze, become pale, sweat and feel dizzy. The heart beat may become so feeble that he may lose consciousness and, unless treated promptly, he may die.

General treatment

If the patient becomes unconscious, place him at once in the recovery position and ensure that breathing is not obstructed. If breathing is weak or stops, give artificial respiration and heart compression if required. The usual 'ABC' applies.

Specific treatment

Give 0.5 ml of adrenaline 1 in 1,000 intramuscularly as soon as possible. If no improvement is observed in 2 to 3 minutes, repeat the injection and move the patient to a hard surface in case he has to be resuscitated.

NOTE: Make very sure that you do not inject adrenaline into a blood vessel. When the needle is inserted under the skin, pull the piston back and ensure that blood does not enter the syringe before adrenaline is injected.

Subsequent management

The patient must be kept in bed and under observation for at least 24 hours following a severe allergic reaction. Treatment should be continued by giving anti-histamines e.g. Astemizole for 5 days, and possibly steroids SEEK RADIO MEDICAL ADVICE. No alcohol should be allowed. It is essential that the patient should understand that contact with the incompatible substance must be avoided in the future and he should be advised to inform his family doctor. The circumstances of the episode should be recorded and the shipping company informed when convenient. A 'MedAlert' bracelet may be advisable in the future.

NOTE: Warn the patient that he may become dizzy or drowsy whilst taking antihistamines. He should not keep watch or work with machinery until the effect of the treatment is known with certainly. Also tell him that alcohol will increase the side effects and should not be taken during the period of treatment.

Lesser allergic reactions

These are usually delayed, any appearance occurring some time within the first day to one month after contact. The skin is usually affected. Slight cases may just show red areas of skin but widespread urticaria, nettle rash, with intense itching may occur. Additional symptoms may be joint pains and fever.

Specific treatment

Give anti-histamines e.g. Astemizole for 5 days.

NOTE: No alcohol should be allowed. This treatment may cause drowsiness and dizziness so the patient should remain off duty until the effect of treatment is known.

Anaemia

Anaemia is a condition which is the result of a reduction in the number of red cells circulating in the body or a reduction in the iron content of these cells.

It can result from haemorrhage of a large volume of blood or from constant loss of small amounts of blood, from destruction of the red cells in certain diseases or from the deficient or defective formation of the red cells.

Anaemia is difficult to diagnose without laboratory facilities but you may notice when you are carrying out your examination of a patient that the membranes of the mouth are pale when compared with those of a healthy person. The colour of the cheeks is no guide as such things as fever and excitement will redden them whilst natural sallowness of the complexion simulates extreme pallor.

The symptoms of anaemia vary but they are best summarised as those of physical weakness and rapid fatigue.

If you think that a person is anaemic, refer the patient to a doctor at the next port of call so that a blood examination can be undertaken, the correct type of anaemia diagnosed and the correct treatment prescribed.

Common cold, cold in the head

Anyone who has a bad cold and a temperature, and who is generally unwell should go to bed until his temperature settles and his nose stops streaming. This may also help to stop the spread of the cold to other seafarers.

Treatment

There is no specific treatment to cure a cold. Any treatment given only aims to make the patient feel better. Simple pain relieving drugs such as paracetamol are useful. Do not give antibiotics. Plenty of fluid should be taken.
Warning: Anyone who is deaf or slightly deaf as a result of a cold should not travel by air or skin dive.

Diabetes

This condition develops when the body is unable to produce enough insulin to cope with the sugar that is taken in with the diet. It is characterised by loss of weight, weakness, excessive thirst, and the frequent passage of large quantities of urine. These symptoms may be modified according to the age of the patient.

In young people the symptoms are present in a more severe form and the disorder may show itself as a rapid, acute illness. In older people, particularly if overweight, it may come on more gradually and only be suspected by the development of thirst and the passing of more urine than usual. In both age groups the disease may show itself by successive crops of boils or carbuncles. Diabetes can be made worse by infection.

If you suspect diabetes, test the urine for sugar about 2 to 3 hours after a large meal. If the test is positive and if the other symptoms of diabetes are present, it should be assumed that the patient is suffering from the disease until proved otherwise.

Treatment

Put the patient on a strict diet avoiding starchy or sugary foods. This will normally avoid complications such as coma (see below) until full diagnosis and treatment can be carried out under medical supervision.
Two kinds of coma can occur in diabetes:

- *Diabetic coma* can occur as the first sign of diabetes in the young person with the acute form of the disease, or develop in the known diabetic when the insulin level is too low and the sugar in his blood has risen too high, especially if they have a concurrent infection.

- *Insulin coma* is seen in the known diabetic who has taken too much insulin or not enough food and whose blood sugar is too low. This can also occur if they burn off too much sugar by more than their usual amount of exercise.

The following table helps to distinguish these two types of coma:

	Diabetic Coma – *High Blood Sugar*	Insulin Coma – *Low Blood Sugar*
Onset	Gradual	Sudden
Temperature	Initially below normal	Normal
Pulse	Rapid, weak	Normal
Respiration	Laboured, deep gasping	Normal or sighing
Skin	Blue tinge, dry	Sweating common
Breath	Smell of acetone (sweet like nail varnish or musty apples)	No sweet smell
Tongue	Dry	Moist
Dehydration	Present	Absent
Mental State	No disturbances	Confusion, sometimes fits
Vomiting	Common	Rare
Urine – **Sugar**	Much present	Trace or absent
Urine – **Ketone**	Present	Absent

If the patient is unconscious you may be able to confirm your diagnosis from clues in his belongings. A known diabetic taking insulin or another diabetic drug may carry a supply of sugar or sweets. He may have an identity card or bracelet or neck chain stating he is diabetic, if not, he should be advised to get one for next time! Treat him as for an unconscious patient and get RADIO MEDICAL ADVICE.

If the patient is passing into a coma but not unconscious and the problem seems to be too little insulin, ask him if he has any insulin and get his advice on how much to give. If he has none, put him to bed, and get RADIO MEDICAL ADVICE. If the problem is too much insulin and he is still conscious then give him four lumps or two heaped teaspoons of sugar dissolved in warm water or milk, at once and keep him under strict observation. If he responds to this then a light carbohydrate meal should be given, such as some sandwiches, to stop the sugar falling again.

If it is difficult to distinguish between the two conditions, give a conscious patient the sugar, as it will do no harm, even if too little insulin is present. Low blood sugar is far more dangerous.

If in doubt, always obtain medical advice.

Note on insulin and other drugs

There are a number of different kinds of insulin which vary in strength and length of action, and all are given by injection. There are also other drugs used to control diabetes and these are in tablet form. If you have to give insulin or other drugs to a diabetic always check the instructions on the container very carefully. Insulin should only be given in accordance with advice from a doctor. Insulin dependant diabetics should not generally be employed at sea – see MSN1712(M).

Drug abuse

It is a matter of great concern that some seafarers obtain and use drugs illegally.

The commonest drug used by seafarers is cannabis or pot. When it is smoked there is an odour of burnt leaves or rope. Attempts will be made to disguise that smell. Pot smoking is more often a communal than a solitary activity.

It is very difficult to identify by inspection the various 'hard' drugs as they are supplied in various shapes, sizes, colours and consistencies.

Prolonged use of any drug results in mental deterioration and personality changes of varying degree. It may be very difficult for a ship's officer to differentiate between the drug user and the person suffering from some form of mental illness.

The signs and symptoms of addiction vary according to the drug which is being used and the picture may be complicated by the user mixing two drugs to obtain maximum effect. The symptoms may be sudden in onset because of overdose or withdrawal, or they may appear slowly during prolonged use.

Here are some indications which may assist in deciding upon a diagnosis of drug abuse:

■ Unexplained deterioration in work performance;

■ Unexplained changes in the pattern of behaviour towards others;

■ Changes in personal habits and appearance, usually for the worse;

■ Loss of appetite;

■ Inappropriate behaviour, for example wearing long sleeved shirts in very hot weather to conceal the needle marks and sunglasses to conceal large or small pupils;

■ Needle punctures and bruises on the skin of the arms and thighs or septic spots which are the result of using unsterile needles;

■ Jaundice (hepatitis) through the use of improperly sterilised syringes and needles.

If you have suspicions, make discreet enquiries of other crew members. These may reveal alterations in behaviour patterns in the patient. There may be rumours of drug problems on board.

Do not accept the patient's word that he is not a drug user as lying, cheating and concealment are all part of the picture.

Treatment

Remove any drugs from the patient and try to identify them and their source.

Always obtain RADIO MEDICAL ADVICE.

If the patient is unconscious, give the appropriate treatment. If the symptoms are those of mental disturbance, read page 158.

NOTE: Police and Customs take a very strong interest in certain drugs and how they come to be on your ship. Any confiscated drug should be clearly labelled and locked away in a secure place and entered in the Official Logbook.

If you are returning to the UK the presence of prohibited drugs on board should be reported to HM Customs who will take appropriate action.

In other countries enquiries as to the proper procedure should be made through the ship's agents.

Hay fever

This condition is caused by an allergy to grass or other pollen. Normally the disease is at its worst during late spring and early summer when the pollen count is at its highest. Seafarers who suffer from hay fever often find that they are free from symptoms while at sea.

The symptoms of hay fever are a running nose associated with itchy eyes, which may become red both from itchiness and from being rubbed. The patient usually knows that he suffers from hay fever.

Specific treatment

The basic treatment is that for lesser allergic reactions. Give the patient anti-histamine until away from the coast. The dose should be adjusted to the degree of allergic reaction and to the side effects of dizziness or drowsiness which may occur.

NOTE: Warn the patient that he may become dizzy or drowsy. He should not keep watch or work with machinery until the effect of the treatment is known with certainty. Also tell him that alcohol will increase the side effects and should not be taken during the period of treatment.

High temperature – hyperpyrexia

See also heat illness and prickly heat.

Hyperpyrexia is the word used to describe too high a body temperature, i.e. one of 40°C or higher. Such temperatures can be dangerous to the survival of the individual and require careful management and nursing. The three main reasons for hyperpyrexia are heat illness, infections which cause fever, and damage to the part of the brain which controls body temperature.

Treatment

Any person who has a temperature of 40°C or more must be cooled rapidly until the body temperature is below 39°C. Tepid sponging (described below) is usually the easiest method. In addition, ice packs or cold wet compresses may be applied to the forehead, armpits and groin and iced drinks given. The air conditioning should be altered and a fan should be used to increase air movement and evaporation from the skin.

If the brain centre which controls body temperature is damaged, heat regulation may be upset for many days. Patients thus affected sometimes need to be surrounded by ice packs or to have frequently changed cold water bottles placed around them. Read the section on fluid balance and on giving fluids to replace loss of salt .

Tepid sponging

If possible get the patient into a bath or under a shower where the water is below normal body temperature. Otherwise, lie the patient down and obtain the equipment required for bed bathing. The temperature of the water in the wash bowl should be noticeably lower than 37°C. Then proceed as follows:

- Take the patient's temperature by rectum and record it.

- Place a sponge wrung out in tepid or cold water in each armpit and another on the forehead. If ice is available put ice bags in the armpits and on the groins. With the patient naked, sponge him all over, using long strokes, with tepid or cold water. It is the evaporation of this water which produces most of the cooling.

- The water which you use for tepid sponging will tend to warm up from the heat of the person being sponged so make sure that it remains noticeably cooler than normal body temperature, 37°C.

- Have a fan blowing over the patient (take care not to touch the fan with wet hands).

- Check the patient's temperature frequently as you cool him. Because this treatment causes rapid cooling of only parts of the body, it is important that the thermometer remains in position for four minutes so that the temperature recorded is that of the body as a whole.

- After tepid sponging, when the person's temperature is down to at least 39°C the skin may be dried and powdered with talc.

- If the patient complains of cold and starts to shiver and his temperature has fallen sufficiently, cover him with a thin sheet.

- As the temperature may well rise again, check the temperature by mouth every 30 minutes with another thermometer until it has been below 39°C for at least an hour; thereafter check the temperature hourly until the fever has disappeared.

Lymphatic inflammation (Lymphangitis)

Lymph is a virtually colourless fluid which circulates in a system of hair-thin tubes called lymph vessels. At certain places in the body the lymph vessels drain into *lymphatic glands or nodes* (Figure 7.11). They are an important barrier to the spread of infection in the body. The glands act as traps for bacteria and other tiny particles and, hence, may become enlarged and tender when the patient is suffering from an infection. When the lymphatic system is infected, lymphangitis and lymphadenitis (see below) appear. Generalised enlargement of the lymph glands is a characteristic of glandular fever, but may be due to blood cancer (Leukaemia).

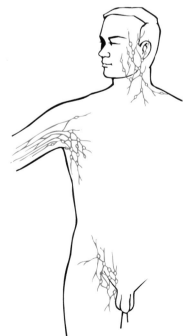

Figure 7.11 The main lymphatic glands.

Lymphangitis

Lymphangitis is recognised by the presence of a red line (the course of the lymph vessel) on the skin spreading from an infected area such as a small boil on the wrist or from an invisible infected prick on the finger. The red line will tend to travel towards the nearest lymph node (gland). In the example of a small boil at the wrist, the line will extend to the gland at the inner side of the elbow and maybe to the glands under the armpit.

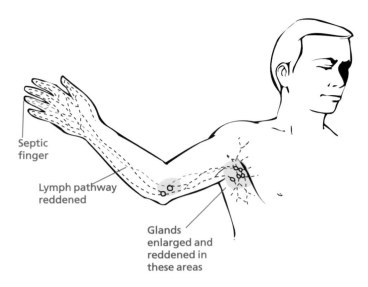

General treatment

Check the patient's temperature, pulse and respiration, and examine the related lymph nodes to see if they are tender or enlarged (Figure 7.12).

Figure 7.12 Lymphangitis, due to a septic finger – usually only one pathway will be so inflamed that it is visible on the skin.

Specific treatment

If the condition is lymphangitis *without* a raised temperature and *without* lymphadenitis (see below), give the standard antibiotic treatment. If the temperature is raised, or if lymphadenitis is also present, or if the patient feels really unwell, give patients not allergic to penicillin one dose of benzyl penicillin 600 mg intramuscularly in addition to oral antibiotic treatment. If the condition does not begin to respond to the treatment after 2 days get RADIO MEDICAL ADVICE.

Lymphadenitis

Lymphadenitis is an inflammation of the lymph nodes. It follows infection elsewhere in the body (see lymphangitis above). It should not be confused with glandular fever.

Lymph node inflammation usually occurs a day or two after the primary infection. If the node suddenly becomes tender and swollen, a rapid spread of infection is indicated. Further effects are a rise in body temperature and the patient feeling ill.

General treatment

Search parts of the body adjacent to the glands for the source of infection. The following table may be of help.

Location of Lymph Nodes	Area to be Searched for Infection
Neck	Scalp, ear, face, forehead.
	Shoulder, neck, mouth, teeth, throat, face, scalp.
Below collar bone	Chest, shoulder
Armpit	Hand, arm, shoulder
Groin	Foot, leg, thigh, genitals, anus, buttock.

Even if you are treating the patient for an infection in one of the areas covered by the inflamed node you should check the other areas as well.

Specific treatment

If the patient seems basically well, has no raised temperature, and the cause of the inflammation is not particularly significant, e.g. a small boil which has already discharged, no antibiotic treatment should be given. Otherwise the treatment is that given for lymphangitis. If the lymphadenitis derives from genital ulcers see Chapter 6.

Oedema (Fluid retention)

Oedema is the name given to the presence of an abnormal collection of fluid in the tissues under the skin. It is not a disease in itself but a sign that there is some underlying condition which causes the fluid to gather.

Its presence can be confirmed by gently pressing the tip of one finger on to the affected part for ten seconds. When the finger is taken away, a dent or pit will be seen in the skin.

Generalised oedema

Generalised oedema occurs in chronic heart failure when the heart's efficiency as a pump is grossly impaired. This condition is not often found on board ships. It can also be found in long-standing disease of certain structures within the kidney. This condition is extremely rare at sea and is beyond the scope of this book.

In all cases of generalised oedema, test the urine for protein. If protein is present in the specimen, give no treatment and get RADIO MEDICAL ADVICE.

Oedema caused by heart disease

In heart disease, the swelling first appears in the feet and ankles and spreads up the legs. If the patient is in bed, the oedema will collect under the skin overlying the lower part of the spine and around the buttocks. The swelling is worse in the evenings or after exertion. In addition, fluid will collect in the lungs causing a cough and breathlessness this is worse on lying down .

General treatment

The patient should be put to bed and a fluid balance chart started. Fluid intake should be restricted.

Specific treatment

If fluid restriction is insufficient to cause a decrease in the amount of the oedema, give frusemide 40 – 80 mg each morning until the patient can be put under medical care. For severe breathlessness oxygen may be required. The patient should be warned that he will pass large volumes of urine at frequent intervals beginning soon after the tablet has been taken and provision should be made for this.

Localised oedema

This condition is much more common on board ships. It can be found:

- in one or both legs where venous return is *sluggish* due to varicose veins.

- in one leg where venous return is *obstructed* because of inflammation of varicose veins.

- at any site in association with boils, abscesses or carbuncles .

It can occur temporarily in the ankles and feet due to long standing in hot climates, sitting in one place as in a lifeboat or in the female just before starting a period.

Your examination will reveal the cause of the oedema, and the appropriate sections of this Guide should be consulted. Relief will be obtained by elevation of the affected part.

Sea sickness

Sea sickness is largely attributable to the motion of ships. Persons unused to the sea are most susceptible, but even experienced seafarers may be affected in rougher conditions.

The effects of sea sickness vary from a slight sense of nausea together with dryness of the mouth and headache to repeated vomiting, giddiness and a greater or lesser degree of prostration. In severe cases, the extent of vomiting can lead to loss of body fluid causing dehydration and general collapse.

Prevention

Hyoscine hydrobromide 0.6 mg should be taken an hour before embarking or in anticipation of need, followed by 0.3 mg every 8 hours thereafter for a maximum of 48 hours. Sea sickness may still develop, but the tablets are far more likely to be effective if taken before symptoms are present. Drowsiness, dry mouth and blurred vision may arise as a side effect, and patients should be warned accordingly.

Treatment

In mild cases, the condition will gradually wear off, perhaps during sleep, and no specific treatment is necessary. More severe cases of prolonged vomiting may be treated by sucking Prochlorperazine 3 mg buccal tablets. However, if this cannot be kept down an injection of Promethazine 25 mg intramuscularly should be administered. Either the tablets or the injection should normally make the patient drowsy and he should be encouraged to sleep to allow the sea sickness to abate. On awakening the patient should drink plenty of fluids (oral rehydration salts can be used especially if vomiting has been severe). In severe cases the dose of medicine may have to be repeated. In any event, normal duties may be resumed 24 hours after the last dose.

Diseases of Fishermen

Infections of the fingers and hands

Fishermen are particularly prone to infections of the hands and fingers because of their working environment and the things that they are required to handle during their work. For instance, they may be injured by fish spines and bones, by broken ends of warps and many other things. Minor cuts and grazes often go unnoticed at the time of injury. Bacteria are carried into these wounds from fish slime and guts and also from pieces of metal etc. Infection then develops with inflammation of the infected area and the formation of pus.

Prevention is always better than cure and it is recommended that Chlorhexidine Gluconate 20% (HIBISCRUB) is used to wash hands and forearms after handling fish of any kind. The Hibiscrub can be used as a soap or in solution.

Hand anatomy is very complex but two features are relevant to fishermen:

- The tissues of the tips of the fingers (the finger pulps) are completely closed off from the tissues of the remainder of the fingers. Because of this, infection and the formation of pus in the finger tip causes a great deal of swelling and pain. This situation is called a pulp space infection.

- The hand tendons (which move the fingers) are enclosed either partially or completely in sheaths (Fig 8.1). A finger infection may spread along the tendon sheath towards the communal sheath in the palm. This is particularly likely when the little finger or thumb is the infected part. Infection of the palm sheath causes severe pain and swelling of the hand. This is a palmar space infection.

Figure 8.1 Tendons of the hand; the tendon sheath does not cover all of the middle three tendons.

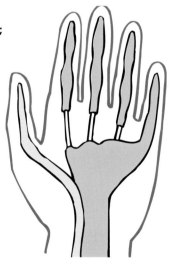

All finger and hand infections are very painful and disabling. Some can cause permanent disability. They should be treated aggressively if they occur but it is preferable to prevent them. Finger and hand infections can be avoided by:

- Thorough washing of the hands at the end of every work period, preferably with chlorhexidine gluconate 20% (HIBISCRUB).

- Prompt treatment and cleaning of all minor cuts, scratches and abrasions.

- Aggressive early treatment including antibiotics if throbbing pain or inflammation is noted anywhere in the hands or fingers

Specific hand and finger infections

Boils

Boils can occur on any part of the hands or fingers. They are often more painful than boils elsewhere on the body because the skin on fishermen's hands is hard and thick and unable to give. Boils therefore take a long time to come to a head and discharge.

To treat boils, a clean, dry dressing should be applied to the area. Antibiotics should be given if there is any evidence of spreading infection (e.g. redness going up the arm)

Pulp space infections

These are usually caused by fish bones or spines or by fragments of wire. They cause severe throbbing pain of the finger tip and require urgent treatment. The patient should be given antibiotics and the pus must be released by incision using a scalpel. If possible the patient should be landed, but if this is not possible, the finger should be numbed using local anaesthetic (Lignocaine 1%) and the palmar surface of the finger incised down to bone in the line of the finger. Pus will be released in this way. The finger should then be dressed and the patient landed.

Nail fold infections

These are also called whitlows. They are usually caused by minor scratches around the finger nails. The skin around the nail becomes painful and swollen. As soon as the infection is suspected it should be treated with oral antibiotics. If the infection comes to a head with pus present, the finger should be numbed with local anaesthetic (Lignocaine 1%) and a small incision should be made in the ballooned skin over the pus. The finger should then be dressed and the patient landed.

Palmar space infections

These are infections of the deep structures of the hand and must be taken very seriously. They are usually caused by an extension of a deep infection of a finger or of an infection of the tendon sheath of the thumb or little finger. They can also be caused by a prick in the palm or a stab wound from a knife in the palm. The most common cause is a finger infection which has been ignored.

The whole hand becomes swollen, there is severe throbbing pain and this is made worse by any movement of the fingers. The patient feels generally unwell, with sweating, shivering, sickness and raised body temperature all being possible. Treatment is urgent to prevent permanent disability. The patient must be put to bed with the hand elevated and arrangements must be made to land the patient as soon as possible. Antibiotics must be given, ideally by injection, until the patient is landed. If in doubt, seek RADIO MEDICAL ADVICE

Lymphangitis

This is infection and inflammation of the lymph channels and commonly occurs as a result of finger and hand infections. It is seen as red lines spreading up the arms. See Figure 8.2 for the pathways along which infection passes up the arms. As well as fiery red lines up the arms the lymph glands at the elbow and in the armpits may become swollen and painful. If lymphangitis appears, there is infection in the hand until proven otherwise and the patient should be given antibiotics even if there is no obvious source of the infection.

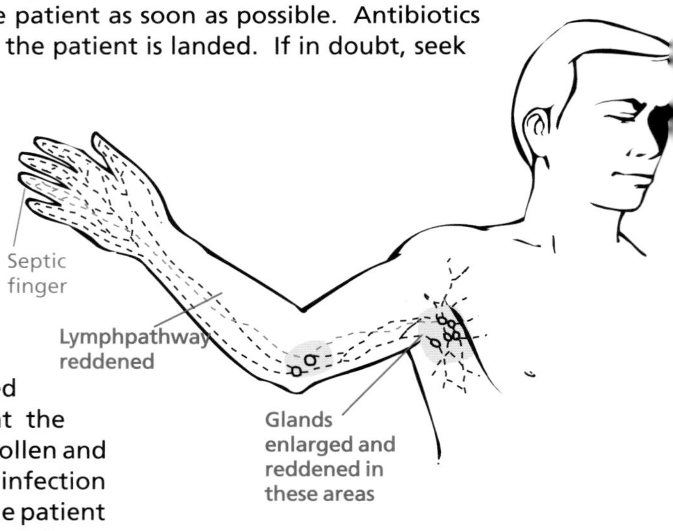

Septic finger

Lymphpathway reddened

Glands enlarged and reddened in these areas

Figure 8.2 Lymphangitis – septic finger.

Haddock Rash

This in an infection of the clefts between the fingers that occurs following gutting white fish, particularly haddock. Untreated it can caused redness, pain and swelling for several weeks. It usually responds rapidly to antibiotics, given for five days.

Cuts to the hands (including tendon injuries)

All cuts to the hands should be taken seriously due partly to the high risk of infection from even minor wounds (see above).

All cuts to the hands and fingers should also raise the possibility of injury to the tendons or nerves. If the patient is unable to move his fingers normally himself or has reduced sensation in a finger, there is possible tendon or nerve damage and the patient needs to be landed for possible surgery.

Salt water boils

These are also called pips or pigeons. They occur because the cuffs of clothing worn by fishermen rub the sand and grit brought up in nets into the skin of the wrists and the back of the hands causing tiny abrasions. The cuffs are usually covered with fish slime from sorting and gutting operations and bacteria in the slime infect the abrasions. Sores appear as small irritating spots which soon become tiny painful septic blisters. Some become large boils and the whole of the wrist and back of the hand may become inflamed, hard and painful.

The sores can be prevented by thoroughly washing the hands and wrists after coming off watch and by frequently scrubbing the cuffs of waterproof coats with soap and fresh water. When sleeve cuffs become cracked and worn, the garment should be replaced.

Once the sores occur, they should be bathed frequently in warm water and covered with a dry dressing. If boils develop the patient should be given antibiotics.

Jumbo Wrist

The medical term for this condition is Fishermen's tenosynovitis of the wrist. It occurs because prolonged repetitive movements of the wrist can cause inflammation of the sheaths through which the tendons around the wrist move. It is fairly common when fishermen are involved in prolonged gutting or when they return to sea after a long period ashore. Wrist movement (as occurs in gutting) causes localised pain and a sensation of fine grating. This grating (known also as crepitus) can be felt by placing the palm of the examiner's hand lightly over the painful place and asking the patient to carry out the painful movements.

The condition can be treated with anti-inflammatory drugs (e.g. Diclofenac or Ibuprofen) but often fails to settle whilst the fisherman continues to work. The most effective treatment is complete rest for a period of 10 – 14 days, preferably with the wrist supported in a splint.

Tit juice conjuctivitis (fishermen's conjuctivitis)

This is an acute inflammation of the conjuctiva (the thin lining membrane over the eyes) due to contact with the juice of 'duffs' or 'tits'. These are marine growths which look like suet dumplings with finger-like growths protruding from them. When they are trawled up they may burst in the cod end of the net and the juice, which contains tiny sharp silicon particles, may be squirted into the eyes of the fisherman. It is very irritant to the eyes, causing redness and inflammation and eventually blistering. The eyes are very painful and this is made worse by exposure to light. If untreated the eyes may close due to swelling.

The treatment is to wash out the eyes with large amounts of clean, fresh water. Relief from the pain can be obtained by instilling eye drops (Betamethasone and Neomycin eye drops four times daily). The eyes must be examined by a doctor on return to port.

Fish erysipeloid (fish poisoning)

This arises from minor pricks or scratches caused by the bones or fins of fish. Particles of fish or infected fish slime are carried into the wounds. Inflammation starts as a small red area, the margins of which become swollen and purple. The inflammation and discoloration spread rapidly up the arms. The margin remains purple and raised whilst the centre appears only mildly inflamed. The whole area is swollen and tender and may itch or burn. Lymphangitis (see above) may occur.

The disease can be prevented by thorough washing with soap and hot water at the end of every watch. When the disease is diagnosed, treatment should be started with antibiotics.

Dogger Bank Itch (curly weed rash)

This is an allergic skin condition caused by contact with a seaweed-like plant, known to fishermen as curly weed, which grows in the shallow waters of the North Sea, especially around the Dogger Bank area. It is also found around Scotland, Norway and Greenland. Not all fishermen in contact with curly weed develop the rash or become sensitised. Sensitisation can be very gradual but once established it requires only contact with nets used in the area to precipitate an attack.

The rash usually appears as a dermatitis on the backs of the hands, wrists and forearms. Once the allergy is established further contact causes the rash to spread to the face and eyes and ultimately to the whole body. The affected parts are itchy, red and swollen. Weeping and drying can cause painful cracks to appear in the skin. When the face and eyes are affected there is marked swelling around the eyes.

The only effective treatment is to remove the patient from all further contact with curly weed. He will need to change to deep water ships. The rash usually clears up on going ashore but in established cases drug treatment may be required. The patient is given antihistamines. These drugs cause sleepiness; the patient must not be allowed to operate machinery whilst on these drugs. Steroid ointment (Hydrocortsone 1% cream) should be applied to the affected parts. Inflammation of the eyes can be treated with eye drops (Betamethasone and Neomycin eyedrops) and the patient should be landed.

Removing a fish hook

Before attempting to remove the hook, the surrounding area needs to be numbed using an injection of local anaesthetic (Lignocaine 1%). Once the area is numb (usually the finger) the hook and the area of skin around it should be thoroughly cleaned with antiseptic solution.

Feel for the position of the barb and make sure that the area is numb, using some more local anaesthetic if necessary. Grasp the shank of the hook firmly in a pair of pliers. Following the curve of the hook, push the barb through the skin until the barb and part of the hook is visible. Clip off the barb and withdraw the hook, again following the curve of the hook.

The patient should be given antibiotics due to the high risk of infection.

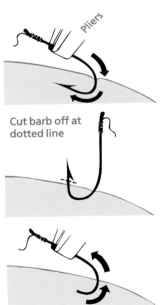

Figure 8.3 Removal of fish hook.

The period and period problems (menstruation)

A woman's period (or menstrual cycle) starts at puberty (11-16 years old) and should occur regularly until the menopause (45–55 years old). The cycle is approximately 28 days and the bleeding last 3–4 days. Individuals will vary widely. Severe generalised illness, severe weight loss, anorexia nervosa, severe stress may all interfere with the cycle, but the most common cause for a missed period is pregnancy.

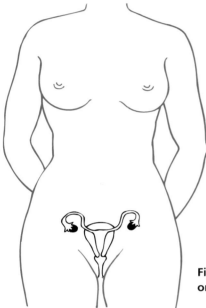

Figure 9.1 Female sexual organs

Painful periods

Many women experience pain with periods. This can range from mild discomfort and a feeling of heaviness, to severe cramping pains, backaches, nausea and even vomiting. It is very individualistic. Paracetamol can be used for the pain and simple measures such as rest, a hot bath or hot water bottle over the lower abdomen all help.

Pre-menstrual tension

The changes in hormones prior to the period can make women more emotionally changeable and alter concentration. However the extremes of the condition are extremely rare.

Pregnancy

As already stated the commonest cause of a missed period in healthy women is pregnancy, especially if the woman has had unprotected sex in the last 2–3 weeks. Suspect pregnancy if the period is overdue by 2 weeks, the woman is experiencing 'morning sickness' i.e. nausea and vomiting on waking which settles as the day progresses, pigmentation of the nipples, and swelling of the breasts. There is usually no sign of abdominal swelling until 16 weeks. A pregnancy test should be sought as soon as possible.

Female disorders and pregnancy

Bleeding during pregnancy or suspected pregnancy

This must always be taken seriously. During the first 6 months it can mean a threatened or inevitable miscarriage. These are most common at 12 weeks. After 6 months it can signify labour or a problem with the placenta. The other important cause is an ectopic pregnancy. See below.

Miscarriage

Threatened miscarriage

There is some vaginal bleeding and there may be some pain (similar to period pain). This should last no longer than 1–2 days. The woman must have bed rest until the bleeding stops and should do no strenuous activity after that until she has seen a doctor for a check-up.

Inevitable miscarriage

More often a threatened miscarriage progresses to an inevitable miscarriage. The bleeding continues, increases and often clots of blood are passed. The pain is worse. The woman must be put to bed, have regular observations performed and all shed blood must be examined for evidence of clots and solid material, which indicate that she has miscarried the foetus. Seek RADIO MEDICAL ADVICE.

If bleeding continues, the pulse rises or she develops a temperature, it can indicate an incomplete miscarriage, i.e. some foetal material still remains inside the womb. Discuss this with your radio medical advisor. She may need Ergometrine 500 mg intramuscularly for continued bleeding and raised pulse rate. She may require antibiotics if she has a raised pulse rate and temperature.

Bleeding after 6 months

This is likely to be the onset of labour , (see chapter 10) or an abnormal position of the placenta causing bleeding. The woman should be put to bed with regular observations until she can be landed. Seek RADIO MEDICAL ADVICE.

Ectopic pregnancy

This occurs when the fertilised egg starts developing outside of the womb, in the Fallopian tubes (the tubes that connect the ovaries to the womb). It is rare. It usually occurs around the 6th week of pregnancy (missed 1 period), but can occur up to the 10th week.

The egg as it grows splits the tube and this can cause severe pain and some bleeding. The sensation of pain is in the lower abdomen, centrally or either side. The blood is often dark in colour. When the tube splits, it can damaged an artery and cause severe bleeding internally, causing very severe abdominal pain and collapse due to shock.

As a rule of thumb – a little pain and lots of blood indicates a miscarriage, a lot of pain and a little blood indicates an ectopic pregnancy. If you suspect an ectopic pregnancy seek RADIO MEDICAL ADVICE at once.

Other vaginal bleeding

This can occur in women after the menopause or in women of childbearing years who are not pregnant and outside of their usual period. If the bleeding is a small amount , she should rest until it stops, and seek medical advice at the next port. If it is a larger amount and continuous, she should be put to bed and observed regularly. If she has significant abdominal pain give intramuscular Morphine 10 to 15 mg. Get RADIO MEDICAL ADVICE.

Vaginal discharge

This is usually due to an infection within the vagina, uterus (womb) or Fallopian tubes. It may be associated with lower abdominal pain (Pelvic inflammatory disease). It can be related to a sexually transmitted disease.

If the discharge is offensive in smell give the antibiotic Metronidazole 400 mg three times a day for 7 days.

If the discharge is white, with the texture of cream cheese, i.e. Thrush., instruct the woman to use a miconazole pessary if available (instructions will be on the packet).

Alcohol must not be drunk whilst taking metronidazole. The patient should refrain from sexual activity, whilst under treatment. She should see a doctor at the next port.

External genital itching. (Puritus vulvae)

A minor degree of itching may occur with menstruation, pregnancy or the menopause. At other times, it can be persistent and troubling. It is usually worse at night, when the patient is warm in bed. If a vaginal discharge is present , treat as above. Ask about any other features such as general health, rash, swelling or redness. Consider problems such as crab lice, scabies, diabetes and threadworm.

Any examination should be restricted to visual only and must be done in the presence of a chaperone, preferably female, to protect yourself as well as the woman. The urine must also be examined for sugar (diabetes) and the faeces for threadworms.

Contraception

There are various methods of contraception, none are infallible. The only absolute way to avoid pregnancy is abstinence.

The Barrier method – Condom, Cap or Femidom

These all prevent sperm reaching the egg. Reliability depends on correct usage. The condom is also useful in preventing sexually transmitted diseases.

The Contraceptive pill

There are many different formulations of pills, but they all work by altering the hormonal balance of the woman's body so that eggs are not released by the ovaries. The pills need to be taken every day as denoted on the packets, at a regular time. For the first month of taking the pill an additional method should also be used, i.e. one of the barrier methods. If a pill is forgotten, as long as it is taken within 12 hours of its usual time, there should be no consequence. If it has been forgotten for a longer period, the woman should continue to take the pills as normal but use additional methods of contraception i.e. a barrier method, for 2 weeks after the missed pill. Similarly if there has been any episodes of sickness, diarrhoea, or a course of antibiotics, the woman should use an additional method for 2 weeks, as all these can interfere with the absorption of the pill into the bloodstream.

Women should have regular monthly bleeds on the pill, and some may experience a small amount of bleeding mid-cycle. This is nothing to worry about.

The coil

This is a small metallic or plastic coil placed inside the uterus, which prevents the egg finding a place to rest. It can cause lower abdominal pain, vaginal bleeding and infection. The woman will need to consult her doctor about suitability or if problems arise.

Post coital contraception 'The morning after pill'

If a woman is able to consult a doctor within 72 hours of unprotected sexual intercourse, a combination of pills can be prescribed which act as a contraceptive. They are not 100% effective and are an emergency measure, not a regular contraceptive method.

CHAPTER 10

Introduction

If a pregnant woman goes into labour whilst at sea, try to get her ashore immediately. If this is not possible, try to get a doctor or midwife to her. If this is impossible, do not panic. The mother does all the work in delivering the baby and mainly needs calm, sensible encouragement.

Most births occur between 38 to 40 weeks after the woman's last period. If earlier than 36 weeks, the baby will be premature. The earlier the delivery, the more the risk of complications and death of the baby.

On average, for a first child, labour takes about 16 hours. Women who have had children before can have a much shorter labour, and most will deliver within 12 hours. There are, however, wide variations.

Stages of labour

There are 3 stages of labour

Stage 1. This stage involves the dilation of the cervix (neck of the womb), so that the baby can pass out of the uterus (womb). See Figure 10.1. It is difficult to say when labour commences exactly. The uterus will start contracting in a co-ordinated, regular pattern with some pains. A discharge of mucus mixed with blood may occur (the show). In the early part, the uterine contractions are relatively painless and occur at 5–10 minute intervals. The membranes, which hold the fluid around the baby in uterus, rupture and the fluid flows out of the vagina. Usually about 250–500 mls. The contractions will gradually get more frequent and stronger.

Stage 2. This stage involves the journey of the baby through the now dilated cervix, down the vagina (the birth canal) and into the outside world. The majority come head first. The pains and contractions will be much stronger, accompanied by a desire to push.

Stage 3. This stage involves the delivery of the placenta (afterbirth).

Childbirth

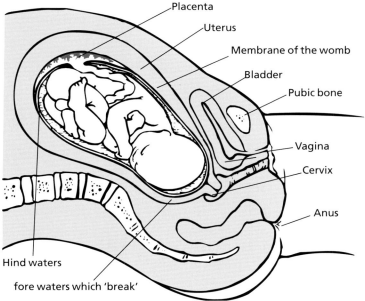

Figure 10.1 Child inside womb.

Preparations

Once it becomes apparent that the woman is in labour, get RADIO MEDICAL ADVICE.
You will need:

- A clean, warm, private room, with a bed ,adequate space to move around and preferably its own toilet and bathroom.

- Clean linen and waterproof sheet to protect the mattress.

- Bed pan.

- 2 pieces of tape about 10 inches long.

- Surgical scissors.

- Sterile dressings.

- Sterile receptacle for the afterbirth, and plastic bag to store it.

- Warmed towels and linen to wrap the baby, and a nappy.

- Something to act as a cot.

- Sanitary towels.

- Clean night dress/shirt for mother.

- Ergometrine 500 mg with needle and syringe.

Onset of labour, Stage 1

Once the contractions are coming regularly, every 10 minutes or so, the woman should be in the room. Allow her to find her most comfortable position, whether on the bed or wandering around. She should be encouraged to empty her bowels and bladder. She can have non-milky fluids (no alcohol) to drink as she wishes, and although traditionally eating is frowned on, if labour is prolonged, light refreshments may help. The pains of contractions are intense, however, do not be tempted to give any drugs unless specifically told to by a doctor. The woman will need a lot of calm reassurance.

The birth, Stage 2 (see Figs 10.2 and 10.3)

Once the cervix is fully dilated the baby is pushed down the birth canal by the contractions of the uterus. These will become stronger, every 2–5 minutes, and last longer. The mother will have the urge to push and should be encouraged to use her abdominal muscles during contractions. It is quite common to hear strong language from the mother. She should be encouraged to sit on the bed propped up at about 45 degrees.

As the baby's head comes through the birth canal it will start stretching the skin between the vagina and the anus, by gently placing a hand there during contractions you may help prevent tearing of the skin, but not always. Do not press on the baby's head. The top of the head appears first and once all the head and face is visible,

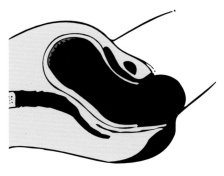

(A) Head delivers 'face down,' ie. looking along baby's shoulder

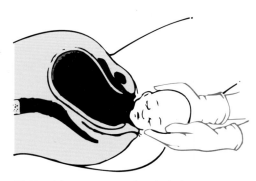

(B) Head then rotates to face baby's front . Support head gently

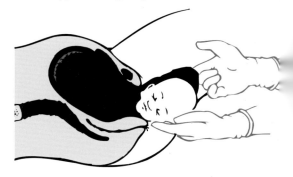

(C) Umbilical cord may be around head or neck – see text

Figure 10.2 Delivery of a baby.

check for and clear any mucus (slime) from the nose and mouth. Also check that the umbilical cord is not around the neck. If tightly round the neck it will have to be clamped and cut now; if loose, it can be slipped over the baby's head.

The head will now rotate and the shoulders deliver next. As soon as these are free the rest of the baby will come very easily. Lift gently, allowing fluids to drain from the face, and check to see that the baby takes a breath, if not try to stimulate it by rubbing. If there is no response refer to 'Problems during birth'.

The baby should be wrapped in the warmed towel immediately to prevent heat loss. Once the cord has stopped pulsating it can be cut. Tie a piece of tape tightly about 5 cm from the baby's abdomen and the other 2 cm further along the cord towards the mother. Cut between the two ties. If there is bleeding from the baby's stump tie a further tie. (see fig. 10.4)

The baby will appear covered in blood, mucus and white flaky material, do not be tempted to wash it. It must be wrapped up warmly, the eyes, nose and mouth given a sterile wipe, and then be given to mother for a cuddle.

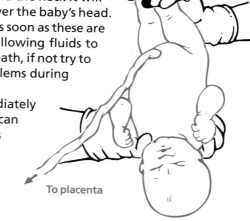

To placenta

Drain baby's throat and nose. Hold carefully, baby is covered in a slippery slime

Figure 10.3 Immediately after birth.

After delivery, Stage 3

Although the baby is now delivered, the placenta (afterbirth) is still attached to the wall of the uterus. It has to separate and then descend through the birth canal. This usually takes about 15–20 minutes. The woman experiences some more contraction pains, more blood and the cut cord lengthens. Do not pull on the cord, the placenta will come naturally. Once delivered, it looks like a small fleshy pizza. It should be put in a bag and stored in a freezer, laid flat until it can be examined by a doctor.

Once the placenta is expelled, give the mother the injection of intramuscular ergometrine. This helps reduce further bleeding from the uterus. If there is a lot of bleeding despite the injection, treat as for shock and get RADIO MEDICAL ADVICE. Occasionally the placenta will not deliver. Get RADIO MEDICAL ADVICE.

The vagina and skin around it should be checked for tears. Some may need stitching, get RADIO MEDICAL ADVICE.

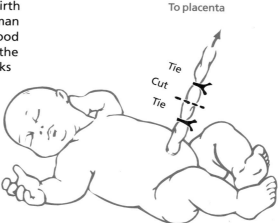

To placenta

Tie
Cut
Tie

Figure 10.4 Tie and cut the umbilical cord.

Subsequent management

Both mother and baby should be landed as soon as possible, and checked by a doctor.

The mother

After the birth, the mother needs to be able to wash, put on a clean night dress, and will need a sanitary towel. She should rest for the first 24 hours, and then she can start gently moving around.

Check her temperature daily, if it rises above 38 degrees centigrade, she will need antibiotics, either Ciprofloxacin 500 mg twice a day or Erythromycin 500 mg 3 times a day for 5 days.

She can eat normally and needs to drink plenty of fluids. She may initially find it painful to urinate and open her bowels. This usually is overcome with encouragement. Trying to urinate initially in a warm bath is often successful. After 3 days if she has not opened her bowels, a mild laxative can be used.

The baby

Once delivered, the cord having been cut and having had an initial cuddle with mother, the baby needs to be gently dried. A sterile dressing must be placed over the umbilical cord stump, a nappy put on and baby warmly wrapped again.

The mother should then have the baby back and attempt to breast feed using both breasts. Initially the breasts give a yellowish fluid, called colostrum, which changes to milk over 48 hours. This is normal. The baby should be encouraged to feed little and often, including during the night. It is best to keep the baby in the same room as the mother, so it can be fed on demand. If there are any problems with feeding, get RADIO MEDICAL ADVICE.

If well, the baby can be gently washed when practical, but keep the umbilical stump dry. The dressing should be changed daily. The cord will shrivel and drop off in about 10 days.

Problems during birth

Different presentations

In some births, it is not the head that comes down the birth canal first, but the bottom. As soon as this is apparent, Get RADIO MEDICAL ADVICE. As soon as the legs and bottom are delivered, do not try and pull the baby, the head is still the biggest part and providing the cord is not tightly wrapped around the neck and it is still pulsating the baby will not suffocate. Wait until the mother pushes the baby out.

Baby not breathing after delivery

This can be extremely distressing. Remove any blood or mucus from the mouth and nose. Rub the baby vigorously to try and stimulate it. If no response, put your own mouth over the baby's mouth and nose and gently blow air in, watching the chest to see if it rises, then allow the air to escape. Ask someone else to do chest compressions over the sternum (breast bone), using two fingers and pressing down no more than 2 cm, at a rate of 100 per minute. Continue doing this until the baby takes a breath or it becomes apparent that the baby is dead. Get RADIO MEDICAL ADVICE.

Obvious deformity or death

If the baby is badly deformed or is still born (born dead), get RADIO MEDICAL ADVICE. Serious abnormalities can often be the cause of premature labour, which may have caused the unexpected delivery.

Survivors

Survivors should be brought on board as quickly as possible since they may be exhausted, nearly drowned, and perhaps injured. They may be in the last stages of exhaustion and totally unable to help themselves. Even a short scramble up rope netting will be beyond their capability and could endanger their life. They will have to be assisted or carried. If possible they should be lifted in a horizontal posture as this reduces the chances of a sudden drop in blood pressure on removal from the water.

Hypothermia

Hypothermia is the term given to the condition when deep body temperature is lowered to less than 35°C. At and below this temperature normal body function will be impaired. Loss of life may occur when deep body temperature falls below 30°C.

Causes

The usual causes among seafarers are immersion in the sea, or exposure to cold air while in a survival craft. In a cold environment body heat production will automatically increase in an effort to balance heat loss, but if the rate of heat loss exceeds the rate of heat production then body temperature must fall and hypothermia will result. The rate of heat loss is many times greater in water than in air. The rate of heat loss will vary depending on the difference in the temperature between the body and the water. Hence in tropical water one may not die of hypothermia for a considerable period of time, whereas in colder water death from hypothermia can occur in less than an hour. In addition, death by drowning is a frequent consequence of weakness caused by hypothermia, before death from hypothermia alone would occur. Almost all seas in the world are at a temperature which can be classed as a cold environment, as heat loss will occur in water at temperatures below 35.5°C.

Diagnosis

Hypothermia should always be suspected in any individual rescued at sea. The three broad categories of uncomplicated hypothermia are illustrated in Figure 11.1

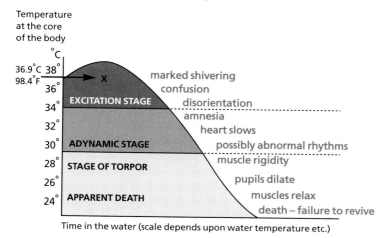

Figure 11.1 Curve representing the change in body temperature during cold water immersion with the associated signs and symptoms encountered at various body temperatures.

The use of a low reading rectal thermometer will be necessary in order to record deep body temperature.

Note that the stage of torpor may terminate in a comatose state which is difficult to distinguish from death. The casualty is unconscious, there are no reflexes and the pupils are dilated. The respiratory rate is very slow with two or three movements a minute. The pulse is imperceptible and heart sounds cannot be heard even with a stethoscope. The condition could suggest death, but the usual criteria for death are not strictly applicable in the case of hypothermia. Death by hypothermia is then defined as being the failure to revive the casualty by re-warming.

Treatment

The treatment for hypothermia will of course depend on both the condition of the survivor and the facilities available. Generally, survivors who are rational and capable of recounting their experiences, although shivering dramatically, merely require removal of all wet clothes and replacement with dry clothes or blankets. Hot sweet drinks and rest in a warm environment not exceeding 22°C (normal room temperature) are also recommended. However, always bear in mind that even conscious survivors can collapse and become unconscious shortly after rescue. They should therefore be laid down and should not be left alone. **NEVER GIVE ALCOHOL** In more serious cases, where the survivor is not shivering and is semi-conscious, unconsciousor apparently dead, slow rewarming is essential. Never attempt rapid rewarming by immersion in a hot bath except on medical advice. The following measures will be necessary to preserve life:

- On rescue always check the survivor's airway and breathing, and then listen for heart sounds. If the survivor is not breathing, ensure the airway is clear and start artificial respiration immediately (mouth to mouth or mouth to nose). Attempts at resuscitation should be continued until medical advice can be obtained, or for at least 30 minutes.

- Prevent further heat loss due to evaporation or exposure to the wind.

- Do not massage the limbs.

- Avoid all unnecessary handling, even the removal of wet clothing. If handling is necessary then be as gentle as possible.

- Enclose the survivor in a plastic bag or blankets or preferably both. It is important that the head, but not the face, is well covered. Place in a warm area with a temperature not exceeding 22°C. Never attempt to give any fluids by mouth to an unconscious casualty. When consciousness is regained never give alcohol. If the survivor is breathing but unconscious, lay him in the unconscious position. When consciousness has been fully regained warm sweet drinks may be given.

- Conscious survivors suffering from hypothermia should be laid on their side and, whenever possible, in a slightly head-down attitude.

- In survival craft, seriously affected survivors should be placed in close proximity to warmer occupants, to permit transfer of body heat.

- When spare clothing or blankets or survival bags are available they should be given to those most affected. Huddling together under blankets or any other covering will conserve heat and permit mutual re-warming.

Freezing cold injury – frostbite

Frostbite is the term given to the condition when tissue fluids freeze in localised areas of the body; the hands, face and feet are particularly susceptible.

Cause

Exposure, particularly of bare skin to sub-zero temperatures, especially when combined with air movement. Look-outs in life rafts or survivors in open boats are particularly prone to this injury. Accordingly, consideration should be given to the length of watch periods and watch keepers should be supplied with any spare clothing.

Diagnosis

The signs are:

- extreme waxy pallor of the skin;
- initial local tingling and stiffness when it is difficult to wrinkle the face or wiggle affected toes or fingers;
- complete absence of sensation in the area affected; and
- local hardness due to freezing of the flesh.

The depth of tissue damage can be graded, like burns, into 1st degree (frost nip), 2nd degree, 3rd degree and 4th degree.

Prevention

If bare skin has to be exposed to the elements, the periods of exposure should be kept to a minimum and freezing winds particularly avoided. Moderate exercise and massage at an early stage will help to prevent the onset of cold injury. Do not smoke; smoking reduces the blood supply to the hands and feet.

Treatment

On detection of the above signs, immediate steps should be taken to re-warm the frozen parts before permanent damage occurs. Get out of the wind. Re-warm the frozen area by applying it to a warmer part of the body, e.g. hands under armpits, cupped hand over cheek, nose, ear, etc. Once freezing has occurred do not rub or massage affected areas. When treatment has been ineffective the skin dies and becomes black. If this occurs dry dressings should be applied to the affected part.

Non-freezing cold injury – Immersion foot

This is a term given to the condition when the temperature of local tissues in the limbs (usually the feet) remains sub-normal but above freezing for a prolonged period. It is commonly encountered by shipwreck survivors who have been adrift and cold for several days. Usually the feet have been wet and immobile, but this injury can occur in dry conditions. Other contributory factors are tight footwear and sitting still with the feet down for prolonged periods.

Diagnosis

Feet become white, numb, cold and frequently are slightly swollen. When returned to the warmth, the feet become hot, red, swollen and excruciatingly painful.

Prevention

Every effort should be made by survivors to keep their feet warm and dry. Shoe laces should be loosened; the feet should be raised and toe and ankle exercises encouraged several times a day. When possible, shoes should be removed and feet kept warm by placing them under the armpits, but outside the clothing, of another occupant of the life-raft or boat. Alternatively, unwanted spare clothing may be wrapped round the feet to keep them warm. Smoking should be discouraged.

Treatment

After rescue every effort should be made to avoid rapid re-warming of the affected limbs. Care should be taken to avoid damaging the skin or breaking blisters. Do not massage affected limbs.

Contamination with oil

Do not clean oil off the skin (except around the mouth and eyes) until the person is warm and comfortable. Survivors who have recovered from hypothermia can be taken to a warm shower or bathroom and should have all their clothes taken off. Then their skin should be wiped with soft cloth and strong paper towels to remove as much of the oil as possible. Injured or burned areas should be wiped with care or not at all. If a strong warm shower is available, mechanical removal of much of the oil can be accomplished by the water jet effect. Hair shampoo will remove oil from the hair and can be used to help remove oil from the body. Then, with time, patience, help, and wiping, and using good toilet soap or shower gel to clean the skin, the rest of the oil can be washed away. Solvents, scouring compounds, kerosene, and other cleaners not designed for skin cleaning must not be used. It is, however, all right to use jellied cleansing agents that are designed for skin cleaning.

Dehydration and malnutrition

Survivors who have been adrift for several days may be suffering from dehydration. If they have been adrift for several weeks malnutrition may also be a problem. Caution should be exercised in trying to reverse either dehydration or malnutrition rapidly. Give sweetened fluids in quantities which will produce a urinary output of one litre per day initially. In temperate climatic conditions (or air-conditioned accommodation) this will usually mean an input of about 2 litres a day. If the weather is warm and the skin is moist or sweaty, higher intakes may be permitted. Initially, a diet of nourishing liquids (sugar and water or milk or soup) will satisfy nutritional requirements and should be given for the first two days. Then small amounts of normal food can be given additionally. RADIO MEDICAL ADVICE should be sought. This diet should continue until either the survivor can be transferred to care ashore or medical assistance is given on board.

Problems in the lifeboat

Vomiting

This may be due to the unusual motion of the small craft (sea-sickness is inevitable in a life raft), or to swallowing fuel oil or sea water. It is unlikely to continue very long. After severe vomiting the patient should lie down and be kept warm with coats or blankets. Seasickness tablets may give relief if taken well before the onset of vomiting. They should be issued at the earliest opportunity after entering a life raft.

Constipation

Action of the bowels is not expected when taking little or no food. No treatment is needed for this condition – in fact laxatives will do harm.

Difficulty in urination

There may be some difficulty in passing urine and the bladder may feel uncomfortably full. In any case, not much water will be passed when the drinking ration is small. The urine may appear dark in colour and thick. This is to be expected and need not cause alarm.

Swollen legs

Swelling of the legs is a common occurrence in the boat and continues for a few days after rescue. The condition subsides without treatment and, by itself, is a matter of no importance but can be partially relieved by the exercises recommended for immersion foot.

The dying and the dead

Care of the dying

There is no stage when nothing more can be done to help a patient. We may be unable to prevent the person from dying, but there remains the task of ensuring that the patient is protected from unnecessary suffering and pain, that he has people around to care for him, and that his dignity as a human being is preserved and respected. If the patient is obviously dying and you believe that death is inevitable, you should make sure that the person remains tranquil in mind and in body during the period of dying. Comfort, companionship, compassion, and the complete relief both of mental and physical suffering, should be the aims. If slight pain is present, it must be relieved by giving simple painkillers. If the patient is suffering from severe pain then morphine is appropriate. Morphine has the added benefit of relieving anxiety. In the event of mental distress, confusion, or behavioural problems consider sedation or tranquillisers. Get RADIO MEDICAL ADVICE.

Signs of death

Never consider anyone to be dead until you and others agree that:

- breathing has stopped. Listen with your ear right over the nose and mouth. You should feel no air coming out and should see no chest and abdominal movement. A mirror held in front of the nose and mouth will be misted by the moisture in the exhaled breath in life, but no misting will occur in death.

- the heart has stopped. No pulse will be felt and no heart sounds will be heard. Put your ear on the left side of the chest near the nipple and listen carefully. If you are not sure what to listen for, listen to the left chest of a living person first. To test that the circulation has stopped, tie a piece of string tightly around a finger. In life the finger becomes bluish, but in death it remains white. Slight pressure on the finger nail or lip in life will cause the area to become pale and when the pressure is released the colour is regained. In death, this will not occur.

- the person looks dead. The eyes become dull and the skin pale. The pupils are large and shining a bright light into the eyes does not make the pupils get smaller.

While none of the signs described above are themselves infallible, taken together there is usually little difficulty in coming to a decision.

Mistaken death – a warning

A person who has taken large doses of certain drugs, usually sedatives or tranquillisers, or who is suffering from hypothermia may look dead, but may still be alive. Mistakes have been made. Check carefully for shallow breathing, for a pulse, for heart sounds, as described above. If you are aware of the possibilities for error you are less likely to make a mistake. The circumstances surrounding the death may help you to decide whether drug overdose or hypothermia may be possibilities.

Cause of death

It is important to try to establish the reasons for death. Causes of death can be ascribed to two main groups:

- natural causes such as illnesses;

- injuries, which may be accidental or non-accidental.

If the person has been ill on board, records of the nature and progress of illness and of the treatment given will have been made. These records should be carefully preserved in case any further enquiries are necessary. Similarly, in case of injuries, the circumstances of the incident which led to injury or injuries should be investigated and recorded. The notes made of the investigations, together with the medical records, should be carefully preserved. It must always be remembered that medico-legal enquiries will subsequently be necessary even when there are, at the time, no apparent criminal or suspicious circumstances surrounding a death. If the circumstances of death are unusual, sudden or unknown, or if there is any suspicion of criminal intent, there must be a post-mortem examination by a pathologist.

Procedure after death

It is usually possible to retain the body until it can be examined by a pathologist at a port. Every effort must be made to retain and preserve the body until the next port of call can be reached. It is vital that as much evidence of what happened is gathered and preserved:

- use a camera to take photographs which might illustrate how the death occurred, this will be helpful in any investigation.

- *Clothing.* Strip the body of all clothing, if possible without tearing or cutting it. Make a brief description of each article and note any initials or names on the garments. Any papers, wallet, money or other articles should be noted on the list. Any articles which are wet should be dried, but not laundered, and should then be put into plastic bags, sealed, labelled, and kept in a safe place for handing over to the British Consul, police or other authorities at the next port. When handing over clothing and other articles, check each item against the list and get a receipt from the person to whom they are delivered. Any other possessions of the deceased should be treated similarly. If there is going to be little delay before reaching port, leave everything undisturbed.

- examine the body. If it is absolutely essential to bury the body before it is examined by a pathologist examine the body carefully (photographs are very helpful) and record the following data:

- race;

- skin colour;

- approximate age;

- height – straighten out the body with the legs fully extended. Make two marks on the deck, one in line with the heels, the other in line with the top of the head. Measure and record the distance between the lines;

- development of the body – note whether fat, thin, wasted, muscular etc.;

- inspect the head and face – record the length and colour of the hair; note the eyebrows and describe facial hair. The complexion should be described (for example, sunburned; pale; florid; sallow). Record the colour of the eyes and the shape of the nose. Open mouth and examine the teeth, noting whether they are sound, decayed, or missing. Dentures should be removed, cleaned and placed with the other articles kept for future examination;

- inspect the rest of the body – record all birthmarks, moles, scars, or deformities from injuries. Note the exact position of all scars and describe their length and width. A diagram will help. Note whether circumcised or not. Vaccination scars should be noted. Tattoos should be described and any words or letters noted. Record the size, position, general appearance, and colour of such tattoos. Wounds and bruises should be noted. You should try to decide whether they could explain the death. Note the exact position, depth and dimensions of all wounds. Describe the character of the wounds – clean cuts as from a knife, or ragged tears, or bullet wounds. Note any skin blackening or singeing of clothing around the entrance bullet wound. Look for an exit wound where the bullet left the body – this is always bigger than the entry wound. Feel under the skin for a bullet which may be lodged there and note the position. Look carefully for signs of bruising round wounds or if there is any escape of blood from the wound as shown by blood clots, blood staining of the surrounding skin, by blood on the clothing or by blood in the area where the body was found. This will help to distinguish injuries caused during life (which bleed) from those caused after death (which do not bleed). Note also any broken bones. External signs of disease such as boils, ulcers, varicose veins, or skin rashes, should be recorded.

■ records. Remember to have all your observational notes countersigned, and to make all appropriate entries in the official log book.

Disposal of the body

Retention for post-mortem examination

Whenever possible a body should be retained for post-mortem examination or for burial ashore. For the sake of the deceased person's relatives and to preserve the body in the best possible condition, if there is going to be any delay in reaching port, thoroughly wash and dry the body all over. Comb out and part the hair and give attention to finger nails. Straighten the arms and legs and interlock the fingers over the thighs. Tie the ankles together to keep the feet perpendicular. Empty the bladder by firm pressure over the lower abdomen. The body should then be put into a body bag and kept in a refrigerator or cold store which will have to be set aside for the purpose. The aim is to store the body at approximately 4°C, it should not be frozen. An alternative, if near port, is to lay the naked body on ice in a bath and to cover the body with lots of ice.

Burial at sea

Only in the most exceptional circumstances (and where there is no suspicion of foul play) might it be appropriate to proceed directly to dispose of the body at sea. Next of kin and/or the seafarer's employing company should always be consulted where possible and advice should be sought on an appropriate commital service or procedure. For burial at sea it is not necessary to do more than to lay the body on a flat surface, straighten the legs and arms and interlock the fingers over the thighs. The hair should be brushed off the forehead, the face washed, and the jaw secured by passing a bandage under the chin and over the top of the head, where it may be tied or clipped. The body should be sewn into a shroud.

Bear in mind that the shroud needs to be made of a very strong material and weighted sufficiently to ensure the rapid sinking and permanent submersion of the body. There should be three or four slits or openings in the material to allow the gases of decomposition to escape and prevent flotation due to trapped air.

Burial should not take place in soundings in any part of the world.

After preparation the body should be placed upon an improvised platform resting on the ship's side rail and a suitable trestle or other support, covered by an ensign, secured to the inboard edge of the platform. Wooden blocks screwed under the platform and resting against the ship's side rail will prevent the platform sliding outboard when the inboard end is raised to allow the body to slide from under the flag into the sea. It is very important to ensure that the whole operation proceeds smoothly and respectfully without unseemly mishaps. If the ship is small and there is a heavy sea, precautions must be taken to ensure that the body will not be prematurely lost and will not fail to drop cleanly into the sea at the right moment. This may warrant fastening guide rails on the platform. The seafarers allocated to perform the disposal must be carefully briefed. At the words of the Committal, and on receipt of a discreet signal, they must raise the inboard end of the platform to allow the body to slide from under the ensign into the sea.

Record the event in the official log book with the exact time and position of burial.

Radio medical advice

This is available by radio telegraphy, or by direct contact with the doctor by radio telephony from a number of ports in all parts of the world. Details of world wide services can be found in the Admiralty List of Radio Signals (ARLS) Vol 1. Satellite telecommunications using facsimile and voice have facilitated this direct contact. Additionally, it may, on occasion, be obtained from other ships in the vicinity who have a doctor on board. In either instance it is better if the exchange of information is in a language common to both parties. Coded messages are a frequent source of misunderstanding and should be avoided as far as possible. However, the medical section of the International Code of Signals should be used whenever appropriate.

Telemedicine systems are in development, exploiting digital image handling and telecommunications technology. As yet they are experimental, expensive and of limited benefit, however, in the near future robust, well supported, effective and affordable systems will emerge.

It is very important that all the information possible is passed on to the doctor and that all his advice and instructions are clearly understood and fully recorded. A comprehensive set of notes should be ready to pass on to the doctor, preferably based on the appropriate format below (one is for illnesses; the other for injuries). Have a pencil and paper available to make notes and remember to transcribe these notes to the patient's and to the ship's records after receiving them. It is a good idea to record the exchange of information by means of a tape recorder if one is available. This may then be played back to clarify written notes. Some countries may not be aware of the contents of your ship's medical chest and it will save time and bother if you have a list of drugs and appliances available (MSN 1726). When contacting British or other doctors who may be aware of the standards required in British ships, be prepared to notify them of the category of medical stores carried and whether there are any deficiencies likely to affect treatment in the particular case.

It may be necessary, under certain circumstances, to withhold the name of the patient when obtaining medical advice in order to preserve confidentiality. In such cases the patient's name and rank may be submitted later in writing to complete the doctor's records. Age, sex and ethnic origin are more important than the patient's name.

Radio medical advice
Medivac service by helicopter
Ship-to-ship transfer of doctor or patient
Communicating with doctors

External assistance

Information to be ready when requesting RADIO MEDICAL ADVICE

Complete the appropriate form or notes before asking for assistance. Give the relevant information to your radio medical adviser. Get any advice you are given down in writing as you receive it, and repeat back to your adviser to avoid misunderstanding.

A. In the case of illness

1.0 *routine particulars about the ship*
1.1 name of ship
1.2 call sign/MMSI/INMARSAT number
1.3 date and time (GMT)
1.4 position, course, speed
1.5 last port of call
1.5.1 port of destination is .... and is .... hours/days away
1.5.2 nearest port is .... and is .... hours/days away
1.5.3 other possible port is .... and is ....hours/days away
1.6 local weather (if relevant)

2.0 *routine particulars about the patient*
2.1 name of casualty (optional)
2.2 ethnic origin
2.3 rank
2.4 job on board (occupation)
2.5 age

3.0 *particulars of the illness*
3.1 when did the illness first begin?
3.2 how did the illness begin (suddenly, slowly, ...)?
3.3 what did the patient first complain of?
3.4 list all his complaints and symptoms
3.5 describe the course of his present illness from the beginning to the present time
3.6 give any important past illnesses/injuries/operations
3.7 give particulars of known illnesses which run in the family (family history)
3.8 describe any social pursuits or occupations which may be important (social and occupational history)
3.9 list all medicines/tablets/drugs which the patient was taking before the present illness began and give the dose(s) and how often taken (see 6.1 below)

3.10 list any known allergies
3.11 has the patient been taking any alcohol or do you think he is on drugs?

4.0 *results of examination of the ill person*
4.1 temperature, pulse and respiration
4.2 describe the general appearance of the patient
4.3 describe the appearance of the affected parts
4.4 what do you find on examination of the affected parts (swelling, tenderness, lack of movement, and so on)?
4.5 what tests have you done and with what result (urine, other)?

5.0 *diagnosis*
5.1 what do you think the diagnosis is?
5.2 what other illnesses have you considered (the differential diagnosis)?

6.0 *treatment*
6.1 list ALL the medicines/tablets/drugs which the patient has taken or been given since the illness began and give the dose(s) and the times given or how often given (see 3.9 above). Do not use the term 'standard antibiotic treatment'. Name the antibiotic given.
6.2 how has the patient responded to the treatment given?

7.0 problems
7.1 what problems are worrying you now?
7.2 what do you think you need to be advised on?

8.0 other comments

9.0 comments by the radio doctor

B. In the case of injury

1.0 *routine particulars about the ship*
1.1 name of ship
1.2 call sign/MMSI/INMARSAR number
1.3 date and time (GMT)
1.4 course, speed, position
1.5 last port of call
1.5.1 port of destination is ....
 and is .... hours/days away
1.5.2 nearest port is ....
 and is .... hours/days away
1.5.3 other possible port is ....
 and is .... hours/days away
1.6 local weather (if relevant)

2.0 *routine particulars about the patient*
2.1 name of casualty (optional)
2.2 ethnic origin
2.3 rank
2.4 job on board (occupation)
2.5 age

3.0 *history of the injuries*
3.1 exactly how did the injuries arise?
3.2 how long ago was that?
3.3 what does the patient complain of?
 (list the complaints in order of
 importance or severity)
3.4 give important past illnesses/ injuries/
 operations
3.5 list ALL medicines/tablets/drugs which
 the patient was taking before the
 present injury (injuries) and give doses
 and how often taken
3.6 list any known allergies
3.7 has the patient been taking any
 alcohol or do you think he is on drugs?
3.8 does the patient remember everything
 that happened, or did he lose
 consciousness even for a short time?

3.9 if he lost consciousness, describe when,
 or how long, and the depth of
 unconsciousness. Use AVPA (see
 Chapter 4) or GCS

4.0 *results of examination*
4.1 temperature, pulse and respiration
4.2 describe the general condition of the
 patient
4.3 list what you believe to be the
 patient's injuries in order of
 importance and severity
4.4 did the patient lose any blood? If so,
 how much?
4.5 what tests have you done and with
 what result (urine, other)?

5.0 *treatment*
5.1 describe the first-aid and other
 treatment which you have carried out
 since the injuries occurred
5.2 list ALL the medicines/tablets/drugs
 which the patient has taken or been
 given, and give the dose(s) and the
 times given or how often given. Do
 not use the term 'standard antibiotic
 treatment'. Name the antibiotic given
5.3 how has the patient responded to the
 treatment?

6.0 *problems*
6.1 what problems are worrying you now?
6.2 what do you think you need to be
 advised on

7.0 *other comments*

8.0 *comments by the radio doctor*

Medivac service by helicopter

Do not ask for a helicopter unless the patient is in a serious situation and never for trivial illness or for your convenience. Remember that, apart from the expense of helicopter evacuation, the pilot and crew often risk their lives to render assistance to ships at sea and their services should be used only in a genuine emergency.

The normal procedure is as follows.

Contact the coast radio station (details in ARLS Vol 1), ask for medical advice and they will normally transfer your call to a doctor. Give the doctor all the information you can so that he can make an assessment of the seriousness of the situation. He will normally give advice on immediate care of the patient. After the link call is over, the doctor will advise the Search and Rescue (SAR) authority on the best method of evacuation and, should helicopter evacuation be thought desirable, the SAR authority will make the necessary arrangements and will keep in touch with the ship.

Do not expect a helicopter to appear right away. There are certain operational matters to consider and although the service is always manned, delay may ensue. Remember that the range of a helicopter is limited, depending on the type in service, and you may be asked to rendezvous nearer land. In bad weather and at extreme ranges it may be necessary to arrange for another aircraft to overfly and escort the helicopter for safety reasons and this aircraft may have to be brought from another base. Arrangements may have to be made for a refuelling stop to be made at say an oil rig so that the helicopter can make the pickup and then fly back without further stops.

All this takes time, and, as it is done with the utmost efficiency, do not keep calling to ask where the helicopter is.

More detailed information is available from the Merchant Ship Search and Rescue Manual (MERSAR) or Volume 3 of the International Aeronautical and Maritime Search and Rescue Manual (IAMSAR).

When helicopter evacuation is decided upon:

- It is essential that the ship's position should be given to the rescuers as accurately as possible. A fix plus the bearing (magnetic or true) and distance from a fixed object, like a headland or lighthouse, should be given if possible. The type of ship and colour of hull should be included if time allows.

- Give details of your patient's condition and report any change in it immediately. Details of his mobility are especially important as he may require to be lifted by stretcher.

- Inform the bridge and engine room watches. A person who is capable of communicating correctly and efficiently by radio should be nominated to communicate with the helicopter.

- Helicopters are fitted with VHF and/or UHF RT. They cannot normally work on the MF frequencies, although certain large helicopters can communicate on 2,182 kHz MF. If direct communication between the ship and the assisting helicopter cannot be effected on either VHF or 2,182 kHz, it may be possible to do so via a lifeboat if one is in the vicinity. Alternatively a message may be passed via a Coast Radio Station or Rescue Co-ordination Centre (RCC) on 2,182 kHz, or on VHF.

- Passenger ships are required to carry radio equipment operating on the aeronautical frequencies 121.5MHz and 123.1 MHz. These frequencies are reserved for distress and urgency purposes and can be used to communicate with the helicopter.

- The ship must be on a steady course giving minimum ship motion. Relative wind should be maintained as follows:

  For helicopter operating area

  - Aft – 30° on Port Bow.

  - Midships – 30° on Starboard Bow.

  - Forward – 30° on Starboard Quarter.

If this is not possible the ship should remain stationary head to wind, or follow the instructions of the helicopter crew.

- An indication of relative wind direction should be given. Flags and pennants are suitable for this purpose. Smoke from a galley funnel may also give an indication of the wind but in all cases where any funnel is making exhaust, the wind must be at least two points off the port bow.

- Clear as large an area of deck (or covered hatchway) as possible and mark the area with a large letter 'H' in white. Whip or wire aerials in and around the area should, if at all possible, be struck.

- All loose articles must be securely tied down or removed from the transfer area. The downwash from the helicopter's rotor will easily lift unsecured covers, tarpaulins, hoses, rope and gash etc., thereby presenting a severe flying hazard. Even small pieces of paper if sucked into a helicopter engine, can cause the helicopter to crash.

- From the air, especially if there is a lot of shipping in the area, it is difficult for the pilot of a helicopter to pick out the particular ship he is looking for from the many in sight, unless that ship uses a distinctive distress signal which can be clearly seen by him. One such signal is the orange coloured smoke signal carried in the lifeboats. This is very distinct from the air. A well trained Aldis lamp can also be seen, except in very bright sunlight when the lifeboat heliograph could be used. The display of these signals will save valuable time in the helicopter locating the casualty, and may mean all the difference between success and failure.

- On no account must the winch wire be allowed to foul any part of the ship or rigging, or the helicopter be made fast to the ship.

- The winch wire should be handled only by personnel wearing rubber gloves. A helicopter can build up a charge of static electricity which, if discharged through a person handling the winch wire, can kill or cause severe injury. The helicopter crew will normally discharge the static electricity before commencing the operation by dipping the winch wire in the sea or allowing the hook to touch the ship's deck. However, under some conditions sufficient static electricity can build up during the operation to give unprotected personnel a severe shock.

- When co-operating with helicopters in SAR operations, ships should not attempt to provide a lee whilst helicopters are engaged in winching operations as this tends to create turbulence.

- The survivor is placed in the stretcher, strapped in such a manner that it is impossible for him to slip or fall out, and both stretcher and crewman are winched up into the helicopter. If the patient is already in a Neil-Robertson type stretcher this can either be lifted straight into the aircraft or placed in the rigid frame stretcher.

- At all times obey the instructions of the helicopter crew. They have the expertise to do this job quickly and efficiently.

Preparation of the patient for evacuation:

- Place in a plastic envelope the patient's medical records (if any) together with any necessary papers (including passport), so that they can be sent with him.

- Add to the medical record, in the envelope, notes of any treatment given to the patient. See that he is tagged if morphine has been given to him.

- If possible ensure that your patient is wearing a lifejacket before he is moved to the stretcher.

Ship-to-ship transfer of doctor or patient

This is a seamanship problem which demands high standards of competence for its safe and efficient performance. There should be no need to advise professional seamen concerning this operation, but this guide may occasionally be in the hands of yachtsmen or small craft operators to whom a few reminders may be appropriate.

A very large tanker or other ship under way at sea may require 30 minutes or more to bring her main propulsion machinery to stand-by, so use your daylight signalling apparatus or VHF as soon as possible. Loaded, large tankers require several miles to take off their headway and are difficult to manoeuvre close to small craft.

Light (unloaded) ships of any type and high-sided passenger ships will make considerable leeway when stopped and must be approached with caution. Some ships may have to turn their propellers very slowly during the operation.

Keep clear of the overhang of bows or stern, especially if there is any sea running. Also beware of any permanent fendering fitted at sides. The general rule is that the ship with the higher freeboard will provide illumination and facilities for boarding and will indicate the best position.

Do not linger alongside for any reason; as soon as the operation is completed use full power to get your craft clear. There may be a suction effect that will hold you alongside and which may be dangerous if you do not use full power. For your own safety, make sure you are seen and your actions are communicated to the Master of the larger ship and act promptly on his instructions.

See section above: 'Preparation of the patient for evacuation'

Communicating with doctors

As a matter of courtesy as well as of information, a letter or form should always be sent with any patient who is going to see a doctor. The crew member will be a stranger to the doctor and there may be a language difficulty. A written communication in a foreign language is often easier to understand than a spoken one. The letter should include routine particulars about the crew member (name, date of birth) and about the ship (name of ship, port, name of agent, owner). The medical content of the letter should follow a systematic approach and should give the doctor a synopsis of all that is known about the person which may be relevant, including copies of any information from doctors in previous ports. This is why the use of a form for this purpose is particularly valuable because the doctor can then be requested to write back to the Master on the form.

Medical Report—Confidential | **3** Doctor's Copy | **2** Medical Records Copy | **1** Master Copy

Part I — To be completed by Master or his Deputy

1 Ship's name | 2 Port of call | 3 Date
4 Surname of patient — Other name(s) | 5 Date of birth
6 Nationality & Language(s) | 7 Job Description | 8 Discharge book number
9 Date illness/injury occurred | 10 Date work ceased on board | 11 Date work resumed on board
12 Details about the illness/injury and treatment on board. (Enclose detailed description or log entry if necessary)
13 Ship's agent — Address — Tel No
14 Ship Master's signature

Part II — to be completed by Examining Doctor

15 To the doctor: Please see this patient and then fill in the form. Retain back copy and return other copies to the Master (or agent).
16 Diagnosis
17 Treatment: Please specify exactly all medicines to be taken the generic name of the medicine, the dose, the frequency of the dose, the way it is to be taken, and any other treatments required.
18 Should he see another doctor? No ☐ Yes ☐ When?
Contagious or infectious disease ☐ ☐ Are any precautions necessary for other crew members?
Estimated duration of illness (days)
19 Fit for normal work now ☐
Fit for normal work from ☐ Date: / /
Fit for restricted work ☐ What restrictions?
20 Unfit for work ☐ For how many days?
Bed rest necessary ☐ For how many days?
Recommended to be signed off ☐
— and be repatriated ☐ Is air transport recommended? ☐ Yes
— and go to hospital ☐ ☐ No
21 The patient was seen — date ...... Charge: ......
— in the doctor's office ☐ Payment received ☐ Yes
— on board ☐ ☐ No
— elsewhere ☐ Specify
22 Doctor's name and address; and Tel No
Doctor's signature:

Part III — Master to complete — Only to be filled in if signed off

23 Port of discharge | 24 Date | 25 Domicile
26 Name and address of next of kin (relationship?) or friend
27 Name of hospital or place where crew member is staying
28 Disposition of effects

ANNEX I

Anatomy and physiology

To provide adequate medical care on board ship there is no need to have a detailed knowledge of anatomy (structure of the body) or of physiology (function of bodily systems). Nevertheless the information provided in this Annex could be useful when examining a patient or obtaining and acting on radio medical advice.

The principal bones of the skeleton and the main muscles of the body are illustrated in Figures I.1 and I.2. The position of the organs in the chest and abdomen is depicted in Plates 14 and 15.

The bone structure

The skeleton, which consists of bones and cartilages, provides a rigid framework. The separate bones and cartilages are held together firmly at the joints by strong bands of connective tissue (the ligaments). Each bone is enveloped in a very tough adherent sheath of fibrous tissue. Between the sheath and the bone surface is a layer of bone-forming cells which can produce new bone in the event of a fracture.

The shaft of a typical long bone has a thick wall of dense bone which forms a hollow cylinder enclosing a central canal containing bone marrow. At each end the shaft is expanded to make the joint surface. These surfaces are covered by a smooth layer of cartilage to permit movements without causing friction.

Voluntary muscles

These form the bulk of the fleshy parts of the body. They are fixed to the bones by blending with the sheaths of fibrous tissue surrounding the bones. Some are attached directly to a wide area of bone surface but others taper to form a strong cord (tendon or leader) which is attached at a specific place on a bone. Muscles, and especially those of the limbs, are arranged in two opposing groups. Contraction of one group in response to an impulse through the nerve supply must be accompanied by simultaneous relaxation of the opposing group, or movement will not take place. These movements are under conscious control.

Involuntary muscles

These are found in the stomach and intestines, in the heart and blood vessels, and also in other internal organs of the body. They continue to work throughout life as part of natural body function outside the control of personal will.

Circulatory system

Blood

The body contains about 5 litres of blood which consists basically of four constituents: plasma; red cells; white cells; and platelet cells.

The plasma is the liquid component of the blood which circulates to all the tissue cells throughout the body. It distributes food, water, salts and heat and collects waste products which are subsequently excreted.

The red cells predominate and give the blood its colour. This colour is derived from a complex iron compound (haemoglobin) which is the main oxygen carrier.

The white cells give protection against infection by attacking and killing bacteria and also by producing substances which are necessary for building up resistance to further infections.

The main purpose of platelets is to assist in the blood clotting mechanism.

The heart and blood vessels

The heart is a thick-walled muscular pump about the size of a clenched fist. It is divided in the mid line into two sides which do not communicate. Each side has an upper and lower chamber which communicate through a main heart valve. The separate chambers are each served by a major blood vessel that either brings blood to the chamber or carries it away. See Plate 15.

The right side receives venous blood which, having been circulated around the body, has given up its oxygen and collected carbon dioxide. This blood is pumped through the lungs where it is replenished with oxygen and discards the carbon dioxide. As purified blood, it returns to the left side to be pumped through the arteries to all parts of the body.

The blood vessels form a closed system of tubes. The arteries, which have to take the full force of the pumping pressure, have thick walls containing muscle fibres and elastic tissue. Each heart beat widens the bore of the arteries to accommodate the surge of blood. Between beats the bore is returned to normal by the action of the muscle fibres and elastic tissue. Where an artery runs close to the body surface, the changing pressures can be felt as a pulse.

The arteries penetrate to all parts of the body, dividing and sub-dividing until they narrow to form very thin-walled vessels (capillaries). The capillaries then join with the venous network which returns the blood to the heart (Figure I.2). The size of veins increases until the heart is reached.

The capillary system is vital to the life of all tissues. The thin capillary vessel wall allows nutrients, oxygen, heat and beneficial chemical substance to enter the cells and, most important, waste products to be passed out into the blood.

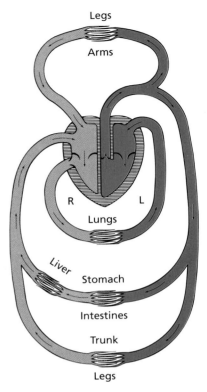

Figure I.1 The heart and the various circulations, diagrammatic

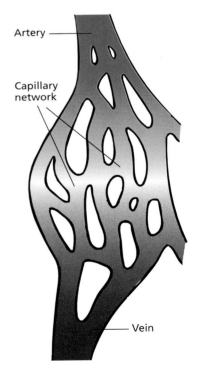

Figure I.2 Capillaries

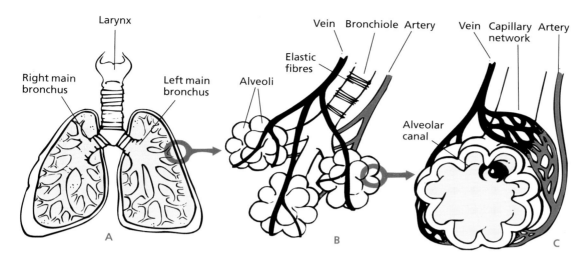

Figure I.3 Lungs, bronchi, and alveoli

Breathing system

Every time a breath is taken in, the air (20% oxygen) passes through the nose or mouth and then past the larynx or voice box into the windpipe (trachea) which is about 12.5 cm long. At its lower end the windpipe divides into two main tubes called bronchi (Figure I.3).

The main air passage in each lung (the bronchus) divides into successively smaller branches which carry inhaled air to all parts of the lung. Each small branch terminates by forming a cluster of very tiny air sacs (the alveoli). A fine network of blood vessels covers the surface of every air sac thereby permitting gas exchange by diffusion. Oxygen from the inspired air passes through the thin tissues to combine with the haemoglobin of the red blood cells. Waste gases, mainly carbon-dioxide, pass from blood into the air sacs and are expelled on breathing out.

> Haemoglobin + Oxygen = Oxyhaemoglobin
> *(purple red colour)*   *(bright red colour of normal blood)*

Whenever the blood is insufficiently oxygenated, as in pneumonia, the purple red hue of the blood shows as a blue tinge of the lips.

Each lung is covered by a lubricated lining called the pleura. The inner side of the chest wall is also covered by a similar lining. These two layers of pleura are in contact and slide smoothly over one another during breathing.

The act of breathing is mainly due to the diaphragm moving up and down. The diaphragm is a large dome-shaped muscle which separates the chest from the abdominal cavity. When the diaphragm muscle contracts, its dome becomes flattened and draws down the lungs, causing air to enter them; when it relaxes the lungs become smaller and the air in them is expelled. The muscles of the abdomen also help in breathing. When they tighten up, they press the abdominal contents up against the diaphragm and help in expelling air from the lungs; when they relax, they assist the diaphragm in drawing down the lungs as breathing in takes place.

The normal rate of breathing at rest is 16–18 times a minute. This rate increases considerably with exertion and also with certain diseases, especially those affecting the heart and lungs.

Digestive system

The abdomen is a cavity shut off from the chest by the diaphragm. The cavity is lined by a sheath of membrane (the peritoneum) which also enfolds some of the abdominal organs. The sheath secretes fluid which keeps the abdominal contents moist and prevents friction.

The digestive tract

This is a passage consisting of the gullet (oesophagus), the stomach, the small intestine, the large intestine, the rectum and the anus.

The gullet is a straight muscular tube which joins the throat to the stomach. It passes down through the back of the chest cavity and goes through an opening in the diaphragm to connect with the upper part of the stomach.

The stomach is a J shaped pouch. It enlarges when food or liquid is consumed. The lower part of the stomach is narrow where it joins with the first part (duodenum) of the small intestine.

The small intestine is a narrow-bore coiled tube, roughly 7.5 metres long, which occupies most of the central part of the abdominal cavity. The internal surface of the wall bears a large number of very small folds which project inwards to increase the surface area in contact with the contents of the intestine. The small intestine joins with the large intestine in the right lower quarter of the abdomen.

The large intestine is a wide-bore tube, roughly 1.5 metres long, which arches upwards and across the abdominal cavity before descending the left side to join with the rectum.

The rectum is roughly 150 mm long and is continuous at its lower end with the very short anal canal which opens to the exterior.

The digestive process

Digestion is the physical and chemical breakdown of food into useful products which are then absorbed by the capillaries of the blood vessels serving the gut. The unwanted residue of food is excreted as faeces.

The digestive tract walls contain involuntary muscle which by contractions moves the contents through the entire length until they reach the rectum where they are stored as faeces prior to evacuation. At certain places such as the entrance and exit to the stomach and at the anus, circular bands of muscle capable of constriction (sphincters) act as valves to shut off the flow.

The physical breakdown of food is accomplished by chewing, by the churning actions of the gut and by the addition of special digestive juices to the food. This begins in the mouth when food is mixed with saliva which contains enzymes. In the stomach, acid gastric juice is secreted by the stomach walls and acts on the food which may be retained there for several hours before passing through the duodenum. Small ducts from the bile system of the liver and also from the pancreas open into the duodenum. These ducts provide juices which are partly designed to neutralise the acid from the stomach juice and thus allow the enzymes secreted by the duodenal walls to act more efficiently. The churning of the gut then ensures a thorough mixing of food and digestive juices throughout the length of the small intestine where most of the chemical breakdown takes place. The main functions of the large intestine are to re-absorb water from the food residue and to reduce the bulk of the faeces.

The liver

The abdominal veins drain into the liver and carry to it the useful products which have been absorbed during the digestive process. One of the main liver functions is to act as a chemical factory which processes these products into substances necessary for nutrition.

Urinary system

The kidneys are located at the back of the upper part of the abdominal cavity, one on each side of the spine (see Plate 14). They are embedded in fat to cushion them from injury.

The main kidney function is to remove water and certain harmful waste products from the blood and, by this filtering process, to form urine. They control total body water and the concentration of various chemical substances in the blood. The kidneys also play an important part in maintaining a steady level of blood pressure.

The urine is carried downward from the kidneys to the urinary bladder by tubes of small calibre (the ureters); one tube for each kidney. The urinary bladder is a muscular bag situated in the front part of the cavity formed by the pelvic bones. The bladder acts as a reservoir where urine collects until it is expelled by voluntary muscular contractions through a tube (the urethra) which leaves from the bladder base.

The male urethra measures 18 to 20 cm from the bladder to the external opening at the end of the penis. A knowledge of this length is important when passing a catheter. The female urethra is much shorter, being about 4 cm in length. It runs embedded in the upper vaginal wall to the external opening just above the vaginal orifice.

Nervous system

Cerebro-spinal nervous system

This consists of the brain, spinal cord and the associated nerves. The brain is in the cavity of the skull. It is the co-ordinating centre for the nervous system, processing incoming information from nerves concerned with sight, smell, taste, hearing, sensation etc. and controlling various parts of the body, particularly muscles by way of out going (motor nerves). Higher functions include intellect, memory, personality etc.

The spinal cord emerges from the base of the brain and leaves the skull into the bony vertebral canal. It is protected by vertebrae throughout its length, and nerves emerge at regular intervals. These nerves control muscles and transmit sensation back through the spinal column to the brain.

Sympathetic nervous system

This is a fine network of nerves not under direct voluntary control influencing the function of various organs, especially gut, bladder, blood vessels and heart.

Skin

This protects and covers the body. It consists of two layers. The outer layer is hard and contains no blood vessels or nerves. This outer layer protects the inner layer, where there are sensitive nerve endings numerous sweat glands and the roots of the hair.

Sweat consists of water, salt and some impurities from the blood. The evaporation of the sweat cools the body, and helps to regulate its temperature.

ANNEX II
Anatomical drawings

FRONT VIEW OF SKELETON

Cranium (skull)

Orbit (eye socket)

Mandible (lower jaw)

Clavicle (collar bone)

Head of humerus articulating with scapula (shoulder joint)

Humerus (upper arm bone)

Ulna (inner bone of forearm)

Radius (outer bone of forearm)

Carpal bones (small hand bones of wrist joint)

Metacarpal bones (long bones of the hand)

Phalanges (bones of the thumb and fingers)

Sternum (breast bone)

Ribs

Costal cartilages (non-bony attachments of ribs to the breast bone)

Floating ribs (not attached to the breast bone)

Ilium (bone of the pelvis)

Ischium (bony part underlying the buttocks)

Pubis (joining the two pelvis bones)

Head and neck of femur forming part of hip joint

Femur (thigh bone)

Patella (knee cap)

Tibia (shin bone)

Fibula

Tarsal bones (small bones of the foot)

Metatarsal bones (long bones of the foot)

Phalanges (bones of the toes)

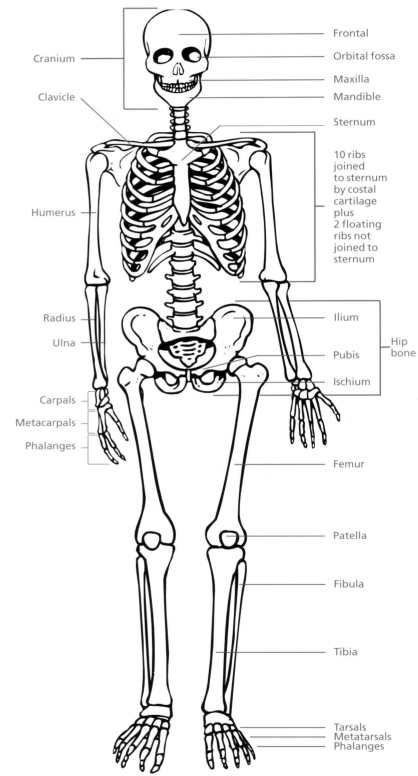

Figure I.1   The skeleton (front)

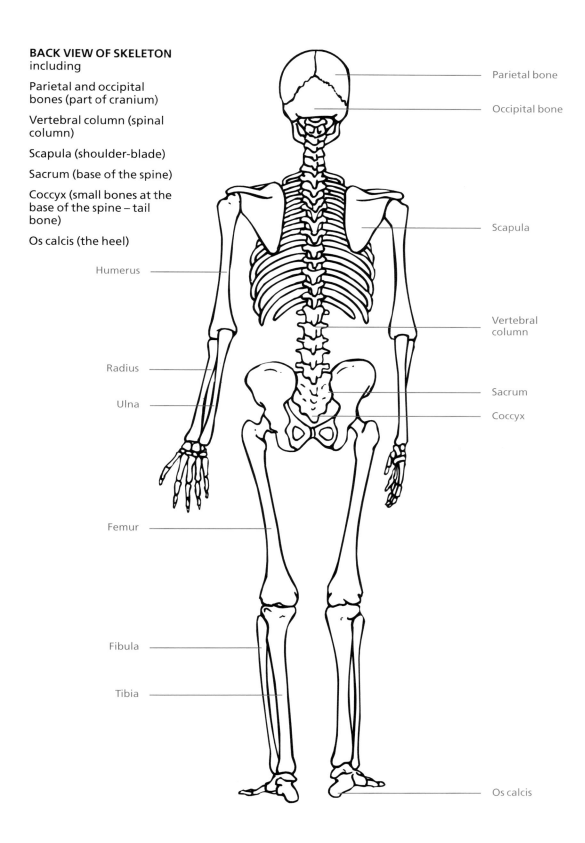

BACK VIEW OF SKELETON
including

Parietal and occipital bones (part of cranium)

Vertebral column (spinal column)

Scapula (shoulder-blade)

Sacrum (base of the spine)

Coccyx (small bones at the base of the spine – tail bone)

Os calcis (the heel)

Parietal bone

Occipital bone

Scapula

Vertebral column

Sacrum

Coccyx

Humerus

Radius

Ulna

Femur

Fibula

Tibia

Os calcis

Figure I.2 The skeleton (rear)

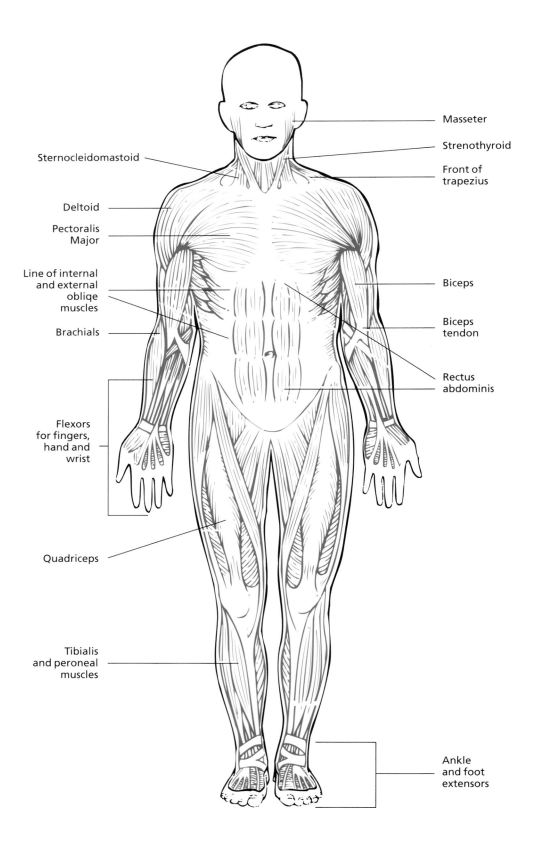

Figure II.3 Main voluntary muscles (front)

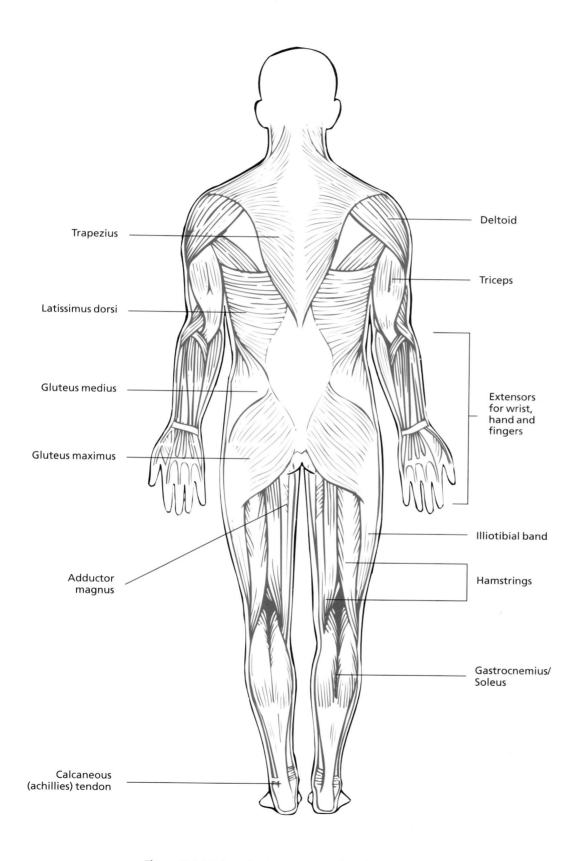

Trapezius

Latissimus dorsi

Gluteus medius

Gluteus maximus

Adductor
magnus

Calcaneous
(achillies) tendon

Deltoid

Triceps

Extensors
for wrist,
hand and
fingers

Illiotibial band

Hamstrings

Gastrocnemius/
Soleus

Figure II.4 Main voluntary muscles (rear)

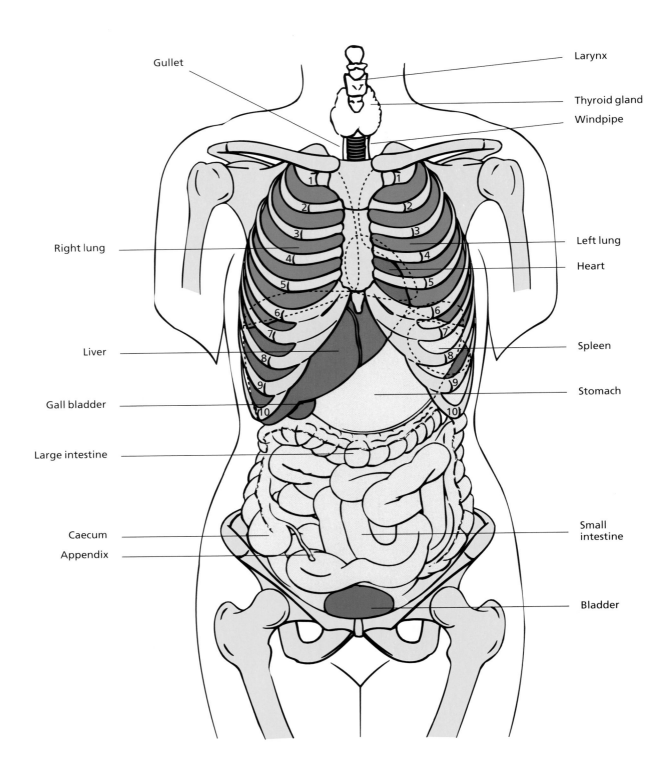

Plate 13   Organs of chest and abdomen (front)

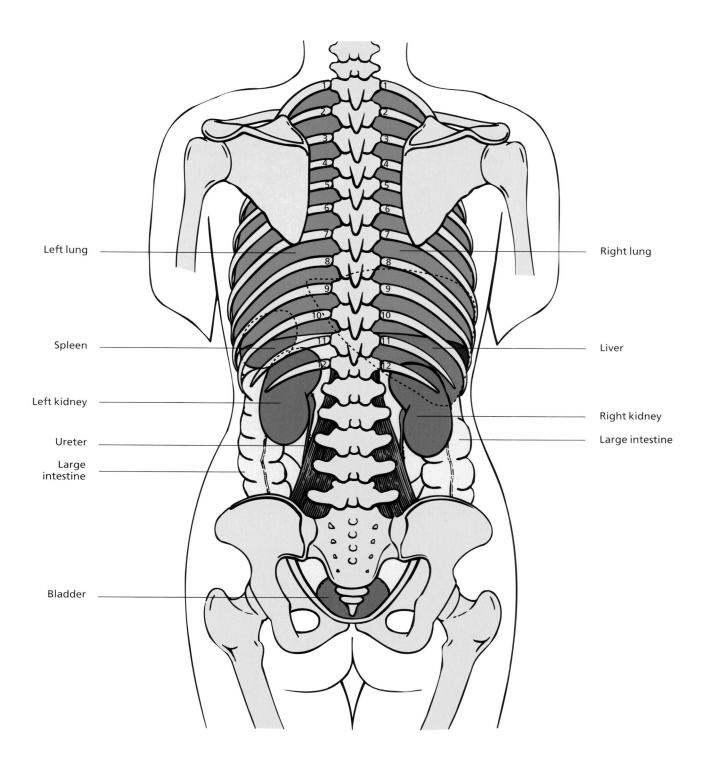

Plate 14 Organs of chest and abdomen (rear)

Index by Dr Olivera Potparic

Notes